Psychological Perspectives on Pregnancy and Childbirth

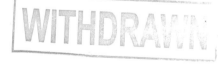

For Churchill Livingstone:

Editorial director: Mary Law
Project manager: Valerie Burgess
Project development editor: Dinah Thom
Design direction: Judith Wright
Project controller: Pat Miller
Illustrator: Keith Kail
Copy editor: Sue Beasley
Indexer: Tarrant Ranger Indexing Agency
Sales promotion executive: Hilary Brown

Psychological Perspectives on Pregnancy and Childbirth

Sarah Clement BSc PhD CPsychol
Lecturer, Department of General Practice,
Guy's and St Thomas's United Medical and Dental School, London, UK

Foreword by
Lesley Page MSc BA RM RN RMT RNT
The Queen Charlotte's Professor of Midwifery Practice,
The Centre for Midwifery Practice, Thames Valley University,
Queen Charlotte's and Chelsea Hospital,
London, UK

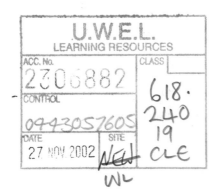

U.W.E.L.
LEARNING RESOURCES
ACC. No.
2306882
CONTROL
0443057605
CLASS
618.
240
19
DATE
27 NOV 2002
SITE
NEW
WL
CLE

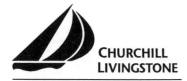

CHURCHILL LIVINGSTONE

EDINBURGH LONDON NEW YORK PHILADELPHIA SAN FRANCISCO SYDNEY TORONTO 1998

CHURCHILL LIVINGSTONE
A division of Harcourt Brace and Company Limited

Churchill Livingstone, Robert Stevenson House, 1-3 Baxter's Place,
Leith Walk, Edinburgh EH1 3AF, UK

© Harcourt Brace and Company Limited 1998

First published 1998

ISBN 0 443 05760 5

British Library of Cataloguing in Publication Data
A catalogue record for this book is available from the British Library.

Library of Congress Cataloging in Publication Data
A catalog record for this book is available from the Library of Congress.

Note
Medical knowledge is constantly changing. As new information becomes
available, changes in treatment, procedures, equipment and the use of
drugs become necessary. The editor, contributors and the publishers have,
as far as it is possible, taken care to ensure that the information given in
this text is accurate and up-to-date. However, readers are strongly advised
to confirm that the information, especially with regard to drug usage,
complies with the latest legislation and standards of practice.

The
publisher's
policy is to use
paper manufactured
from sustainable forests

Produced through Longman Malaysia, PP.

Contents

Contributors

Hazel Baslington MA MPhil

Formerly Researcher, Centre for Reproduction, Growth and Development, University of Leeds, UK

With Janet Warrilow, Hazel Baslington has recently carried out a research study examining women's views and preferences in relation to antenatal care. This qualitative study also examined women's knowledge about maternity care and about the training and skills of staff providing care.

Sarah Clement BSc PhD CPsychol

Lecturer in Health Services Research in the Department of General Practice, Guy's and St Thomas's Medical and Dental School, London, UK

After completing her PhD in psychology, Sarah Clement has worked as a research fellow and lecturer researching various psychosocial aspects of maternity care. She is the author of *The Caesarean Experience*. She also helps to run STaRNet, the South Thames Primary Care Research Network.

John Coleman BA PhD

Director, Trust for the Study of Adolescence, Brighton, UK

John Coleman trained as a clinical psychologist and is now a chartered psychologist. He has written a number of books including *The Nature of Adolescence* and is editor of the *Journal of Adolescence*. He teaches psychology at the Institute of Education and at the University of Sussex, where he is a Visiting Fellow.

Catherine Dennison BSc PhD

Research Psychologist, Trust for the Study of Adolescence, Brighton, UK

The Trust for the Study of Adolescence is an independent applied research organization based in Brighton. During the past 5 years, Catherine Dennison has been involved in research into a number of issues concerning young people's lives. She now coordinates a Carnegie Trust and Baring Foundation funded research project examining the family relationships of young mothers.

Therese Dowswell PhD

Senior Research Fellow, Department of Psychology, University of Leeds, UK

Therese Dowswell has extensive experience as a health service researcher with a particular interest in maternity services.

Natalie Fenwick MA

Research Associate, Department of Public Health Medicine, Guy's and St Thomas's Medical and Dental School, London, UK

Natalie Fenwick studied psychology at Edinburgh University before carrying out research in the field of education, and more recently health services. Her research interests currently concern professional attitudes and patient evaluation of services.

Jenny Hewison MA MSc PhD

Senior Lecturer, Department of Psychology, University of Leeds, UK

Jenny Hewison specializes in the psychology of health and health care. She has research interests in maternity care, genetics, and in the growth and development of children.

Janet Hirst MSc RGN SRN

Lecturer in Midwifery, School of Health Care Studies, University of Leeds, UK

Janet Hirst has 12 years of clinical experience in the NHS and has spent the last $4\frac{1}{2}$ years as a research midwife. Her interest particularly lies in the way in which the maternity service is organized and how this affects the quality of care for women.

Patricia Hughes MBChB MSc FRCPsych

Senior Lecturer and Consultant Psychotherapist, St George's Hospital Medical School, London, UK

Patricia Hughes is an associate member of the British Psychoanalytic Society. Her research interest is in security of attachment in young children, and in particular in the effect of the mother's experience of stillbirth on her relationship with the next child.

Suzanne Lyons BA DipClinPsychol

Clinical Psychologist, West Dorset Psychology Services, Dorchester, UK

Suzanne Lyons works in the area of mental health, with a special interest in psychological problems following childbirth. She has worked and undertaken research in the field of maternal health, including a study of the factors influencing the development of post-traumatic stress disorder following childbirth.

Anne McFadyen MBChB MSc MRCPsych

Senior Lecturer in Child and Adolescent Psychiatry, Leopold Muller Department of Child and Family Mental Health, The Royal Free Hospital School of Medicine and The Tavistock Clinic, London, UK

Anne McFadyen's research interests include the impact of illness and disability on family functioning and the development of research methods which encompass the meaning of individual and family experience. She is the author of *Special Care Babies and Their Developing Relationships*.

Jane Ogden BSc PhD (Psychol)

Senior Lecturer in Health Psychology, Department of General Practice, Guy's and St Thomas's Medical and Dental School, London, UK

Jane Ogden teaches health psychology to medical and psychology students and is currently involved in projects examining predictors of a range of health behavious such as diet, smoking and safer sex, with a particular focus on women's health. She is the author of *Fat Chance: the Myth of Dieting Explained* and *Health Psychology: a Textbook*.

Jane Podkolinski BA(Econ) MSc SRN SCM DPSM

Midwife, Salisbury District Hospital, Salisbury, UK
Jane Podkolinski trained as a nurse, and then a midwife. She qualified in midwifery in 1979 and has been working in all aspects of clinical midwifery in both the hospital and community settings since then. She has recently completed a Master's degree in Midwifery Studies at South Bank University, London.

Jim Sikorski BA MRCP MRCGP DRCOG

General Practitioner; Honorary Research Fellow, Department of General Practice, Guy's and St Thomas's Medical and Dental School, London, UK
Jim Sikorski has a particular interest in researching aspects of community-based maternity care and led the team which undertook the Antenatal Care Project (a randomised controlled trial comparing two schedules of antenatal visits).

Mary Smale BA PhD CEd

Breastfeeding Counsellor and Tutor, National Childbirth Trust, Beverley, East Yorkshire, UK
Mary Smale is involved in training health professionals in breastfeeding as well as writing and editing. She wrote *The NCT Book of Breastfeeding* in 1992 and her PhD is about the experiences of breastfeeding women.

Jo Sullivan-Lyons BSc PGCE

Research Psychologist, School of Sciences, University of Greenwich, London, UK
Jo Sullivan-Lyons graduated from the University of Reading in 1991 with a BSc(Hons) in Psychology. She trained as a teacher and worked for two years teaching in nursery and infant schools. In 1994, she began working as a research psychologist at the University of Greenwich, examining sex differences in psychological well-being.

Janet Warrilow BSc(Psychol)

Research Assistant, Centre for Reproduction, Growth and Development, University of Leeds, UK
With Hazel Baslington, Janet Warrilow has recently carried out a research study examining women's views and preferences in relation to antenatal care. This qualitative study also examined women's knowledge about maternity care and about the training and skills of staff providing care.

Jane Weaver BSc SRN SCM

PhD student, Department of Psychology, University College London, UK
Jane Weaver trained as a midwife at West Cumberland Hospital, Whitehaven and practised as a hospital and a community midwife between 1976 and 1991. She has a first degree in Psychology and is currently working towards her PhD. Her area of research is control in childbirth.

Sandra Wheatley BSc(Psychol)

Research Associate, Academic Psychiatry, Leicester General Hospital, Leicester, UK
Sandra Wheatley has been a researcher for the University of Leicester working in the
Academic Department of Psychiatry at Leicester General Hospital as coordinator of the
Perinatal Research Team since 1995. She is currently a doctoral student at the University of
Leicester having gained her BSc(Hons) in Psychology at Royal Holloway, University of
London. Her past and current research interests include postnatal depression, social support,
and the practical application of preventative health psychology interventions.

Jennifer Wilson BSc MSc RGN RM
Research Midwife, Department of General Practice, Guy's and St Thomas's Medical
and Dental School, London, UK
Jennifer Wilson is a part-time Research Midwife working on the Antenatal Care Project
Follow-up Study at Guy's and St Thomas's Medical and Dental School. She has a first degree
in Mathematics and Statistics from the University of Exeter and Master's degree in Health
Promotion from Brunel University. After training as a nurse and a midwife, she spent two
years in Thailand running the Mother and Child Health Service in a Cambodian refugee
camp.

Foreword

The quality of care of a mother, her baby and family around the time of birth will affect the health and happiness of the individuals and family concerned for many years to come. The time around birth is a critical and sensitive time, which may affect not only the physical health, but also spiritual and emotional health in a profound way. Maternity caregivers, who in today's world often act as substitute kinfolk of mother and baby, hold tremendous power to affect those in their care for better or for worse. Negative care will cast a long shadow forward into the life of the individual and the family. Sensitive and supportive care will cast a light, enhancing the ability of parents to cherish and to confidently care for their baby into adulthood.

For some time now, it has seemed that all that mattered in the care of mothers and babies was to have a live mother and baby. Emotional trauma and morbidity was ignored. Paradoxically, at a time in which birth has never been safer, the focus on the risk of birth has led to the reduction of birth to a medical event in which the woman has become a passive recipient of care. The shift of birth to the hospital has created systems in which mothers and their carers, and mothers and their babies, are alienated from each other, and in which the mother may actually be prevented by the health-care system from receiving the kind of supportive care which is so neccessary to emotional health.

In the hospital system, birth becomes separate from the woman's everyday life. The lack of extended family, small nuclear families, and the lack of cohesive communities are characteristics of modern society, which often mean that mothers and their families are left to cope without support for the demands of parenting. Such a situation makes it more crucial than ever that everything possible is done to support emotional well-being and self-confidence, and to support the growth of love between parents and baby. A loving attachment is a bond which ties and protects even in the most challenging circumstances. It is the most protective and enriching part of family life.

There is a growing consciousness that the goal of our care is far more than having a live mother and baby leave our care on discharge. This is a minimum and inadequate standard. Instead we should seek to have family leave our care with their personal and family integrity intact, feeling cherished by their carers, knowing the full extent of their love for their baby, and able to cope with the rigours and demands of parenting. Pregnancy and birth are far more than a physical experience. The transition to new roles and responsibility require a social and emotional adaptation which is one of the most crucial of human life.

This book will go a long way to helping maternity carers provide the kind of sensitive and informed care which is so essential to this broader goal of care. It is a highly readable, thought-provoking book. The authors are multi-disciplinary. The topics dealt with are key to modern day maternity services. Sarah Clement describes herself as an outsider to care, yet she has brought tremendous insight to care through the topics selected, and the thoroughness with which they are treated.

The book provides a clear theoretical base, and clear advice for practical application. I found many of my beliefs challenged. The psychological perspective of pregnancy and birth is a new and crucial dimension for exploration in our modern-day maternity services. This thoughtful exploration will do much to help maternity care professionals, and consumers of the service, understand that dimension and treat it with due respect.

1997   Professor Lesley Page

Preface

This is a book about the psychological journey women make when they become pregnant, give birth and adjust to life after childbirth. Women's own experiences are the primary focus for the majority of the chapters in the book. However, women do not have babies in a social vacuum, and are not the only people involved. Partners, families, the baby, and health care professionals all have key parts to play, and their experiences are presented too.

In charting this journey, the contributors have focused on three main issues:

- What is the experience like for women, their families and caregivers?
- What are the psychological needs of women and their families at this time?
- How can caregivers best meet these psychological needs?

To answer these questions the contributors have presented findings from their own research studies and evidence from the existing literature. They draw upon a wide variety of disciplines and methodologies, viewing the journey from particular vantage points, and interpreting what they see differently depending on the insights gained from their own professional and personal backgrounds. By seeing pregnancy, childbirth and the postnatal period from these multiple perspectives we are able to build up a clearer picture of parents' experiences. Although each contributor has approached the time around childbirth from her or his own unique perspective, a number of common themes have emerged from the different perspectives presented. These themes are the cornerstones of good psychological care around childbirth, and are outlined in the Introduction to the book.

At a time when practitioners are keenly aware of the need to base practice on sound research evidence, there is a danger of over-focusing on purely clinical aspects of care, to the detriment of a more woman-centred, psychosocial approach. There is, however, a mass of research evidence about psychosocial aspects of care, and one of the objectives of this book is to help caregivers to tap into this wealth of evidence. Although the evidence is often less accessible, more diverse and perhaps more complex than clinical evidence, the findings of psychological research can provide an important foundation for reflective practice.

My aim in bringing together the contributions in this book is to provoke thought, discussion and debate about the psychological side of maternity care, with the hope that this will ultimately enhance the psychological care that midwives, general practitioners, obstetricians and other caregivers are able to provide to women and their families before, during and after childbirth.

London 1997   Sarah Clement

Acknowledgements

Authors often compare the process of writing a book to the experience of pregnancy and birth, describing the book's lengthy gestation, and their long, hard labour, culminating in the arrival of their 'baby'. Editing a book is different and perhaps more akin to the role of a midwife. All midwives need people helping and supporting them, so they can help and support the women they care for. Like a midwife, there have been a number of people who have helped and supported me in my task of facilitating the safe arrival of this book. I would like to thank:

- The chapter authors for their insightful contributions
- Maureen Statham for her excellent secretarial assistance
- The staff at Churchill Livingstone for guiding me through this work
- Steve, Joel and Calum Bowen for their support, patience and understanding.

Lastly and most importantly, I would like to thank all the parents and caregivers who took part in the research studies presented in this book for generously sharing their experiences of pregnancy, childbirth and the early postnatal period.

Introduction

Sarah Clement

This book is about psychological perspectives on pregnancy and childbirth. It does not attempt to cover every aspect of pregnancy, birth and early parenthood, as to try to do so in a book of this length would result in superficial coverage of each aspect. Instead I have asked the contributors to focus in depth on one particular aspect. The main criterion I used when choosing the topics to be covered was their current relevance to maternity caregivers, topics which were identified after discussion with midwifery colleagues and friends.

I have endeavoured to avoid the *problem-orientation* of some other books on the psychology of pregnancy and childbirth, which seem to present the whole experience as a catalogue of potential problems. To present pregnancy and childbirth in this way gives an inaccurate picture of women's experiences by over-focusing on illness and difficulties. So, for example, rather than having chapters on antenatal and postnatal depression, there are chapters on the psychological support women may need at these times. The emphasis is thus on what caregivers can do to prevent problems and promote health rather than on the problems *per se*.

The book takes a multidisciplinary approach. I believe that psychologists are not the only people who have something important to say about psychological aspects of pregnancy, childbirth and early parenthood. The contributors include midwives, a general practitioner, a breast-feeding counsellor, psychotherapists and psychiatrists, as well as psychologists.

The contributors have drawn on their diverse professional/academic backgrounds to address the topics from a variety of perspectives. The contributors have used several different theoretical approaches and methodologies. Many of the contributors have taken a qualitative approach and presented quotations or case studies to illustrate and animate their findings. Others have presented statistical findings which can also inform our understanding of pregnancy and childbirth.

Despite this diversity, there is one section that is common to all the chapters, *Key points for caregivers*. The contributors have outlined the main messages of their chapter which may have implications for professional practice. The key points are not offered prescriptively, but rather as issues for consideration and reflection. Caregivers are invited to decide for themselves what implications the key points might have for their own practice.

I would like to say something here about my position as a non-caregiver editing a book aimed primarily at caregivers. There are two people with central roles in maternity care: the midwife/general practitioner/obstetrician and the pregnant/labouring/newly delivered woman. I have personal experience of one of these roles, but not the other. I therefore have an outsider's perspective on caregiving. My perspective may well be different from that of a practitioner, but I believe that both insider and outsider perspectives can make a valuable contribution to our understanding of the psychological side of pregnancy and childbirth.

The chapters are presented in broadly chronological order, from pregnancy, through childbirth, to early parenthood, ending with two chapters examining the experiences of different groups (fathers and teenagers) across these three periods.

The first chapter is by Jennifer Wilson, Jim Sikorski and myself, and presents findings from our research on women's experiences of ultrasound scans. Although we focused on one particular technology, many of the issues that emerged may also apply to other technologies used in screening for fetal abnormality. Such screening has come to play an increasingly prominent role in antenatal care, and has the potential to cause psychological harm, particularly if women's psychological needs around screening are not understood or met.

The second chapter is by midwifery lecturer Janet Hirst and her colleagues in Leeds, and addresses the question *What do women want from their antenatal care?* The chapter highlights the complexities of choice and some of the difficulties of incorporating users' views into changes in the structure and process of antenatal care.

The next chapter is by Sandra Wheatley and looks at psychosocial support in pregnancy. The chapter provides a useful overview of theories of social support and its association with psychological well-being. Sandra is part of a team currently evaluating an antenatal social support intervention designed to help prevent postnatal depression, and she describes this innovative work.

The fourth chapter is unique in that it focuses solely on the experiences of the providers, rather than the users, of maternity care. Natalie Fenwick reports the findings of her in-depth study of two midwifery group practices and explores the difficulties, dilemmas and delights of providing continuity of carer. This work clearly highlights the fact that midwives have psychological needs too, and that these must be recognized and met if midwives are to be able to provide optimum care to women.

In the next chapter Jane Weaver, who is both a midwife and a psychologist, explores the complex issues of choice, control and decision-making in labour. The three C's of choice, control and continuity are supposed to form the bedrock of current maternity care in Britain, but offering choice and control is not straightforward as these concepts have different meanings for different women. By mapping out some of these meanings, Jane's work suggests ways in which caregivers can work towards giving women real choices and a sense of control.

The next chapter stays with the theme of intrapartum care, and looks at women's decisions about, and experiences of, giving birth at home. Jane Ogden takes a long-term perspective and presents qualitative data from women who had homebirths 3–5 years earlier. This research shows that the physical context of childbirth can have important and lasting psychological ramifications for women.

Whilst Jane Ogden's chapter is largely about the positive long-term consequences of childbirth, the next chapter focuses on potential negative consequences, and examines post-traumatic stress disorder following childbirth. Clinical psychologist Suzanne Lyons describes what post-traumatic stress is, its causes and consequences, and how it might be prevented, identified and treated. There is currently a great deal of interest in this topic amongst maternity caregivers and Suzanne's chapter provides an excellent overview of relevant theoretical and practical considerations for everyone working with childbearing women.

In Chapter 8 consultant psychotherapist Patricia Hughes examines one of the most tragic aspects of childbirth, namely stillbirth and neonatal loss. Patricia explores the processes of grief, mourning and depression and how women integrate and adapt to their loss. Like several of the other contributors, Patricia describes what caregivers can do to minimize psychological difficulties and maximize the emotional well-being of the families they care for.

In the next chapter Anne McFadyen looks at the particular needs of parents of babies in special care baby units, the needs of the babies themselves and of the professionals caring for them. Anne takes a psychodynamic approach and presents in-depth case studies demonstrating how existing and earlier relationships shape experiences of special care. An understanding of these relationships will help to sustain caregivers working in the emotionally challenging environment of special care.

Mary Smale examines the psychosocial context of breast-feeding in the next chapter. Although breast-feeding is a biological process, it takes place in, and is shaped by, the psychological and social context. This context can facilitate or impede breast-feeding. Mary has drawn upon her experience as a breast-feeding counsellor and upon her doctoral thesis on women's experiences of breast-feeding to extend our understanding of this topic, and will help those working with breast-feeding women to provide sensitive and appropriate care.

The last chapter on early parenthood looks at women's experience of postnatal support. Midwife Jane Podkolinski asked women to keep diaries of their experiences in the first 28 days after birth, and found that support was vitally important to all the women in her study. Jane highlights the need to consider the transition to parenthood in terms of loss as well as gain. She also explores and questions the concept of postnatal depression.

The penultimate chapter, by Jo Sullivan-Lyons, looks at the experiences and needs of men as they become fathers. Although several of the other chapters consider aspects of men's experiences, this chapter explores these issues in some detail. Jo focuses on men's emotional well-being and how men differ from women in the ways in which they express emotional distress.

The last chapter, by psychologists Catherine Dennison and John Coleman, describes the experiences of teenage women during pregnancy and after childbirth. They challenge many of the myths and stereotypes surrounding this group. Catherine and John focus in particular on the relationship between the teenagers and their parents, and how everyone's roles are changed with the arrival of the new baby.

Although the chapters are diverse in their subject matter and methodologies, a number of common themes run through them. These common themes are outlined below, as the main messages of this book:

- Pregnancy, childbirth and the puerperium are biopsychosocial events, and by considering psychological and social, as well as biological, aspects we can gain a better understanding of these processes.
- Women's experiences at the time around childbirth cannot be viewed in isolation, as they are embedded in a network of social relationships.
- Pregnancy and childbirth are life events. The way in which they are experienced will be influenced by past events in women's lives. Experiences in pregnancy and childbirth will, in turn, influence women's future life experiences.
- Women, and their families vary enormously in their psychological needs and resources, and care should be tailored accordingly. It is necessary to talk with women about their individual needs, rather than make generalized assumptions based on a woman's social group.
- Psychosocial support is a key component of psychological care before, during and after childbirth. As well as providing direct support, caregivers can usefully help women to tap into other sources of social support. The right kind of support will help women to become confident and self-reliant rather than dependent.
- Offering choices, facilitating informed decision-making and respecting decisions made give women a sense of control and enhanced emotional well-being.
- Technology, such as ultrasound, intrapartum interventions and special care, brings costs as well as benefits. Caregivers face the challenge of minimizing these costs through good psychological care.
- Caregivers have psychological needs of their own that must be recognized, acknowledged and met. By attending to their own needs caregivers will be better equipped to meet the needs of the women and families they care for.

FURTHER READING

Clement S 1995 'Listening visits' in pregnancy: a strategy for preventing postnatal depression?
    Midwifery 11: 75–80
Clement S, Elliott S 1998 Psychological health before, during and after childbirth. In: Marsh G,
    Renfrew M (eds) Community-based maternity care. Oxford University Press, Oxford
Clement S, Sikorski J, Wilson J, Das S 1997 Planning antenatal services to meet women's
    psychological needs. British Journal of Midwifery 5: 298–305
Hunter M 1994 Counselling in obstetrics and gynaecology. BPS Books, Leicester
Niven C A, Walker A 1996 Conception, pregnancy and birth, psychology of reproduction
    series. Butterworth-Heinemann, Oxford
Raphael-Leff J 1991 Psychological processes of childbearing. Chapman & Hall, London
Riley D 1995 Perinatal mental health: a sourcebook for health professionals. Radcliffe Medical
    Press, Oxford
Sherr L 1995 The psychology of pregnancy and childbirth. Blackwell, Oxford

1

Women's experiences of antenatal ultrasound scans

Sarah Clement   Jennifer Wilson   Jim Sikorski

INTRODUCTION

The aim of this chapter is to describe women's experiences of antenatal ultrasound scans, and to suggest ways in which caregivers can best support women and their partners before, during and after this procedure and facilitate informed decision-making.

Ultrasound scanning is currently an almost universal feature of antenatal care in industrialized countries, with many women having more than one scan. Scanning serves a number of clinical functions: scans can be used to date a pregnancy, detect a low-lying placenta or multiple pregnancy, and to give an indication of fetal growth, for example. Scans may also detect fetal abnormality, and this is the main clinical justification given for scans undertaken in the 18–20th week of pregnancy. The routine use of ultrasound in the first half of pregnancy has been shown to increase the number of terminations for fetal abnormality and to reduce the number of inductions for 'post-maturity', but does not appear to improve perinatal mortality or any other infant health outcomes (Neilson 1997). Scans cannot detect all major fetal abnormalities (Ewigman et al 1993), and can occasionally give a false diagnosis of major abnormality when no abnormality, or only a minor one, is actually present (Brand et al 1994).

Scanning is increasingly being used as a screening tool to gauge the risk of fetal abnormality as more structural markers of chromosomal abnormality are being discovered and evaluated. These markers include: nuchal translucency (the presence of a thickening of the tissues overlying the skull at the back of the baby's neck; choroid plexus cysts (cysts in the baby's brain); and dilatation of the fetal renal pelvis (swelling of the part of the kidney which collects urine). These are often termed 'soft markers' (Whittle 1997), a term which highlights the fact that they are relatively weak predictors of fetal abnormality. These markers do not indicate that there *is* a problem with the baby, but merely that there *may* be a problem. Consequently, some women will experience false positive results, being told that their baby may have a problem and often undergoing invasive tests and weeks of anxiety only to be told that there was nothing wrong with the baby after all. It is in the nature of screening that some women also receive false negative results; that is, they will be told that the scan indicates that all is well, but will discover after the baby is born that he or she has an abnormality. When scans are used to screen for fetal abnormality this adds a new dimension to women's experiences.

Lying, sometimes rather awkwardly, alongside these clinical functions are the psychosocial functions or meanings of ultrasound for women and their families. To explore the meaning of scans to women and the nature of women's experiences we draw upon the existing literature and findings from the Antenatal Care Project, our study of women's experiences of antenatal care.

The data and research findings we present relate only to abdominal scans. However, transvaginal scans are becoming more common, particularly when detailed anomaly screening in early pregnancy is indicated. We were unable to locate any research evidence on women's experiences of vaginal scans, but we speculate that women will feel differently about vaginal scans than abdominal ones, given that many women find vaginal examinations difficult or distressing (Clement 1994).

WOMEN'S EXPERIENCES OF ULTRASOUND
Seeing is believing: positive experiences

Women's experience of ultrasound scanning is, on the whole, very positive. When women in the Antenatal Care Project were asked what was the best thing about their antenatal care the second most common response was the ultrasound scan (see Table 1.1). Scans did not appear at all in the top six answers women gave when asked what was the worst thing about their antenatal care (see Table 1.2). Women's enthusiasm for scans was also evident in our finding that 30 women stated that they would have liked more scans:

[The worst thing was] only getting one ultrasound scan.

I think it would have been nice to have more than one scan. Friends who have been to other local hospitals for their antenatal care have had at least three scans.

Everything has been brilliant apart from the scans. I was very disappointed you only got one scan. I feel you should at least have three to see the progress of your baby.

THE ANTENATAL CARE PROJECT

The Antenatal Care Project was a randomized controlled trial comparing different patterns of antenatal care (Sikorski et al 1996). The project involved 2794 women receiving maternity care at one of three hospitals in South East London or the surrounding community sites between June 1993 and February 1995. The women were socially and ethnically diverse. All were considered to be at low risk for antenatal complications generally, although none of our exclusion criteria related to fetal abnormality.

For women in the Antenatal Care Project, like most other women in Britain, ultrasound scanning was almost universal, with 99% (2634/2663) of women having at least one scan. 47% (1251/2663) of women had more than one scan, and the total number of scans received ranged from 0 to 9. The most common scan received by women in the Antenatal Care Project was a fetal anomaly scan at 18–20 weeks of pregnancy, and consequently this chapter focuses mainly, but not exclusively, on this type of scan.

In this chapter we present some statistical data relating to ultrasound scanning. We also report some qualitative findings resulting from a content analysis of women's written responses to three open-ended questions in a questionnaire sent to women in the 34th week of pregnancy. These questions were: 'What was the best thing about your antenatal care?', 'What was the worst thing about your antenatal care?' and 'Is there anything else you would like to tell us about your antenatal care?'. Our qualitative analysis was confined to a subsample of 700 women who returned questionnaires between December 1993 and June 1994, and who wrote something in response to at least one of these questions. Responses ranged from single words to two-page accounts of women's views and experiences.

Because examining women's experiences of scans was not a primary aim of the Antenatal Care Project, and because our questionnaires did not contain any questions specifically about scans, readers should bear these limitations in mind when reading the chapter. We see our chapter as providing some important initial insights into women's experiences of scans, and hope it will lead to further research investigating the issues it raises more directly.

One woman said that the best thing about her antenatal care was discovering that she had a low lying placenta, because this meant that she would have another scan!

Previous research has attempted to elucidate what it is that parents like about scans. In a detailed qualitative study of middle-class American parents, Sandelowski (1994) describes how parents see scans as a pleasurable early

Table 1.1 Perceived best things about antenatal care: top responses of 700 women in the Antenatal Care Project

Best things about antenatal care	Number of comments
Reassurance	213
Ultrasound scan	193
Positive qualities of caregiver	168
Listening to baby's heartbeat	111
Continuity of carer	44
Antenatal classes	41

Table 1.2 Perceived worst things about antenatal care: top responses of 700 women in the Antenatal Care Project

Worst things about antenatal care	Number of comments
Long waits at antenatal clinics	151
Lack of continuity of carer	60
Negative qualities of caregivers	56
Short/rushed consultations	41
Administrative problems/disorganization	30
Not enough antenatal visits	30

meeting between parent and child; an opportunity to become acquainted with the baby; to appraise, admire and claim it as their own; or as a picture-taking session celebrating family life.

In our more socially diverse British sample, we saw some evidence of this desire to 'meet' with the baby:

[The best thing was] the ultra scan when you see the baby, it makes you feel very happy.

[The best thing was] having my baby's picture taken at the scan.

[The best thing was] the scan check – actually seeing a little body moving around.

The scan gives parents visual access to their baby. Parents have a profound curiosity about the fetus, as the baby is someone who will have a central role in their future lives, and yet is hidden from view. For some women, simply glimpsing the baby – their first encounter – brings enormous pleasure. As one commentator has put it, in scanning 'the fetus, from being something nebulous, comes sharply into focus as a living individual' (Furness 1990).

However, for women in our sample, the desire for an antenatal encounter was matched, and to some extent overshadowed, by two other needs or desires: to have the emotional reality of the pregnancy confirmed by the scan and to obtain general reassurance about fetal well-being.

For some women, the main psychosocial benefit of the scan was that it gave them visual evidence that they were actually pregnant. These women generally had no intellectual doubt that they were carrying a baby, but emotionally they did not feel pregnant, particularly before they felt the baby's movements. The scan confirmed that they were truly pregnant, and this was something that women appeared to value:

[The best thing was] having the ultra scan, until then I didn't really feel like I was having a baby because I couldn't see it.

The best part or thing about the antenatal care I received must be the day my boyfriend and I saw our baby on the scan screen. It was a small comfort to us both as I did not carry big with the baby, and it was nice to see that even though I looked as though I were not pregnant, there actually was a baby inside me.

[The best thing was] being able to see baby on the ultra scan. I found this very emotional and it gave me the realization that something *is* actually there.

The other major psychosocial function of scans for women in our sample was ultrasound's apparent ability to reassure parents about fetal well-being:

[The best thing was] having my scan at 22 weeks. Knowing my baby has all its bits and pieces.

The ultrasound scan was incredibly reassuring, to see arms, legs, face, heart, spine, etc. with your own eyes.

The best thing so far has been the scanning of the baby and also hearing the baby's heartbeat, which reassured me that he/she is alive.

The ultrasound scan was the thing that put my mind at rest that the baby was developing properly.

Our qualitative findings clearly show that women generally *perceive* scans to be reassuring, but, although the vast majority of women in the Antenatal Care Project had at least one scan, 81% (1488/1839) of women still reported having some worry about fetal abnormality towards the end of their pregnancies. One in five women rated this concern as being 'a really major worry'. Furthermore, when presented with a list of 16 potential sources of worry in pregnancy, women rated concern about fetal abnormality as their second biggest worry, exceeded only by anxiety about the forthcoming birth. Other studies have also found no evidence that scanning reduces anxiety (Baillie et al 1996).

It is difficult to explain this paradox that women perceive scans as being very reassuring but are not apparently truly reassured by them. It is, however, a paradox that arises in many areas of health care with many diagnostic and screening tests being sought for reassurance but leaving patients with residual anxiety even after a supposedly 'reassuring' result (Fitzpatrick 1996). In the context of scanning, the paradox might be explained by our finding that women tend to see their scans as providing a global view of fetal well-being – whether the baby is alive, growing and developing – as well as information about whether the baby has any specific abnormalities. Unlike fetal abnormality, the general well-being of the fetus is changeable. A scan indicating that all is well at 18 weeks will be temporarily reassuring, but if women are seeing the scan as an indicator of general well-being, this reassurance will be transitory, and will begin wearing off after a few weeks when the woman begins to wonder whether the baby is *still* all right:

Not having a scan again did make me feel anxious about the development of the baby.

I would also like to have had a second scan of my baby later in pregnancy, i.e. 30–35 weeks . . . I'm sure it would let us relax a little more to see for ourselves that our baby is growing in the normal way.

It would be great if you had the option of having a further scan, perhaps at 33–38 weeks, when you feel most apprehensive about size and position of the baby.

The very direct and dramatic view of apparent fetal well-being that the first scan generally provides seems to fuel a desire for more scans. One woman wrote how she saw scans as being 'incredibly seductive' (Kuba 1995) and another described her 'craving for an ultrasound fix' (Sandelowski 1994).

The evidence discussed so far appears to suggest that women have a different agenda from the main medical one of detecting specific fetal abnormalities. For women, scans seem to be about giving emotional confirmation that there is a baby inside them, showing them that the baby is healthy and thriving, and providing the opportunity to see their as yet unknown closest of relatives (Raphael-Leff 1991). Scans appear to provide reassurance, but this reassurance can be temporary, and may create an enthusiasm for scans in situations where there is no clinical indication for ultrasound.

Some commentators have written dismissively about 'ultrasound for entertainment' (Furness 1990), but our research suggests that women value scans for reasons far less superficial than entertainment. Women's needs for reassurance about fetal well-being, for emotional confirmation of the pregnancy, and for making contact with their babies are important and should not be dismissed. Raphael-Leff (1991) has written evocatively about the pregnant woman's thirst for information about her baby, and her need to know: 'How is her baby doing? What is her baby doing? . . . How big is her baby? and how happy – does s/he like it in there? . . . Who is living in her womb? Who will her baby be' (Raphael-Leff 1991). The mother–baby relationship 'happens in the dark . . . through an enigmatic veil obscuring sight, hearing, smell, and direct contact' (Raphael-Leff 1991). Ultrasound seems to light up this darkness for a moment, providing some partial answers to parents' pressing questions about the baby.

Whilst accepting the validity of women's psychosocial needs outlined above, we question whether scans are the only way of meeting these needs, and suggest that the needs may be met, to some degree, by other means. Perhaps caregivers could help satisfy these needs by encouraging women to become more attuned to the baby's movements and activity patterns; by involving women more when palpating their abdomens, pointing out different parts of the fetus and teaching women to recognize the parts through touch; by using an ordinary stethoscope to enable women to hear their baby's heartbeat; and by helping women to feel, or maybe even measure, their own abdomens to see for themselves that the baby is growing well. Although these methods cannot easily compete with the powerful images scans provide, such strategies merit consideration in the difficult on-going debate about the provision of routine ultrasound scans (Neilson 1997).

Scanning as a family and cultural event

Ultrasound does not simply involve the pregnant woman and her sonographer, but often becomes a family event. Partners are frequently present, and sometimes the baby's siblings or grandmother are also there:

[The best thing was] if this can be included in this category it would be the early scan as it enabled my husband and older children (as well as myself) to 'see' the baby.

I have enjoyed all the antenatal care, in particular the scan at approx. 20 weeks. My husband and mum-in-law came with me and it was a brilliant experience.

Women report that the scan makes the pregnancy seem more real for their partners and others, who do not have the physical experience of pregnancy to convey the baby's reality to them.

Scan pictures appear to be highly valued, and are often placed in a handbag, on a mantelpiece, or as the first picture in a baby's photo album. The picture is shown to family, friends and work colleagues, and the baby's features commented upon in much the same way as if it were a photograph of a newborn baby. Women sometimes wish to make their own video recording of the baby on the ultrasound screen, and in America and the Netherlands there are advertisements inviting parents to have 'Baby-look' or 'Fun-ultrasound' sessions (Keirse 1993), and to 'Have a videotape of your unborn baby made in your own home' (Furness 1990).

An Australian scientist has recently developed a technique for creating an exact plastic replica of the fetus's face using the ultrasound scan recordings. A televised documentary showed a ghostly fetal face emerging as the plastic gradually took on its final form. The scientist then presented this tiny plastic face to the baby's mother. She seemed slightly bemused and uncertain about this object, and later reported that she had given it to her mother-in-law as a gift (Tomorrow's World, BBC1, 11 November 1996, 8 p.m.).

In a recent television soap opera a man took the scan picture of his child and had it reproduced and emblazoned on a T-shirt, which he excitedly gave to his wife as a present (Brookside, Channel 4, 15 April 1997, 8.30 p.m.). The fuzzy ultrasound image of the fetus has acquired a firm place in popular culture, as an icon signifying pregnancy.

Do scans facilitate maternal–fetal bonding?

Many commentators have noted the apparent potential of scans to facilitate or bring forward bonding between the mother and her fetus (e.g. Fletcher & Evans 1983). However, when researchers have critically reviewed existing research in this area, it seems that there is no evidence for such an effect (Baillie et al 1996, Green 1990). Interestingly, although many of the women in the Antenatal Care Project commented that having a scan made their babies seem more real to them, none said that scans made them feel closer to their babies. A further finding from our study also contradicts the view that scans improve attachment between mother and fetus. We found a significant correlation between the number of scans received and having a negative attitude to the pregnancy ($r = 0.11$, $p < 0.001$) where negative attitude was the sum of women's ratings of how *stressed*, *worried*, *uncertain* and *depressed* they felt about their pregnancies. This finding can probably be explained by the fact that women experiencing pregnancy problems are likely to have more scans, and it is the anxiety caused by the problems, rather than the number of scans, that is making women feel more negative about their pregnancies.

Even if scans did bring about the earlier onset of maternal–fetal bonding we cannot assume that this would necessarily be beneficial. Perhaps the very gradual onset of attachment to the fetus over the course of pregnancy has an important function in minimizing psychological trauma if the fetus is subsequently lost through miscarriage, for example. Research suggests that for some women who lost their babies in this way, having had a scan does indeed add to women's anguish by heightening the reality of what had been lost, although other women in the same situation can find having had a scan helpful and see their memory of the image of the baby as a gift (Black 1992).

When a fetal abnormality has been diagnosed, the powerfully emotive ultrasound image of the fetus may increase the anguish of parents making decisions about termination.

'I felt as if I was going crazy. We watched our baby on the screen sucking her thumb while we tried to cope with the devastating news we had just been given.' (Kuba 1995).

Some have speculated that ultrasound might have a beneficial effect on health-related behaviour, by reducing the prevalence of smoking, for example. However, two randomized controlled trials comparing routine and selective scanning found no evidence that scans reduce smoking (Newnham et al 1993, Saari-Kemppainen et al 1990).

Knowing too little and too much: negative experiences

Although women's experiences of, and attitudes towards, ultrasound were generally very positive, 23 women in the Antenatal Care Project mentioned some aspect of scanning as being the worst thing about their antenatal care.

Sometimes this was a feeling of disappointment that they did not see the baby as well as they had hoped:

[The worst thing was] that I was not told how much fluid to drink when I went for my scan. I therefore could not see my baby very well and felt like a failure.

I think that I should have had more than one scan and that's not because I'm worried about the baby, it's that I should be entitled to see the baby a bit more because my picture wasn't clear enough.

I wasn't pleased with the one scan I had at 18 weeks. I was expecting to have more than one, since the picture was not very clear.

Others were unhappy about impersonal care received during the scan:

I would like to say that I received cold treatment on that day by the doctor or radiographer who undertook the scan. I was very upset and . . . my husband was disappointed and upset too.

[The worst thing was] the bluntness of the consultant who performed the detailed scan, who needs to be more sympathetic and understanding because of the traumatic time it causes and the dilemma the parents are left in.

Some women expressed anger at not being given enough information during their scan:

[The worst thing was] when I had my scan, I felt it was very rushed, hardly anything was explained to me when I did ask a simple question 'Can you see the arms?', the reply was 'We can't go that much into detail', which upset me very much.

Some women were upset when they felt that information about the baby's sex had been withheld from them:

The only thing I was not happy about with the antenatal check-ups was the sex of my child I requested to know but I was not told. Whereas in other hospitals, if you ask they will tell you. In near future, I think it is better if someone asks for the sex of the child, they should tell the person.

I was very disappointed in the doctors who scanned me and said that they haven't time to tell me the child's sex. It would be a lot easier for me to know in that buying baby items as I'm unemployed I have to spread the cost throughout pregnancy. Although there are far more important things, i.e. health, it would make a big difference.

However, other women were angry about being told the baby's sex when they had not wished to have this information before the birth:

One person started calling the baby 'her' when I did not really want to know the sex before!

One concern, mentioned in other studies, but not by women in the Antenatal Care Project, was that the scan was intrusive, giving them access to information that perhaps ought not to be known before birth, 'like finding out what you're getting for Christmas before Christmas' (Sandelowski 1994).

Other women feel that the scan invades the baby's privacy, and makes the baby 'public property' (Lumbley 1985).

Risks and dilemmas

The research evidence on the safety of scans is generally reassuring, although not definitive (Neilson 1997). No women in our study expressed any concerns about the safety of scans. Other research confirms that, in general, women have few concerns about potentially harmful effects of ultrasound (Tsoi & Hunter 1987). However, some women have noticed their babies making violent movements during scanning and have interpreted these as a sign of distress (Beech & Robinson 1993, Sandelowski 1994). Also, in a study comparing women's perceptions of routine antenatal scanning with their perceptions of cerebral scanning of the baby's head postnatally, Thorpe and colleagues (1993) found that women were less likely to accept postnatal scans than antenatal ones, and that this was often due to an undercurrent of uncertainty about the safety of ultrasound. It appeared that when ultrasound is presented in a routine context, and where it has a large psychological pay-off, such as seeing the baby and being reassured that he or she appears healthy, women tended to minimize or dismiss concerns about safety. However, anxieties about safety can apparently be raised, even in a routine antenatal context, by media scares, for example (Hyde 1986).

When ultrasound is used either as a formal screening procedure looking for structural markers of chromosomal abnormality, or as a more general procedure for detecting a variety of fetal problems, there is the potential for false positive findings. A false positive is when a woman is told there may be a problem when in reality there is not. False positive findings can create immense anxiety. For women in the Antenatal Care Project the major drawback of scans was their ability to throw up false positive findings:

[The worst thing was] knowing at the first scan that the radiographer wasn't happy about something, but not knowing what, and waiting until the second scan when everything proved to be OK.

Having my scan was quite upsetting as I was told they could not measure the spine as baby moved but all else was well, had to wait 1 week for next scan this time told baby's thigh bone was too short, had to worry for 1 more week to go to hospital then they told me all was well, so I had 2 weeks of worry which really upset me. I think it should have been dealt with much quicker to save a lot of upset.

I had an appointment at the hospital, where I was told the baby could be abnormal, that I needed a scan that day. Appointments for a scan were full, so the doctor said he would call me in the following week at short notice for one. I was then left to worry for 2 weeks after, before another scan was done. Fortunately, everything was fine.

Although little research has looked specifically at the long-term impact of false positive scan results, we know from studies on other prenatal screening tests that for some women anxiety about the baby's health can persist even after a diagnostic test has revealed that the baby is normal (Marteau et al 1988, Statham & Green 1993).

Furthermore, when scans raise suspicions of abnormality this can herald a cascade of invasive diagnostic tests such as amniocentesis. One woman described this 'prenatal roller coaster' as 'the scariest ride of her life' (Kuba 1995). Having an amniocentesis test is invariably a difficult experience for women and their partners. The decision to have the test can be anguishing as parents have to weigh up the small risk of miscarriage and the potential loss of a healthy baby against their need to know whether the baby has an abnormality. After the test has been undertaken there is a wait of 2–3 weeks where women have very high levels of anxiety as they inevitably dwell on the possibility of the termination of a wanted pregnancy or the difficulties of bringing up a handicapped child. It is difficult to know whether the anxiety of the many parents who go through this process, only to discover that there was no fetal abnormality after all, is offset by the benefit for a small number of parents who discover true abnormalities and consequently have the opportunity to terminate the pregnancy or prepare for a child with special needs.

Indeed, the small minority of women who are found to be carrying babies with serious or lethal abnormalities may see the scan as a necessary intervention that enabled them to make their subsequent decisions. Of those who decide to continue with the pregnancy, some are grateful for the forewarning provided by the scan which enabled them to prepare for the birth of a handicapped child or the loss of a child whose abnormality is lethal (Chitty et al 1996). However, some parents wish they had not known about their babies' problems in advance, and find that the knowledge of an abnormality created a fearful image of the baby as a 'monster', their imagined baby always being far worse than the reality (Turner 1994).

Scans cannot detect all fetal abnormalities, and so can give false negative as well as false positive findings. In one large study, scans undertaken before 24 weeks' gestation were only able to detect 17% of the fetal abnormalities present (Ewigman et al 1993). This suggests that the majority of women giving birth to a child with an abnormality will have been scanned, and may have been falsely reassured by that scan. At present we have no evidence about the psychological consequences of such scenarios.

THE CAREGIVER'S ROLE

Providing information

The provision of information is an important prerequisite of informed decision-making. If women and their partners are to make informed decisions about scanning they need information about the purpose of the scan, what will happen during the scan, the fact that the scan is optional, and information on the effectiveness of scans, as well as details about practical matters such as when and where to attend. When scans are used in a screening context there is also a need for information relating to screening. It could be argued that such information should be presented before any type of scan, as all scans have the potential to reveal abnormalities, even if this is not the primary purpose of the scan. Abramsky (1994) has listed some of the types of information parents need when deciding about screening tests:

- information on what conditions are being tested for and what conditions the test cannot detect
- the implications of the conditions for babies
- how, when and where the test would be done, and what it would feel like
- how accurate the test is
- the possible consequences of receiving the information the test provides.

A recent survey of 94 British maternity units suggests that information provided about scans in many maternity units is woefully inadequate (Proud & Murphy-Black 1997). For example, a quarter of units provided no information other than the appointment time, and less than half (48%) of the units surveyed reported providing any information indicating the scan's potential to pick up fetal abnormalities. Similar findings were reported by Smith & Marteau (1995) in their observational study of 215 consultations in six different maternity units. They found that fetal anomaly scans were presented as being optional to only 11% of women; in only a third (37%) of the consultations was there any mention of what a fetal anomaly scan might detect; and in none of the consultations were the possibilities of false positive or false negative scan results mentioned.

Reviewing research in this area, Marteau (1995) concludes that there are five main reasons why caregivers tend to give minimal information about screening tests: lack of time, lack of knowledge, lack of skill in imparting information, the tendency to underestimate women's information needs, and women not requesting more information.

When discussing structural markers for chromosomal abnormality, caregivers have the difficult task of conveying quite complex risk information to women. However, the problem is not just one of communicating complex concepts. Research has shown that the way caregivers present risk information may be influenced by their own beliefs (Marteau et al 1993). Further research is needed about the best way to present risk information and what women understand by it.

Researchers are beginning to investigate the relative merits of different methods of providing information about screening. One study compared leaflets, videos and an early antenatal class as possible formats for the provision of screening information, and found that the video was rated as being more helpful and easier to understand than leaflets (Fairgrieve 1997).

The antenatal class was not well attended, a finding echoed by other researchers (Thornton et al 1995) who found that more women attended individual information sessions about screening.

In a pilot study exploring women's views about an *Informed Choice* leaflet on routine ultrasound (MIDIRS/NHS Centre for Reviews and Dissemination 1996) it was found that the leaflet which detailed a number of potential drawbacks of having a scan did not deter any women from having scans. The authors concluded that, although some women regarded the information in the leaflet as disturbing, more commented on the importance of ultrasound in allowing them to see their babies and to feel reassured that they were all right, and these positive aspects overshadowed the potential disadvantages of scanning mentioned in the leaflet (Oliver et al 1996).

Similar findings come from the study of Thornton and colleagues, in which the offer of extra information increased women's understanding and their satisfaction with the amount of information received, but had no effect on the proportion of women (99%) who accepted the offer of a scan (Thornton et al 1995). The authors speculate that this is because ultrasound is valued for non-medical reasons and is chosen even by informed people who decline other screening tests.

Women's comments presented earlier in this chapter also highlight the fact that women appreciate detailed information and feedback during and after scans, a finding that is echoed by other research (Neilson 1995).

Facilitating decision-making

As well as providing information, caregivers wishing to facilitate informed decision-making will also counsel women to help them to come to their own decisions. This involves listening to women's concerns and priorities; acknowledging these; providing further information if necessary; clarifying women's feelings about what would be the best course of action for them; and discussing the consequences of different courses of action (Hunter 1994).

It is generally agreed that counselling should be non-directive; that is, that caregivers should not impose their own views or advise a particular course of action (Abramsky 1994). In practice, however, non-directiveness is difficult to achieve. In a recent survey around a third of women said that they felt that they had not been given any choice about whether or not to have a scan (Audit Commission 1997). Comments like 'The other thing you should have done is a scan' and 'You have to make an appointment with the scan department. It's between 18 and 23 weeks' bring directiveness into the consultation (Smith & Marteau 1995). Another form of directiveness occurs when caregivers state what they would do in a similar situation. What the caregiver would do is irrelevant as it is not their baby and they would not have to live with the consequences of any decisions made (Abramsky 1994). The whole area of decision-making is a complex one, as discussed in Chapter 5.

The issue of directiveness is relatively unproblematic when the woman and the caregiver share the same view about whether or not to have a scan, but difficulties arise when differing views are held. We have anecdotal evidence that women declining scans often find it difficult to have this decision accepted and respected by caregivers, although we were unable to locate any research evidence on this.

However, other caregivers are now questioning the advisability of routine ultrasound and may find it hard to be non-directive when discussing ultrasound with women who want a scan without a specific clinical indication. Even where caregivers support the policy of routine screening they may be faced with women requesting further scans that they believe to be unwarranted. At a time when there is a strong movement within health care to increase evidence-based practice, given a cash-limited National Health Service, and given that no research has, as yet, conclusively proven scans to be safe (Neilson 1997), scanning in the absence of a specific clinical indication becomes problematic. It presents a particular dilemma because many women want scans and gain satisfaction from them. Those concerned to provide a woman-centred service may advocate scanning on maternal request, in the absence of a clinical indication, often using the argument that scans may improve maternal psychological health or facilitate bonding, but as we have seen there is little research evidence to support either of these propositions. However, as discussed earlier in this chapter, women's desire for scans is not trivial; it reflects important underlying needs for reassurance, information about the baby, and confirmation of the emotional reality of the pregnancy. We have questioned whether scans are the only way to meet these needs, but this is a complex debate and there are no easy answers.

When scans are being used in a screening context, caregivers need particular skills in facilitating informed decision-making. Caregivers often assume that there is no point in undergoing screening if the parents would not terminate a pregnancy where the fetus has a major abnormality. However, many women appear to see the main purpose of screening, and scanning in particular, to be to provide reassurance to them that all is well, and so could rationally decide to have screening despite not being willing to consider termination in the event of a major abnormality being detected (Green et al 1993). Therefore, caregivers need to be aware of, and to acknowledge, women's own agendas when discussing screening with them.

The need to facilitate informed decision-making is paramount when a diagnosis of a major or lethal fetal abnormality is made. Research has shown that, in this situation, caregivers often become prescriptive rather than presenting information and supporting parents to come to their own decisions. For example Marteau et al (1994) report that obstetricians, geneticists and genetic nurses tend to be directive and advise termination for fatal conditions such as anencephaly. Chitty et al (1996) describe the experiences of one woman carrying a baby with a fatal condition who reported that there was no discussion of options, she was simply booked in for an 'induction' at 21 weeks' gestation. It was only on arrival at the labour ward that the implications of the induction became apparent and she chose to continue with the pregnancy.

Caregivers will inevitably bring their own beliefs, values and experiences to any encounter. It can be helpful for caregivers to consider and explore their own beliefs around scanning, screening, disability and termination as an awareness of these may help caregivers to minimize their influence on the counselling situation (Isle 1995).

Training can also help caregivers to improve their ability to support parents in making informed decisions about screening. A 1-hour training session involving small group discussions focused around a video and the provision of individual feedback to caregivers on their consultations before and after training have both been shown to improve caregivers' information-giving and communication skills in prenatal screening (Smith et al 1995).

Giving support

It is clear from the literature that women value and benefit from psychological support at all stages of scanning. Support should involve listening to women, acknowledging their feelings and responding to their wishes and needs as individuals. Supportive care is of greatest importance for women who are told their baby has, or may have, an abnormality.

It is wrong to assume that any one package of supportive care will be appropriate for all women whose scan reveals a suspected or actual abnormality. Individuals differ widely in their needs and wishes, even when faced with the same situation. The only way to find out what is the most appropriate care for any parents is to talk with them, and to listen carefully as they articulate their needs and preferences. There are, however, some needs common to all parents in this situation. These include privacy, continuity of caregiver, empathy, and respect for any decisions made.

When an abnormality is diagnosed some parents will choose to continue with the pregnancy. Such parents need a high level of supportive care, with continuity of carer and sensitivity from all the staff they encounter during their maternity care. Many women will appreciate being seen outside normal antenatal clinics, and having a separate room on antenatal and postnatal wards (Chitty et al 1996). Parents will also have an ongoing need for support after the birth. Women who decide to terminate their pregnancies also need the highest level of supportive care before, during and after the termination.

BROADER ISSUES

The widespread and routine use of ultrasound in pregnancy, and its increasing role in screening for fetal abnormality may have ramifications beyond those discussed above. Pregnancy may seem shorter with increasing numbers of women apparently not announcing their pregnancy until after scanning and other screening tests in case they may terminate the pregnancy (Rothman 1994). Rothman believes that this has led to the 'tentative pregnancy' in which women hold back from becoming attached to their fetus until after the results of screening to protect themselves against the pain they anticipate if an abnormality is found and the pregnancy is terminated. Rothman also speculates that this has contributed to the view that babies are *products* and that only *perfect* babies are acceptable.

We also speculate that the introduction of scanning and other screening tests may have created a more anxious experience of pregnancy. We have no direct evidence about this, but in a study carried out in the 1960s only 17% of pregnant women reported being concerned about fetal abnormality (Royal College of Midwives 1966) whereas in the Antenatal Care Project 81% of women reported having at least some worry about fetal abnormality.

The increased use of screening tests for fetal abnormality also has implications for the way people see people with disabilities. Marteau & Drake (1995) presented health professionals and lay people with information about a woman who gave birth to a child with Down syndrome, and when the scenario described also included the information that the woman had declined the offer of a prenatal screening test, both health professionals and lay groups said that the woman was in part to blame for the child's condition. It seems that the availability of screening tests reinforces the view that children with disabilities should not be born and have no rightful place in society. For example, in one early survey 41% of obstetricians thought that the State should not be expected to pay for the specialized care of children with severe handicaps if parents had declined the offer of prenatal diagnosis (Farrant 1985). One of us has previously pointed out some of the dangers inherent in some medical attitudes to screening for fetal abnormality and has highlighted the need to value and support the lives of handicapped children and those who care for them (Sikorski 1989). The mother of a daughter with spina bifida not diagnosed during a scan makes a similar point when she reports her anger at the many friends and health professionals who commented 'Why don't you sue, you could get compensation for them missing it?', comments which reflect their apparent perception of her daughter as an unfortunate mistake of the health care system rather than 'a happy baby girl who happens to have been born with some disabilities' (Lindsay 1994).

We have endeavoured to present some of the complex, paradoxical, and potentially far-reaching issues surrounding antenatal ultrasound scanning and women's experiences of scans. We hope that our findings will provoke discussion amongst caregivers about how best to meet women's needs in relation to scanning.

Key points for caregivers

- In general, pregnant women appear to be very positive about their experience of antenatal ultrasound scanning. The antenatal scan seems to give reassurance, confirm the reality of the pregnancy and act as a significant 'first meeting' with the baby.
- Despite the significance of antenatal scans to women and their partners, caregivers should be aware that scanning has not been shown to reduce anxiety and should be careful to explore antenatal worries. Caregivers should be aware that scans, like other screening tests, may, in spite of normal findings, paradoxically increase anxiety. This may need to be discussed with women in some circumstances, for example when a woman requests further scans for reassurance.
- Women's comments remind caregivers of the paramount importance of sensitivity and information-giving in undertaking the antenatal scan.
- Maternity caregivers should be aware of the limitations of scanning technology and in particular its ability to create anxiety through false positive results.
- Caregivers should aim to provide accurate information on the purpose, benefits and disadvantages of antenatal scanning and to present scanning as an optional, rather than mandatory, investigation.
- Caregivers involved in facilitating decision-making in relation to information obtained from scanning should ensure that they possess appropriate counselling skills.

ACKNOWLEDGEMENTS

We would like to thank all the women who took part in the Antenatal Care Project and shared their experiences with us. Our thanks also go to our colleagues on the Antenatal Care Project: Sarah Das, Nigel Smeeton, Maureen Statham and Becky Green. The Antenatal Care Project was funded by the NHS Executive, South Thames.

REFERENCES

Abramsky L 1994 Counselling prior to prenatal testing. In: Abramsky L, Chapple J (eds) Prenatal diagnosis: the human side. Chapman & Hall, London, ch 5

Audit Commission 1997 First class delivery: improving maternity services in England and Wales. Audit Commission, London

Baillie C, Hewison J, Mason G 1996 The psychological potential of routine ultrasound scanning: a systematic review of the evidence. Journal of Reproductive and Infant Psychology 14: 324

Beech B L, Robinson J 1993 Jumping babies. AIMS Journal 5: 15–16

Black R B 1992 Seeing the baby: the impact of ultrasound technology. Journal of Genetic Counselling 1: 45–54

Brand I R, Kaminopetros P, Cave M et al 1994 Specificity of antenatal ultrasound in the Yorkshire region: a prospective study of 2261 ultrasound detected anomalies. British Journal of Obstetrics and Gynaecology 101(5): 392–397

Chitty L, Barnes C A, Berry C 1996 Continuing with pregnancy after a diagnosis of lethal abnormality. British Medical Journal 313: 701–702

Clement S 1994 Unwanted vaginal examinations. British Journal of Midwifery 2: 368–370

Ewigman B G, Crane J P, Frigoletto F D et al 1993 Effect of prenatal ultrasound screening on perinatal outcome. New England Journal of Medicine 329: 821–827

Fairgrieve S 1997 Screening for Down's syndrome: what the women think. British Journal of Midwifery 5: 148–151

Farrant W 1985 'Who's for amniocentesis?': the politics of prenatal screening. In: Homans H (ed) The sexual politics of reproduction. Gower, London

Fitzpatrick R 1996 Telling patients there is nothing wrong: unless their true fears are addressed, diagnostic tests may leave them more anxious than before. British Medical Journal 313: 311–312

Fletcher J C, Evans M I 1983 Maternal bonding in early fetal ultrasound examinations. New England Journal of Medicine 308: 392–393

Furness M E 1990 Fetal ultrasound for entertainment? Medical Journal of Australia 153: 371

Green J M 1990 Calming or harming? A critical review of psychological effects of fetal diagnosis on women. Galton Institute, London

Green J M, Snowdon C, Statham H 1993 Pregnant women's attitudes to abortion and prenatal screening. Journal of Reproductive and Infant Psychology 11: 31–39

Hunter M 1994 Counselling in obstetrics and gynaecology. BPS Books, Leicester

Hyde B 1986 An interview study of pregnant women's attitudes to ultrasound scanning. Social Science and Medicine 22: 587–592

Isle S 1995 Precious lives, painful choices: helping parents who have abnormal prenatal test results. Journal of Perinatal Education 4: 11–18

Keirse M J N C 1993 Frequent ultrasound: time to think again. Lancet 342: 878–879

Kuba L M 1995 The prenatal testing roller coaster: one mother's story. Journal of Perinatal Education 4: 19–22

Lindsay Y 1994 'Why don't you sue?' British Medical Journal 308: 1377

Lumbley J 1985 Ultrasound debate. New Generation 4: 5–6

Marteau T M 1995 Toward informed decisions about prenatal testing: a review. Prenatal diagnosis 15: 1215–1226

Marteau T M, Drake H 1995 Attributions for disability: the influence of genetic screening. Social Science and Medicine 40: 1127–1132

Marteau T M, Kidd J, Cook R et al 1988 Screening for Down's syndrome. British Medical Journal 297: 1469

Marteau T, Plenicar M, Kidd J 1993 Obstetricians presenting amniocentesis to pregnant women: practice observed. Journal of Reproductive and Infant Psychology 11: 3–10

Marteau T, Drake H, Bobrow M 1994 Counselling following diagnosis of a fetal abnormality: the differing approaches of obstetricians, clinical geneticists and genetic nurses. Journal of Medical Genetics 31: 834–867

MIDIRS/NHS Centre for Reviews and Dissemination 1996 Ultrasound screening in the first half of pregnancy: is it useful for everyone?. MIDIRS, Bristol

Neilson J P 1995 High versus low feedback to mother at fetal ultrasound. In Enkin M W, Keirse M J N C, Renfrew M J, Neilson J P (eds) Pregnancy and childbirth module of the Cochrane Database of Systematic Reviews. Update Software, Oxford

Neilson J P 1997 Routine ultrasound in early pregnancy. In Neilson J P, Crowther C A, Hodnett E D, Hofmeyr G J, Keirse M J N C (eds) Cochrane Database of Systematic Reviews. Update Software, Oxford

Newnham J P, Evans S F, Michael C A et al 1993 Effects of frequent ultrasound during pregnancy: a randomised controlled trial. Lancet 342: 887–891

Oliver S, Rajan L, Turner H, Oakley A 1996 A pilot study of 'Informed Choice' leaflets on positions in labour and routine ultrasound. NHS Centre for Reviews and Dissemination, York

Proud J, Murphy-Black T 1997 Choice of a scan: how much information do women receive before ultrasound. British Journal of Midwifery 5: 144–147

Raphael-Leff J 1991 Psychological processes of childbearing. Chapman & Hall, London

Rothman B K, 1994 The tentative pregnancy: amniocentesis and the sexual politics of motherhood. Pandora, London

Royal College of Midwives 1966 Preparation for parenthood. Royal College of Midwives, London

Saari-Kemppainen A, Karjalainen O, Ylostalo P et al 1990 Ultrasound screening and perinatal mortality: controlled trial of systematic one-stage screening in pregnancy: the Helsinki ultrasound trial. Lancet 336: 387–391

Sandelowski M 1994 Channel of desire: fetal ultrasonography in two-use contexts. Qualitative Health Research 4: 262–280

Sikorski J 1989 Prenatal diagnosis and genetic screening. British Medical Journal 299: 1033

Sikorski J, Wilson J, Clement S, Das S, Smeeton N 1996 A randomised controlled trial comparing two schedules of antenatal visits: the antenatal care project. British Medical Journal 312: 546–553

Smith D K, Marteau T M 1995 Detecting fetal abnormality: serum screening and fetal anomaly scans. British Journal of Midwifery 3: 133–136

Smith D K, Shaw R W, Slack J, Marteau T M 1995 Training obstetricians and midwives to present screening tests: evaluation of two brief interventions. Prenatal Diagnosis 15: 317–324

Statham H, Green J 1993 Serum screening for Down's syndrome: some women's experiences. British Medical Journal, 307: 174–176

Thornton J G, Hewison J, Lilford R J et al 1995 A randomised trial of three methods of giving information about prenatal testing. British Medical Journal 311: 1127–1130

Thorpe K, Harker L, Pike A, Marlow N 1993 Women's views of ultrasonography: a comparison of women's experiences of antenatal screening with cerebral ultrasound of their newborn infant. Social Science and Medicine 36: 311–315

Tsoi M M, Hunter M 1987 Ultrasound scanning in pregnancy: consumer reactions. Journal of Reproductive and Infant Psychology 5: 43–48

Turner L 1994 Problems surrounding late prenatal diagnosis. In: Abramsky L, Chapple J (eds) 1994 Prenatal diagnosis: the human side. Chapman & Hall, London, ch 9

Whittle M 1997 Ultrasonographic 'soft markers' of fetal chromosomal defects. British Medical Journal 314: 918

FURTHER READING

Abramsky L, Chapple J (eds) 1994 Prenatal diagnosis: the human side. Chapman & Hall, London

Green J M 1990 Calming or harming? A critical review of psychological effects of fetal diagnosis on women. Galton Institute, London

Hyde B 1986 An interview study of pregnant women's attitudes to ultrasound scanning. Social Science and Medicine 22: 587–592

Proud J, Murphy-Black T 1997 Choice of a scan: how much information do women receive before ultrasound. British Journal of Midwifery 5: 144–147

Sandelowski M 1994 Channel of desire: fetal ultrasonography in two-use contexts. Qualitative Health Research 4: 262–280

Thorpe K, Harker L, Pike A, Marlow N 1993 Women's views of ultrasonography: a comparison of women's experiences of antenatal screening with cerebral ultrasound of their newborn infant. Social Science and Medicine 36: 311–315

2

Antenatal care: what do women want?

Janet Hirst   Jenny Hewison   Therese Dowswell
Hazel Baslington   Janet Warrilow

INTRODUCTION

In Britain over the last 5 years those involved in the provision of maternity services, that is National Health Service (NHS) purchasers and providers, have required more information regarding women's views of their maternity care for planning and evaluation purposes. Of course none of this is new to those organizations that have sought the views of women for years, such as the National Childbirth Trust, Community Health Councils, the Maternity Alliance and Maternity Service Liaison Committees. The apparent demand for information by the providers (NHS trusts providing maternity services) and the purchasers of maternity care (NHS health authorities) has been attributed to 'Changing Childbirth', the report of the Expert Maternity Group (DoH 1993). But it is plausible that the need to consult the users of the health service is part of a much broader development within the NHS which coincides with several reports (DoH 1991, 1993).

For us to understand the implications of what women want from their antenatal care it is helpful to know who it is that wants to know and what type of antenatal care women already receive. Of course antenatal care cannot be considered entirely in isolation from intrapartum and postpartum care, as a change in one part of the service will affect the available resources in another. Some of these issues will be discussed in the following sections. Firstly we consider why there is such an interest in the views of women, what type of antenatal care women generally receive, what antenatal care is really about and how it is documented. We then discuss whether all women want the same things, how this may cause a dilemma for the carers of women and how changes in the structure of antenatal care may, or may not, provide what women want. The first and the subsequent antenatal visits are considered separately because there is specific information available about the first visit that challenges the current trend in the provision of that first contact. The type and gender of the professional, and the number and location of antenatal visits are discussed after a short consideration of the impact of offering a choice. The last section before our concluding discussion considers whether knowing a carer is enough and what other attributes of the carer women would like.

WHAT DO WOMEN WANT? WHO WANTS TO KNOW?

During the late 1980s rapid changes occurred within the NHS that altered the way in which the service thought, planned and operationalized in both hospital and community settings. The trust status of hospital and community care endorsed a more business-like approach towards health care and an interest in the quality of that care. Quality assurance management and surveillance began to incorporate user satisfaction questionnaires to assess and develop health care services. The maternity services were well ahead in their thinking about assessing users' views of their care, along with mental health and paediatric services, compared to other fields within the NHS. A survey manual commissioned by the Department of Health (Mason 1989) containing standard questionnaires, helped providers and purchases of maternity care to evaluate their local service and assess local needs. This was the first comprehensive guide available for the evaluation of maternity care. The manual has been adapted for local use by many maternity services and purchasers and although it can produce healthy response rates as a postal survey, or in one-to-one interviews, using this very structured questionnaire would not allow women to talk easily about their own priorities.

In conjunction with quality assurance surveillance, other information has been obtained by the providers of health care to complement the views of users and to help with the future planning of the service. Detailed workload analysis, mainly in the clinical nursing and midwifery areas, became widespread within many trusts. The amount of time spent on direct patient care, such as physical observations and medication, and indirect patient care, such as documentation and answering the telephone; provided specific profiles of ward activity by the type of tasks being undertaken and by whom.

In theory, women's views of their antenatal care, that is their preferences for and satisfaction with care, along with the workload analysis could direct planned changes within the maternity services. Such a straightforward market strategy, however appealing to the purchasers of maternity care, is of course not that easy to implement. Firstly, finding out what women want is not straightforward as there are financial and resource constraints that need to be considered.

As the NHS organizational changes were well under way several government reports, e.g. the Winterton Report (House of Commons Health Committee 1992) and 'Changing Childbirth' (DoH 1993), also began to challenge the way in which the maternity services were delivered. Women's views of their maternity care were now not only important locally, but also of national interest. Purchasers and providers were urgently called upon to find out and provide what women want during their maternity care, in particular where care should take place and who should provide it. The concepts of choice and women-centred care, as emphasized in 'Changing Childbirth' (DoH 1993), has increased the need to obtain and use users' views.

WHAT DO WOMEN GET? THE ORGANIZATION OF CARE

Generally, women tend to have about 15 clinical antenatal checks during their pregnancy (Bull 1990, Dowswell et al 1995, Steer 1993). Most of the antenatal care takes place in the community setting (within the general practice surgery or health centres) and the responsibility has traditionally been shared between the hospital consultant and the general practitioner. Ultrasonography is mainly located at the hospital, but there is an increase in the number of community ultrasound facilities sometimes in conjunction with a community consultant antenatal clinic. These facilities may be found where women have a long or difficult journey to the hospital or where the uptake of the services can be significantly increased by making such facilities more easily available. There has been a general increase in the amount of antenatal care taking place in the community, although this has not always been accompanied by a reduction in the amount of hospital antenatal checks. Dowswell et al (1995) found that in six districts in the Yorkshire region the number of hospital antenatal visits excluding the booking visit and scans ranged from 1.9 to 4.6. In addition to these visits, the community antenatal visits ranged from 7.8 to 11.8. There are a minority of women who have part or all of their antenatal care at home. This is mainly women receiving care from pilot schemes of new ways to organize care, e.g. midwifery group practices, or women intending to have a home birth.

Although it is generally believed that a good outcome for mother and baby is dependent upon good antenatal care, this is not necessarily the case. No relationship was found in a large UK birth cohort study between delayed antenatal attendance (after 28 weeks of pregnancy) and any important indicator of pregnancy outcomes (Thomas et al 1991). What constitutes good antenatal care may be thought of as the optimum number of antenatal visits at the most appropriate place to provide the content needed for each individual woman. This varied and flexible service is sometimes difficult to maintain for women with diverse needs and sometimes compromises have to be made. For example, some non-English speaking women may prefer to attend a place for their antenatal care where they are most likely to have the benefit of a linkworker. This may prove to be the hospital or a health centre rather than a general practice surgery or, if this means that the woman has further to travel, even at home.

WHAT IS ANTENATAL CARE ABOUT?

There is little doubt that for most women antenatal care does some good and the benefits include the prevention and detection of pregnancy-related problems, education and psychological support. The extent to which these issues need to be addressed vary from woman to woman, but there has been a general view that the content of antenatal checks is mainly about clinical screening purposes. Indeed the documentation is geared to make the routine physical checks easy to record. These endless measurements such as blood pressure, weight, urinalysis and fundal height are challenged as having limited obstetric value and therefore the need to continue doing them, as often or at all, has been questioned (Steer 1993). Steer has suggested that the number of antenatal visits is more to do with the fact that women find them reassuring. But women do not only get reassurance from the physical checks during their antenatal care. They also have contact with their carers and with other pregnant women which may help them to feel confident about being pregnant and becoming mothers. In addition to these positive feelings women may also become frustrated, anxious and irritated by their maternity care experience. Over the years women have repeatedly raised concerns such as impersonal 'conveyor belt' care or lack of continuity (Reid & Garcia 1989). It is not uncommon for women to become frustrated and irritated by long waiting times in antenatal clinics or conflicting advice. One woman has said: 'but I just feel that they are like rushed, and they've got so many things and they're waiting for the next patient to come in and it doesn't relax you' (Dowswell et al 1996).

Apart from the process of antenatal care causing these feelings, pregnancy itself can arouse feelings of happiness and, at the same time, uncertainty. For example, first time mothers may be more anxious than women having their second or third baby, as past experience plays an important part in influencing how women feel and what women want.

Steer also suggest that *practitioners* find antenatal checks reassuring because the process minimizes the chance that they have overlooked something and reassures them that the pregnancy is progressing as it should. If this is the case it would be difficult for practitioners to reduce the number of antenatal visits without raising anxiety within themselves. Also, it has been found that carers feel that they have less opportunity to get to know the women that they care for when they are seen less often (Sikorski et al 1996). So, it is not only the content, but also the number, of antenatal checks that are under question. In 1980, Hall and colleagues reviewed the effectiveness of antenatal care. Their study concluded that the number of antenatal checks could be reduced without any detrimental effect on the detection and diagnosis of pregnancy-related problems such as intrauterine growth retardation, malpresentation and pre-eclampsia. What we need to know, however, is how women feel about fewer antenatal visits, and this is discussed later in this chapter.

When we also consider other types of contacts many women have with the maternity services, such as ultrasound scans on different days from antenatal checks, parentcraft sessions, home assessments, ad hoc contacts with their midwife or their general practitioner and telephone communication, it is easy to see that some women have many more contacts during their antenatal care than is documented in their casenotes. It is not clear why there are so many contacts, but if some of them are provided on the grounds of reassurance, perhaps it is worth remembering the fact that the process of antenatal care makes some women feel anxious as well as reassured. This is particularly true as far as ultrasound screening for fetal abnormality is concerned. Women's experiences of scans are covered in a separate chapter. However, other aspects of antenatal care can also cause anxiety, such as concern about fetal size which turns out to be unfounded. So we can see the very process of antenatal care can affect what women want in different ways. One thing that we are sure about is that women want reassurance and it is likely that most practitioners are more than happy to provide it.

ANTENATAL DOCUMENTATION

The type of maternity documentation available makes it difficult to prove that any of the antenatal checks undertaken are on the grounds of anything other than physical checks even though psychosocial aspects of care are legitimate parts of antenatal care. Obstetric and midwifery casenotes record antenatal clinic visits by responding to a physical check list. Practitioners do not tend to be explicit when recording the original reason for the antenatal check and the precise content, both of which are needed for the accurate assessment of what happens during an antenatal check. The words 'reassured' or 'anxious' may be found written in the casenotes but this does not explain to us the amount of counselling time or the type of care that a woman may have needed. One of the reasons for this could be that most women keep their own antenatal casenotes with them whilst they are pregnant. To try to ensure confidentiality, some details such as sensitive psychological or social information may appropriately be withheld from the records. The routine audit of antenatal care, which is becoming widespread in all maternity services, will become more sensitive to the actual process of antenatal care when the documentation is explicit and complete. Until then practitioners will be criticized for providing endless ineffective clinical care even though we know for some women this may not be the main reason for, or content of, their antenatal check.

A CAREGIVER'S DILEMMA

There is a constant conflict facing the caregivers within maternity care to juggle with what women want and what the caregiver feels might be best overall. In addition, professionals have difficult decisions to make about what choices can be offered in the context of finite resources. Also, choices that are available need to be accessible to all women to provide equitable maternity care. The problem does not end here for carers. Carers may discover that some aspects of clinical care which they believed were effective, and which they may have been undertaking for the last 20 years, have no proven clinical benefit. For example, to find out that weighing women routinely at antenatal visits is not clinically worthwhile can be profoundly unsettling, in that to accept this, caregivers must also accept that they have been wasting their time carrying out an unproductive procedure for many years. This conflict between the new information and the old belief is referred to as cognitive dissonance. There has been a belief about antenatal care by both women and caregivers that if carers are doing something, then it must be worth doing. Such examples of cognitive dissonance have maintained many common practices within the maternity services for decades. Dedicated well-meaning carers are now trying hard to accept that many established practices are being shown by research not to be worthwhile. Nevertheless, although it may not be clinically worthwhile to weigh women at each antenatal visit, some women find it reassuring to find that their weight gain is within the normal range. For such a woman, it has become another piece of the jigsaw of information that suggests that what she is doing is all right, and that her pregnancy is progressing well.

DO ALL WOMEN WANT THE SAME TYPE OF CARE?

Finding out what women want can, at a first glance, seem fairly straightforward. Today the majority of women are happy to share their views and postal surveys are successful at obtaining the views of most white middle-class women, but are less successful at reaching women from lower socio-economic groups, minority ethnic groups, travellers, teenagers and substance abusers. However, the views of women from these groups can be successfully obtained by one-to-one interviews either at their home or at a mutually convenient place. Overall there appears to be a general consensus that there are some fundamental commonalties in what women want, such as being able to understand, to communicate, to express their wishes and to be treated with respect. However, the way in which these fundamental needs are met may differ for individual women. Indeed these needs can only be met if there are resources available to do so. A study that asked the views of black and ethnic minority women found that 40% of the women that were interviewed said that they had difficulty being understood (Leeds FHSA 1992). Carers need to maintain a flexible approach to be able to continuously adapt to what individuals want. For example, some women want to be involved with the decisions about their care whereas others are happy for the practitioners to take the lead. Whilst some women want to understand the smallest details about their care, others only want basic information but prefer not to worry about what they may not need to know. Some women need interpreters to explain to them what they need to know and others who are indigenous still may not feel that they understand. Conversely, some practitioners feel that women do not understand and yet the women may feel that they do.

STRUCTURES AND PROCESSES OF CARE

What does seem to matter to women is the quality of the service in terms of who provides antenatal care, where such care is provided and the technical and psychological support given. An efficient administration may also matter. When we are considering what women want from their maternity care we need to be clear about what is part of the structure of the service (where care takes place and by whom) and the processes of care (what is being done and how it is being done). The structure of a service facilitates the process of care and we need to recognize that if we bring about a change in the structure of the service, such as where care takes place, we cannot assume that this will improve the quality for women. We also need to be clear about how the process of care has been affected.

Women have a variety of complaints about their maternity care and some of them are about the interaction between one person and another. When we change the structure of a service those people who are energetic, confident and competent often take the lead to bring about the change. The new structure may leave untouched some of the things that the women previously complained about, such as discourteous behaviour at one of the antenatal clinics. An example of such behaviour is as follows:

After she saw me she told me to go and get my blood taken so she handed the card into the woman, you know, who takes the blood and this woman were calling everybody else apart from me so I ended up waiting a whole hour. Right, in the end, when I went over and said 'Well you haven't called me out for my blood to be taken', she says 'Oh I finish at half past four' and she locked up and that, so I had waited there for an hour for nothing basically (Dowswell et al 1996).

If an evaluation of care is undertaken that focuses upon the structure of antenatal care, and does not include the process of care, important factors, such as discourteousness, will not be assessed. Hence the new structure may appear better than it actually is because women will still encounter the same interpersonal problems as they did before. So we need to be clear when women are telling us about the structure of care and when they are telling us about other attributes of quality.

What a good deal of work in organizational psychology shows is that organizational structures can affect the ability of staff to offer a person-centred type of service and be responsive to what women need. The car manufacturer, Volvo, found that production lines were not good for productivity in car manufacture, because the workers on the line did not care about the quality of their products (Gyllenhammar 1977). Antenatal clinics have been compared to production lines. If the main benefit of delivering maternity care is psychological, then it makes no sense to deliver that type of care through structures (production lines) that make psychological benefits such as reassurance and support harder to deliver.

DO WOMEN WANT CHOICE?

There is strong evidence that women want choice about many aspects of their antenatal care which include the setting, the caregiver and the tests available. As we have mentioned, sometimes women choose to leave many decisions to their carer because the carer is the 'expert' or because they just do not know what to do for the best. For example, there is an increase in the number of women who carry their own casenotes and this is often supported by local policy. It has been shown that not all women want to do this and one study has found that 15% of women wanted the midwife to keep their maternity records (Gready et al 1995).

Women can only make choices where they are offered a choice and some choices are more easily available to some women than others. One woman was annoyed because the choice that she wanted was initially withheld. When she commented upon her ultrasound experience she said: 'I was irritated because they don't tell you the sex of the baby and they evade the question as if it is not important and they get haughty about it. I'm sure they know, my consultant said that if I wanted to know he would recommend it. I wanted a choice' (Hirst et al 1997).

We should remember that for some women offering choice can have its downside. For example, antenatal visit schedules can be reduced and women invited to attend for unscheduled visits if they feel that they need to do so, either for a physical problem or because they are worried or need support. This can be seen as increasing women's choice, which is generally considered a good thing. However, for some women there may be a stigma attached to the psychological aspects of care. It may be all right to tell your partner or employer that your antenatal check is for you and your baby's health but it is less easy to say, even to yourself, that you need that antenatal care for psychological reasons. This type of behaviour has some similarities with the social science research on sick roles. If you are ill you can get off some of your obligations and even pass them on to someone else in the home and at work. Of course treating pregnancy as an illness has lots of problems, but for some women it may have its advantages.

THE FIRST ANTENATAL VISIT

Many satisfaction surveys repeatedly show that most women are satisfied with their maternity care and there is evidence that when women are asked about their care that they tend to like the type of care they get (Porter & MacIntyre 1984). More recent research has shown that although women generally do like what they get, this is not always the case and that some women prefer some types of care more than others. For example, a study conducted in the Yorkshire Region (Dowswell et al 1996, Hirst et al 1996) found that although women's preferences did appear to be shaped by what they had experienced, the extent to which women prefer the care they experienced depends upon which type of carer they saw.

Table 2.1 shows who the women in this study would have liked to have seen and who they actually saw at their first antenatal visit. As we can see most women saw the midwife only, general practitioner (GP) only or the midwife and GP. However, when these women were asked who they would have liked to have seen, more of them chose the combination of midwife and GP than just one caregiver. So, although many women did see their preferred carer (59%) many did not.

The right-hand column of Table 2.2 shows the number of women who saw each carer. The diagonal bold type shows the number of women who not only saw this carer but also preferred to do so. The table (horizontal rows) also shows the other carers that some women would have liked to have seen instead.

What Table 2.2 clearly tells us is that a combination not only of the midwife and GP, but also of the hospital doctor and midwife, was preferred by more women to a single carer. To explain further, of the 139 women who saw the midwife only, 64 (46%) of these women actually preferred to do so. Similarly of the 142 women who saw the GP only, 78 (55%) preferred to do so. In contrast, of the 118 women who saw the midwife and GP, 88 (75%) preferred to do so. A chi-squared test on the first four rows of this table indicates that

Table 2.1 The type of caregiver women would have liked to have seen and who they actually saw at their first antenatal visit (n = 520)

Carer	Would have liked to have seen	Actually saw
Midwife only	97 (19%)	139 (28%)
GP only	99 (20%)	142 (28%)
GP and midwife	193 (38%)	118 (24%)
Hospital doctor only	19 (4%)	22 (4%)
Hospital doctor and midwife	81 (16%)	75 (15%)
Midwife, GP and hospital doctor	12 (2%)	3 (0.6%)
GP and hospital doctor	2 (0.4%)	4 (0.8%)

Table 2.2 Who did these women see? Who preferred these carers? For those who did not see their preferred carer who would they like to see instead? (Hirst et al 1996, with permission)

Caregiver seen	Preferred caregiver							
	MW	GP + MW	GP	MW + HD	MW + GP + HD	GP + HD	HD	Total
MW only	64	51	4	16	2	0	2	139
MW + GP	10	88	13	3	2	0	2	118
GP only	13	41	78	4	4	0	2	142
MW + HD	7	10	1	54	0	0	3	75
MW + GP + HD	0	1	1	0	1	0	0	3
GP + HD	0	0	0	1	1	2	0	4
HD only	3	2	2	3	2	0	10	22

Key: MW = midwife; GP = general practitioner; HD = hospital doctor

this pattern could not have occurred by chance, i.e. the carer women preferred to see differed significantly from the carer women actually saw (chi-squared $= 27.7, p < 0.0001$). We must be careful in how this message is understood. The information tells us about who these women would like to see at their first antenatal visit (structures) but not about the content of the visit or the roles of the carers (processes). We must not assume that this means women want to see a combination of carers for the same things or even together in the same room. It is much more likely that many women find that there is an advantage to seeing different types of carers at the same visit to answer different types of questions.

WHICH PROFESSIONAL DO WOMEN WANT TO SEE FOR SUBSEQUENT ANTENATAL CARE?

Most of the evidence around preference of carer is about which staff women would like to see during their intrapartum care (Green et al 1990). For many women, preference of carer is a conditional preference that is influenced by many other factors such as who they know, their past obstetric experience, the gender of the carer, the place they can see carers, the language that they speak and other resources that are available (such as linkworkers, crèche facilities, bus connections and parking). It is not unusual for women to apply conditions to who they want to see for their antenatal care such as: 'Anyone as long as it's a lady' or 'Anyone as long as they know what they are doing' or 'Not any midwife, my midwife' or 'Any midwife as long as there is a linkworker' (Hirst et al 1997). It is not yet clear how women make a choice about what they want or whether they have sufficient knowledge about the respective roles and training of midwives and medical staff to make this choice. Sometimes a single carer is favoured. In a London study, seeing a midwife for most of their antenatal care was favoured by women who had one-to-one midwifery care and women receiving care shared between the doctors and midwives (McCourt & Page 1996). Other women have said they like a midwife 'because it's their job and no one can take their place' (Hirst et al 1997). However, whatever care package is available it is likely that most women will see the midwife most of the time as there are proportionately more midwives per pregnant woman than GPs or obstetricians. Other women value having a mixture of professional carers. In the London study (McCourt & Page 1996) nearly a third of women who were receiving shared care liked it. Other women have reported the benefits of seeing a mixture of carers such as: 'They check for things at different times and so you feel more confident if the GP and hospital doctor can see you now and then to check you over' (Hirst et al 1997).

Women with no past experience of maternity care rely on their carers to inform them of the benefits of seeing the midwife, GP or obstetrician. Some women say that they would like to meet an obstetrician at least once during their antenatal care, so that if anything goes wrong later in their pregnancy or labour they would have a familiar carer. However, in the event of a problem at a later point there is only a small chance that these women would see the obstetrician that they had actually met. Others have argued that all women (irrespective of risk) should see an obstetrician in pregnancy and labour (Walker 1995). A study in Oxfordshire found that women allocated fewer antenatal visits with an obstetrician were more likely to be satisfied with their care than those women who had the usual regime (Hill et al 1993). However, this does not tell us very much about women's views on not seeing the obstetrician at all. A study in Scotland compared routine antenatal visits by the GP and midwife only with shared care led by an obstetrician for women with normal pregnancies. They found that women were highly satisfied with both types of care even though more women in the GP and midwife group maintained a better continuity of carer and fewer antenatal visits (Tucker et al 1996). There were no additional benefits for the women in the obstetric shared care group. It would be difficult therefore for GPs and midwives to advise women with normal pregnancies to see the obstetrician on clinical grounds. However, women in the shared care group were highly satisfied which adds to the debate the fact that, for women, there is more to antenatal care than clinical outcomes.

Of course antenatal care does not have to be divided up among the midwife, GP and obstetrician. Midwifery managed care has been found to be clinically safe and women report high levels of satisfaction. A comparison of women receiving care from a midwifery development unit (MDU) and routine shared maternity care found that both groups of women were satisfied with their care. However, women who received the MDU style of care were more highly satisfied with all aspects of their care. Also more of the women receiving MDU care would recommend it to their friends than those receiving shared care (Turnbull et al 1996).

WHICH GENDER OF CAREGIVER DO WOMEN WANT TO SEE?

It is not clear the extent to which gender of carer is an issue for women during the antenatal period. When a pregnancy is progressing normally most women will see a female midwife most of the time. When a pregnancy is not progressing well it is likely that a preference for a male or female carer will be less of an issue and this preference would be traded for expert care. Many women assume that midwives are female and may choose a midwife because they think that this person will undoubtedly be a woman. During the antenatal period having a male midwife may not matter; as one woman said, 'It doesn't matter they are doing the same job' (Hirst et al 1997). The interaction at the antenatal visit is not just about the gender of the professional, it includes other factors such as the carer's personality and ability to communicate. For some women gender does matter. Dowswell et al (1996) found that 30% of women in their survey preferred a female carer for their antenatal care. It is well understood that Asian women, particularly Muslims, generally prefer a female carer for their maternity care. Most Asian women have a male general practitioner and are probably quite happy with this, but if their consultation with the carer involves an intimate discussion or examination most Asian women would prefer a female (Gatrad 1994).

'There are certain situations where you can't actually talk to the doctor because it's embarrassing, but being with a lady midwife you can say whatever you want' (Hirst et al 1997).

For Asian women an Asian female would generally be preferred to an English female but an Asian male would not be preferred to an English male. Here the Asian women would trade enhanced communication for a more embarrassing encounter. This is not to say that to see an English male is less embarrassing but he is less likely to know about Muslim customs and religion and therefore not be aware that a Muslim woman should not be examined by a male.

WHERE DO WOMEN WANT TO HAVE THEIR ANTENATAL CARE?

The setting of antenatal care has shifted from the hospital to the community setting over the last 10 years. For most women this change will be more convenient but for others it may limit access to resources such as interpreters and linkworkers. Whether women want their community antenatal care in their home or at the local surgery or health centre seems to vary from woman to woman. There are times when undoubtedly an antenatal visit in the home would be prudent for women, such as when they are heavily pregnant, when the weather conditions are poor or when they have difficulty arranging care for their other children. Some women who have experienced home visits as a regular part of their antenatal care have found that they like it (McCourt & Page 1996). It may be that home visits are more personal, convenient and longer. Women may feel more relaxed in their home environment which could encourage communication and improve the overall relationship between the woman and the midwife. For other women it may be inappropriate. Not everyone has privacy in their homes to discuss sensitive issues and sometimes the home environment can make a physical examination seem out of place and embarrassing. It is important to note that home antenatal visits incur a greater cost to the health services, such as greater mileage claims and use of midwives' time. The place where women want to have their antenatal care, therefore, will use the available resources differently, and may have implications for other areas of maternity care.

HOW MANY ANTENATAL VISITS DO WOMEN WANT?

It is likely that different women will have different views about the number of antenatal visits they would like. Some women in a recent survey have said: 'I will come whenever they call me' (Hirst at al 1997). Other women wanted a different number and frequency of antenatal visits. One of the women who was asked how many antenatal visits she would choose said: 'every three weeks then every two weeks for the last ten weeks. Six and five weeks is too long I feel neglected if it's too long, there are things to ask and be reassured more often really' (Hirst et al 1997).

A randomized trial comparing traditional and fewer antenatal visits has provided a new perspective in that women were more dissatisfied with the reduced number of antenatal visits than with the traditional schedule of visits (Sikorski et al 1996). This challenges other work that has found that women tend to like whatever form of care that they get. The trial by Sikorski and colleagues also found that women who had the reduced number of antenatal visits were more worried about their baby and more likely to perceive their babies more negatively. However, many of these same women said that they would choose this reduced pattern of care in a future pregnancy. There seems to be a difference between what women like in their current pregnancy and what they would choose in the future. Perhaps this is a trade-off that these women would make between their own gain from attending for an antenatal check and managing other commitments in their lives such as work, homes and families. Women may presume that such commitments will be greater in a future pregnancy when they will have two or more children to care for. It is also possible that women presume that their need for reassurance, information and support provided at the antenatal visits will be less in a future pregnancy, when they have the experience of at least one pregnancy and birth.

IS KNOWING THE CARER ENOUGH?

It is well recognized that many women want to know or get to know the caregiver who provides their antenatal care. This is not only important for women during the antenatal period, but during the birth as well. Many women like to know beforehand the carer who will be with them during the birth. Gready and colleagues found that nearly half the women in their survey wanted this (Gready et al 1995). However, this is not the whole story. Women want to see a carer that they like, one that is accessible and available, and one with whom they can communicate easily. Even if you know the midwives, seeing too many different ones can have its problems:

I would liked to have seen the same one, I said before I wasn't bothered about different ones but as I got on it mattered. One of them was a bit abrupt, I wouldn't have wanted her . . . the antenatal visits were OK, they weren't worthwhile when you see different ones it's like a conveyor belt . . . they don't seem that interested in you, you're in and out in two minutes (Hirst et al 1997).

For some women there is a trade-off during their antenatal care because to increase the chance of knowing their midwife during their labour and the birth of their baby they need to meet a team of seven or eight midwives during their pregnancy. Therefore continuity of antenatal care is reduced to increase the chance of continuity at the birth. However, for most women, friendliness, kindness and how knowledgeable a caregiver is are the most important characteristics of caregivers (Dowswell 1996). This probably describes most practitioners, but sometimes the environment in which caregivers are working is so uncomfortable that it becomes difficult for them to be kind and friendly. One woman has described such an experience:

I wasn't very happy with the woman I saw at all. I think they were very rushed. The sister was trying to get this massive form filled in while the consultant was waiting to see me, and she was rushing and she was extremely short on temper. She was abrupt to say the least. I don't really blame her, it was just the circumstances. She was trying to rush and she came across as being quite unpleasant, but I am quite sure she is not usually (Dowswell et al 1996).

The provision of antenatal care cannot be considered in isolation from intrapartum and postnatal care because they are all utilizing the same resources. Limited resources raise some important questions, such as: *Is it wise to provide aspects of care that some women want when other women are indifferent to them?* An important example would be: if it is more costly to provide what some women want (such as the same midwives during their antenatal care and delivery) than to provide what is acceptable to many (such as having the same midwives during the antenatal and postnatal time but not necessarily knowing the carer at delivery), then perhaps it is logical to provide the latter. Furthermore, if providing high antenatal–intrapartum continuity results in shortages of staff and/or a high caseload this can tip the scales for any practitioner so that he or she is working in an anxious state and perhaps incapable of providing what all women want – a kind, competent and helpful caregiver.

DISCUSSION

We have said that there is a general consensus that fundamentally all women want the same things from their antenatal care, that is to be able to understand, communicate and express their wishes. We also know that the way in which these needs are met vary from woman to woman. As we find out more about what women want from their antenatal care we can see that the way in which women decide what they want is not straightforward. There are many influencing factors such as past experience, personal commitments, family influence, the setting of antenatal care, the type of carers, the skills that carers possess and the gender of carer. The choices that women make are not always straightforward either. For example, some women will want a carer that they know, but they will also want to like that person; some women will see any carer as long as she is a woman; some women will see any carer as long as the caregiver is perceived to be competent. Women also differ in their need for psychological support. Women with good existing social support networks may want little support from their antenatal carers, whereas other women may want higher levels of support. So, it is not sufficient for providers of care to ensure that the structural resources that women want are available, such as the type of carer or setting of antenatal care; the process of care must also be of a good quality. This includes good technical, interpersonal, administrative and support skills. To enable carers to use good interpersonal skills, we have shown that the environment in which carers work needs to facilitate and not hinder this interaction.

As we can see, finding out about what women like will not necessarily translate easily into services that women want or that they would choose. To find out what type of care women actually want we need to ask specific questions, such as:

- If you could choose, who would you like to see for your antenatal care?
- If you could choose, how many antenatal checks would you like?
- If you could choose, where would you like to have your next antenatal check?

Only then can we provide what women want. However, when women actually receive the aspects of care that they said they wanted this may not ensure that they are satisfied with what they get and we cannot necessarily assume that a quality service is maintained. We have shown that many women like the care that they receive, some women like some things more than others and some women would choose something else in the future. We should not underestimate women's ability to assess their antenatal care on a multidimensional level, taking all aspects into consideration.

Providing what women want during their antenatal care on an individual basis can prove to be difficult to organize, particularly if what women want is very diverse, is wanted by a minority of women, or is something that consumes a disproportionate amount of resources, such as regular home antenatal visits. This raises the question: 'If women want it can they have it?' To answer this question antenatal care needs to be considered in the context of the maternity services as a whole. For example, there are many women who want to develop a relationship during their antenatal visits with the carer who will be with them when they give birth. For some women knowing their carer at the birth enables them to feel more relaxed, more able to ask questions, less embarrassed, and they may enjoy giving birth more. Women who know the carer who will come to see them at home after the birth may also feel more positive such as feeling more confident about going home, more comfortable about contacting their carer and may look forward to their postnatal visits more. So we can see that some of the things that women want during their antenatal care, they may also want during their entire maternity experience. Of course, not all women will choose exactly the same things. This is where carers need to be vigilant about obtaining the views of women in their care and avoid stereotyping groups of women as wanting the same type of care, whatever their background. Many women are asked by their carers what they want. Delivering this is not always straightforward for caregivers if local policy prevents them from doing so. Such an example is that some women wish to know the sex of their baby during ultrasound scans, and sometimes local policy dictates that caregivers are not permitted to give this type of information.

The purchasers and providers of maternity care plan and implement local policy. To do this the views of women are being sought. If users' views are assessed effectively, purchasers and providers will discover that antenatal care is not and should not be just about endless clinical checks. Reassurance, support and confidence-building affect how women feel about their birth and postnatal experience. In addition these psychological aspects of care may have long-term psychological benefits for how the mother feels about herself and her baby. As we have shown, the resources that women need to enable them to understand, communicate and express their wishes vary and we have mentioned several studies that have compared different ways of delivering maternity care and have highlighted women's views about their care (Hill et al 1993, McCourt & Page 1996, Sikorski et al 1996, Tucker et al 1996, Turnbull et al 1996). These studies have also addressed other important issues such as the views of the carers, evaluation of clinical outcomes and comparison of the cost of different ways of providing care. When policies are being developed these other issues also need to be addressed, alongside the important question of 'What do women want?'

Key points for caregivers

- To find out what type of antenatal care women want, we need to ask specific questions; for example, 'If you could choose, who would you like to see for your antenatal care?'
- Caregivers need to be realistic about the type of care they are offering, and consider whether they can really meet the demand.
- Providing what women say they want will not necessarily guarantee a good quality service.
- Offering choice can have it's downside, some women do not want the responsibility of making a choice. Carers need to consider how they can help women make a choice, if that is what women want to do.
- Women fundamentally want the same things in their antenatal care; that is, to understand, to communicate and to express their wishes. Caregivers might usefully consider how they address these needs for individual women?
- It is wrong to assume that all women want to receive care in the same way whatever their background. An individual approach is required.
- It may be useful to document why antenatal checks are being undertaken and what happens during these visits other than clinical care. This will help researchers to find out from the maternity casenotes what antenatal care is really about.
- Women and practitioners like to be reassured that a pregnancy is progressing well, but it is debatable whether routine antenatal checks always tell us this. There may be other, more effective ways of providing the reassurance, information and support women need.
- The structure of a service facilitates the process of care and we need to recognize that if we bring about a change in the structure of the service, such as where care takes place, this may improve the quality for women, but we cannot assume that this will be the case.

REFERENCES

Bull M J V 1990 Maternal and fetal screening for antenatal care. British Medical Journal 300: 1118–1120

Department of Health 1991 The patients' charter. HMSO, London

Department of Health 1993 Changing childbirth: report of the Expert Maternity Group. (Cumberlege Report) HMSO, London

Dowswell T, Hirst J, Piercy J, Hewison J, Lilford R J 1995 Patterns of maternity care and their consequences. Report to the Northern and Yorkshire Regional Health Authority, Institute of Epidemiology and Health Services Research, University of Leeds, Leeds

Dowswell T, Baslington H, Warrilow J, Hewison J, Hirst J, Holt A, Leach J 1996 Explaining consumer preferences for staff providing maternity care: the maternity caregivers project. Report to the Northern and Regional Health Authority. Centre for Reproduction and Development, University of Leeds, Leeds

Gatrad A R 1994 Attitudes and beliefs of Muslim mothers towards pregnancy and infancy. Archives of Disease in Childhood 71: 170–174

Gready M, Newburn M, Dodds R, Gauge S 1995 Birth choices: women's expectations and experiences. Report of a research project Choices: childbirth options, information and care in Essex. National Childbirth Trust and North Thames Regional Health Authority, London

Green J M, Coupland V A, Kitzinger J V 1990 Expectations, experiences and psychological outcomes of childbirth: a prospective study of 825 women. Birth 17: 15–24

Gyllenhammar P 1977 People at work. Addison Wesley, Reading, Massachusetts

Hall M, Chng P K, MacGillivray I 1980 Is routine antenatal care worthwhile? The Lancet ii: 78–80

Hill A M, Yudkin P L, Bull D J, Barlow D H, Charnoch F M, Gillmer M D 1993 Evaluating a policy of reduced consultant antenatal clinic visits for low risk multiparous women. Quality in Health Care 2: 152–156

Hirst J, Dowswell T, Hewison J, Lilford R J 1996 Women's views of their first antenatal visit. British Journal of General Practice 46: 319

Hirst J, Hewison J, Kauser Z 1997 Assessing the quality of the maternity services for Pakistani women and indigenous white women: a report to the Northern and Yorkshire Regional Health Authority. Centre for Reproduction, Growth and Development, University of Leeds, Leeds

House of Commons Health Committee 1992 Health committee second report: maternity services. (Winterton Report) HMSO, London

Leeds FHSA 1992 Research into the uptake of maternity services as provided by primary health care teams to women from black and ethnic minorities. Leeds Family Health Services Authority, Leeds

McCourt C, Page L 1996 Report on the evaluation of one-to-one midwifery. Wolfson School of Health Sciences, Thames Valley University, London

Mason V 1989 Women's experience of maternity care: a survey manual. HMSO, London

Porter M, MacIntyre S 1984 What is, must be best: a research note on conservative or differential responses to antenatal care provision. Social Science and Medicine 19: 1197–1200

Reid M, Garcia J 1989 Women's views of care during pregnancy and childbirth. In: Chalmers I, Enkin M, Keirse M J N C (eds) Effective care in pregnancy and childbirth. Oxford University Press, Oxford, pp 131–142

Sikorski J, Wilson J, Clement S, Das S, Smeeton N 1996 A randomised controlled trial comparing two schedules of antenatal visits: the antenatal care project. British Medical Journal 312: 546–553

Steer P 1993 Rituals in antenatal care: do we need them? British Medical Journal 307: 697–698

Thomas P, Golding J, Peters T J 1991 Delayed antenatal care: does it affect pregnancy outcome? Social Science and Medicine 32: 715–723

Tucker J S, Hall M H, Howie P W 1996 Should obstetricians see women with normal pregnancies? A multicentre randomised controlled trial of routine antenatal care by general practitioners and midwives compared with shared care led by the obstetricians. British Medical Journal 312: 554–559

Turnbull D, Holmes A, Shields N et al 1996 Randomised control trial of efficacy of midwife-managed care. Lancet 348: 213–218

Walker P 1995 Should obstetricians see women with normal pregnancies? British Medical Journal 310: 36–38

FURTHER READING

Garcia J, Kilpatrick R, Richards M 1990 The politics of maternity care. Oxford University Press, Oxford

Gready M, Newburn M, Dodds R, Gauge S 1995 Birth choices: women's expectations and experiences. Report of a research project Choices: childbirth options, information and care in Essex. National Childbirth Trust and North Thames Regional Health Authority, London

Kroll D 1996 Midwifery care for the future: meeting the challenge. Baillière Tindall, London

McCourt C, Page L 1996 Report on the evaluation of one to one midwifery. Thames Valley University, London

3

Psychosocial support in pregnancy

Sandra Wheatley

INTRODUCTION

This chapter aims to introduce the main theories of psychosocial support and its importance during pregnancy, as at all other times in our lives. The chapter begins with a brief review of the psychosocial support literature, including the potential types and sources of support that may be available to a person, and how to quantify the psychosocial support an individual has access to. The potential influences of psychosocial support, and lack of support on pregnant women are examined. The chapter then discusses the support provided by and for partners. Finally, antenatal psychosocial interventions designed to reduce the negative outcome of poor quality psychosocial support are explored; such outcomes include antenatal and postnatal depression and low emotional well-being. It is these psychological outcomes and their relationship with psychosocial support that are the focus of this chapter. The possible implications of this research for health professionals working with pregnant women are also outlined.

GENERAL THEORIES OF PSYCHOSOCIAL SUPPORT

Psychosocial support has been defined by Cobb (1976, p. 300) as 'information leading the subject to believe that he [sic] is cared for and loved . . . esteemed and valued . . . [and] that he belongs to a network of communication and mutual obligation'. A definition which is more appropriate to this chapter's perspective of psychosocial support is that of Schumaker & Brownell (1984,

p. 13), who define psychosocial support as 'an exchange of resources between at least two individuals perceived by the provider or the recipient to be intended to enhance the well-being of the recipient'. The emphasis on the exchange of resources between two individuals, and the perception of that exchange, was an important development in this area of research. The result was that the myriad of combinations of supportive human relationships were studied in detail to give a more accurate reflection of supportive interactions.

As is explained below, psychosocial support is thought to protect against, or at least lessen, the negative effects of psychosocial risk factors. Culpepper & Jack (1993) divided psychosocial risk factors into three categories. The first was demographic or social characteristics, such as being young or old, poorly educated or living in inadequate housing. The second category was psychological factors like stress and/or anxiety and previous or ongoing psychiatric problems. The final category was adverse health habits, such as smoking, drinking, drug abuse, and being over- or underweight. This chapter will focus upon the psychological factors, in particular, the area of poor social support and its interaction with stress/anxiety.

As all of us are individuals, we each have our own optimum level of support that keeps us emotionally healthy. By the same token, what is good for one is not necessarily good for another. Therefore, there is not one inclusive theory that can account for everyone's experiences or can predict what will make us happy or unhappy, whatever stage we are at in our lives.

There are two general explanations of how psychosocial support reduces stress and ultimately protects one's mental health from, for example, anxiety or depression. The *Main* or *Direct effect* model suggests that psychosocial support is a protective factor in all situations, not just during periods of perceived stress. However, this model has been rejected by the consensus of psychologists on various grounds and so is no longer widely supported. The current school of thought tends toward the *Buffering* hypothesis. This theory proposes that psychosocial support buffers individuals from stressful events as and when they occur, i.e. support is only functional in its protective role when stress is experienced and not as an ongoing barrier to stress as in the Main or Direct effect model (Champion & Goodall 1994, Cohen & Wills 1985).

THE TYPES OF PSYCHOSOCIAL SUPPORT

Various types of psychosocial support have been identified and categorized, for example esteem support, informational support, tangible support, and social companionship. However, Power et al (1988) suggest that the general categories of emotional and practical support, which incorporate the types of support given as examples above, are sufficient to assess the quality of a persons' significant relationships.

Emotional support can be defined as all those instances where reassurance, intimacy and the knowledge that one is loved and cared for are received, when advice is either sought from or offered by someone who can be confided in and relied upon to help.

Practical support covers all aspects of help that involves aiding an individual with a problem in a physical or 'doing' capacity, for example lending money or helping to carry out tasks that the individual is unable to do alone.

SOURCES OF PSYCHOSOCIAL SUPPORT

Psychosocial support may be *available* in different amounts from different sources and some sources may be more *acceptable* for the individual to receive support from regardless of whether the support was either sought or offered. The sources of psychosocial support that have the greatest influence on individuals are the people closest to them, for example their partners, relatives and good friends, collectively known as their significant others.

All the possible sources of psychosocial support individuals have available to them are known as a social network. A person's social network can be broken down into primary and secondary sources. Primary sources include partners, close relatives, good friends, and, with reference to pregnancy, may include health professionals such as the woman's general practitioner, her midwife, or her obstetrician. Secondary sources include, for example, friends and relatives who are not so close, acquaintances and perhaps work colleagues. Which individual in the social network a person turns to or gains support from, will depend on the person's perception of not solely the availability of the support, but also the acceptability of support from that particular source for the particular type of support sought.

Psychosocial support can be either costly or beneficial to an individual, be the person a source or a recipient of the support. How psychosocial support influences, or is likely to influence the person, is weighed up prior to either seeking or offering support. This can play a major part in the acceptability of psychosocial support. The person's perception of the combination of availability and acceptability is built up from previous experience of problems or difficulties. For example, when problems or difficulties have arisen in the past, if someone has shown that he is willing and able to help in an emotional crisis, the person will have learnt that she can turn with confidence to that source of support, who can and will help her to the best of his ability.

It is, however, very rare that a source of support will only offer either emotional or practical support. Nevertheless, it may be that one particular source is much better at giving practical support than he/she is at giving emotional support. This will also influence the acceptability of that source's psychosocial support.

It has been argued that it is the *quantity* of a person's relationships with significant others that positively influences the individual's *physical* health (Oakley 1992). Of more importance to this chapter, with its focus on psychological outcomes, is the *quality* of a person's relationships. It is the *quality* of the support offered or received that is believed to have an effect on *emotional* health (Oakley 1992). That is to say, if people have sources of support who are acceptable and available, they are more likely to be emotionally satisfied. Quite simply, a great quantity of psychosocial support may be available to people but relatively little of it is acceptable to them. Whether it is enough for them will be determined by their individual differences (for example personality traits, coping styles, and problem-solving abilities), the situation which they are presently facing, and the culture and society in which they live.

QUANTIFYING AND ASSESSING PSYCHOSOCIAL SUPPORT

An individual's available sources of psychosocial support are represented as a social network. This allows the measurement of how the quantity of psychosocial support is related to areas such as physical and emotional health.

It may be easier to represent the idea of a person's social network as an image. Imagine a central figure surrounded by two rings. The inner ring consists of the primary sources and the outer ring consists of the secondary sources. The distance between the central person and a source represents the potential acceptability of that particular source's support to the recipient in the centre. The greater the distance, the less acceptable that source's support, be it predominantly practical or emotional, is to that person. The fact that they are available to support the central figure is indicated by their presence in either ring. The rings will not be geometrically perfect and will change over time as life experiences alter the central figure's perception of need. For instance, if this image were to be separated into two – one for the social network of the person seeking practical help, and another for the same person seeking emotional advice – the same social network would take on a different shape even with the same sources present in the inner primary and the outer secondary source ring. It can now be seen how a person's social network alters structurally over time and/or with different problems even if the content of the network, i.e. the sources, remains the same.

An example of a pregnant woman's social network for seeking practical help, for instance child care arrangements upon her return to work, may include in the inner primary source ring her partner, midwife, mother, and best friend, and in the outer secondary source ring her mother-in-law, and sister-in-law. The same pregnant woman's social network for seeking emotional advice, for instance how to deal with the difficult feelings she may have about leaving her baby to return to work, may then include in her inner primary source ring her partner, best friend, and sister-in-law, and in the outer secondary source ring her mother, midwife and mother-in-law. A similar social network is thus differently arranged depending on the emphasis of the support being sought.

A social network can be objectively measured in such a way as to quantify the psychosocial support of an individual. Various tools have been devised to assess psychosocial support in the form of social networks. For example, the Interview Measure of Social Relationships (IMSR) has been developed by Brugha and colleagues (1987) to measure the network density (quantity) of a person's psychosocial support sources, and also, in part, satisfaction with the support received (quality).

Measuring the *perceived adequacy* of psychosocial support, that is the availability and acceptability of the support to the individual in question, can highlight any unrealistic expectations that a person may have. For example, Arieti & Bemporad (1978) proposed that individuals with depression have unrealistically high expectations of others and themselves, which was seen in their work as the large difference between their actual and ideal ratings of the support they required and received.

Another measure, the Significant Others Scale (SOS) (Power et al 1988) has proven to be a useful tool for assessing the support available not only to individuals suffering from depression, but also to members of the general population. This measure differentiates between ideal and actual support, indicating the perceived adequacy and therefore quality and acceptability of support. As previously mentioned, it is an important step forward for this topic as the quality of support appears to be more influential for emotional health than the quantity of support.

It may be that the person is receiving too much emotional support from one particular source which will then make this support unacceptable. Or, she may receive too little practical support from a different source, again making the support unacceptable. In both instances the psychosocial support is available but the differentiation between ideal and actual support ratings allows a more accurate inference about acceptability to be made. Therefore, when assessing a person's psychosocial support those measures which investigate the perceived adequacy of psychosocial support are recommended, particularly when the individual may be feeling depressed.

THE POSITIVE INFLUENCE OF PSYCHOSOCIAL SUPPORT IN PREGNANCY

It is a widely held opinion by health professionals that psychosocial support has a positive influence upon mental health throughout the life span of an individual. During pregnancy its presence has been shown to significantly enhance women's emotional well-being. To identify what particular aspects of support play pivotal roles, the term support has been dismantled into its constituent parts and studied in detail. One such aspect is that of the function of psychosocial support.

Schumaker & Brownell (1984) identified three functions of support which they called health-sustaining. The first is *gratification of affiliative needs* and is described as psychosocial support confirming that the person belongs to a group and is accepted within their norms. The second is *self-identity maintenance and enhancement*, where individuals learn through interactions with others how they are perceived via feedback about the appropriateness of their behaviour; this may result in negative or positive self-identities for different areas of ourselves. The third function of psychosocial support is thought to be *self-esteem enhancement* as it conveys reassurance of our value to others and confirmation of ourselves as being OK. These functions are thought to promote well-being in the absence of stress. Although Schumaker & Brownell labelled these functions as health-sustaining, they could in fact be relabelled as the *emotional health*-sustaining functions of psychosocial support.

Schumaker & Brownell (1984) also categorized the factors that can influence the effects of psychosocial support. They identified four main factors, which are:

- person–environment fit
- perceptions of the exchange
- the resources exchanged
- short-versus-long-term effects.

Firstly, the person–environment fit can be thought of as the difference between the acceptability and the availability of support from the source. Secondly, the perceptions of the exchange may differ between the source and the recipient which could lead to the support being rejected or the recipient feeling let down because the support given was not sufficient. Thirdly, the resources exchanged may not be efficient in the long term, as practical help received at the time may solve the immediate problem, but could be creating the secondary problem of dependency on that source in the event of future difficulties. Finally, the short-term effects may differ from the long-term effects, as illustrated above, in such a way that support producing immediate positive effects may in time produce negative effects, and vice versa. These four points could almost be considered as warnings of how even the best-intentioned help can be misconstrued or that the effect the help has may alter over time.

When there is a good person–environment fit, similar perceptions of the exchange are held by both the source and the recipient. With a good fit, the resources exchanged are the most effective and the most suitable to provide the desired length of effect; that is, immediate or prolonged. In these situations psychosocial support will have a positive influence upon the person's emotional well-being. The woman will feel more in control, prepared for both the best and the worst scenarios, and more content if there is a good person–environment fit. If there is a poor fit, when the perception of the quality of support being sought is fundamentally different from the perception of the quality of the support being offered, this can result in low emotional well-being during pregnancy and after childbirth. If the support encourages dependence on particular sources for particular types of support;

and/or the support does not have the expected effect for the desired time period, this may result in the woman's emotional health suffering and may eventually lead to postnatal depression.

The range of psychological outcomes that psychosocial support during pregnancy may influence positively, if the support received is perceived as adequate by the individual in question, includes the following:

- a reduction in anxiety
- a reduction in antenatal as well as in postnatal depression
- an increase in the woman's self-esteem and confidence as a mother.

LACK OF PSYCHOSOCIAL SUPPORT IN PREGNANCY AS A FACTOR IN POSTNATAL DEPRESSION

Poor social support, in particular, where a woman lacks a warm confiding relationship with her partner, and/or with her parents, has been identified in numerous studies as a factor associated with postnatal depression (Ball 1987, Elliott 1989, Oakley 1992). The influence of a lack of support is not confined to postnatal depression. Many studies have shown that it is associated with depression at other times in women's lives (Brown & Harris 1978) and also with depression in men. However, postnatal depression is particularly problematic as it occurs at a time when enormous demands are placed on a woman, and it can have long-term effects on the woman and her family.

The symptoms of postnatal depression include:

- difficulty sleeping
- early morning wakening
- loss of appetite and weight
- difficulty in thinking
- feelings of guilt, inadequacy and worthlessness
- severe hopelessness and despair
- loss of ability to feel pleasure – particularly with the baby
- feeling that everybody would be better off without them.

Although there is some debate about the term postnatal depression, and the concept itself (see Ch. 11 for an example), its consequences can be serious. Elliott (1989, p. 879) states that depression after childbirth may:

- Fundamentally and enduringly undermine a woman's self-esteem, particularly her confidence in her ability to be a 'good enough' mother.
- Be a permanent and well-remembered source of regret, since women describe having 'missed the first year' of their child's life.
- Delay the development of mother–infant attachment and mutually satisfying interactive behaviours.
- Lead to long-term effects on the child's behaviour or cognitive ability, as well as the mother/child relationship, if the mother's 'withdrawal' is not adequately compensated for by the father or other suitable persons.
- Lead to marital stress and, if this remains unresolved, eventually divorce.

A lack of adequate social support (as perceived by the individual using her own terms of availability and acceptability) from significant others such as her partner, parents, best friend(s), and professional caregivers, has been found to have the effect of low emotional well-being (Oakley 1992). This could lead to postnatal depression, and continue for 1 year or more after the birth of the child if adequate support was lacking before and/or after the baby was born.

PARTNERS AND PSYCHOSOCIAL SUPPORT

One influential source of psychosocial support that is potentially available to the majority of pregnant women is that of the partner. The possible reasons for a partner's lack or loss of support at this time have recently been explored by researchers. A number of studies (described below) have addressed the issue of why men may not fulfil their partner's needs during pregnancy. How this could be prevented from damaging their relationship and the couples collective emotional well-being is discussed.

Palkovitz (1992, p. 141) found that 'the typical first-time father and mother undergo significant drops in their beliefs about the importance of father–infant bonding across their first transition to parenthood'. However, it is not known whether this is a normal behaviour pattern or exceptional to this sample as no other studies have been carried out in this area. Future research may help to clarify whether positive attitudinal changes and the enhancement of individuals' adaptation to first-time parenthood could be brought about by reducing negative attitudinal changes. For example, Palm & Palkovitz (1988) found that men have less nurturing experience and caregiving knowledge than women. If these areas were targeted for enhancement during pregnancy, men may feel more confident about fatherhood, which may enable them to support their partners more effectively. Thus, psychosocial support in pregnancy need not be completely focused on the mother.

Men's readiness for parenthood can have an important influence on the emotional well-being of the new family. Rankin et al (1985, p. 145) found that 'men's readiness for the pregnancy predicted their satisfaction with the partner relationship during pregnancy' and implied that 'men's readiness for a pregnancy may be more intimately tied to the marital relationship than women's'. In a different study (May 1982a) men identified the following factors as contributing to readiness for fatherhood:

- their intention to have children
- a sense of stability in the couple relationship
- relative financial security
- a sense of closure to the childless part of the couple relationship.

These four factors were found to have differing effects on the ambivalence of the father-to-be to the birth of his first child. Men who perceived a difficulty in any one of the second, third, or fourth factors tended to become more positive with time. Men who perceived a problem in more than one of the second, third, or fourth factors, *or* never intended to have children, tended to have a continuing difficulty with the idea of being a parent and this may, in time, lead to an irretrievable breakdown of the partner relationship.

May (1982c) identifies three phases of father involvement in pregnancy. These she terms: an announcement phase, a moratorium, and a focusing phase. The critical phase would appear to be the second, moratorium, phase. The length of time he spends in the moratorium phase is related to his perception of his own readiness for the pregnancy – the shorter and less stressful this stage, the more ready he feels he is to become a father. May (1982b) also suggests that first-time fathers have individual needs, as do first-time mothers, and if they feel that they can find their optimum level of involvement then this will enhance their emotional well-being and possibly make their adjustment to fatherhood smoother. If the father can achieve his optimum level of involvement, this should in turn reduce stress upon his partner and thus increase her emotional well-being. Future research in this area could inform the design of future antenatal interventions, which have tended to focus solely on the woman. Group interventions involved in educating both pregnant women and their partners could help each partner to understand how the other feels. This may not solve the problem completely but it does allow more scope for effective social support between them and should also encourage them to feel that they can turn to others too, be they close relatives, good friends, or health professionals.

Although the idea that a lack of adequate social support from a partner may be associated with postnatal depression has been extensively researched, though by no means completely, it may not provide an account of some women's postnatal depression or postpartum low emotional well-being. The possibility that *too much* social support can be as problematic as *too little* is beginning to be investigated. For example, in a study I carried out ('Partners in Parenthood: Who Needs Them?', presented at the British Psychological Society Annual Conference, Brighton, April 1996) with a group of 48 first-, second- and third-time mothers randomly drawn from the general population, women who reported receiving *lots* of emotional and practical support from their partner during pregnancy were significantly more likely to experience levels of *low* emotional well-being postnatally. Possible explanations for this surprising finding include women feeling let down by their partner after the birth, women accumulating 'caring debts' which they feel they can not repay, and/or that the level of expressed emotion from their partner was inappropriate to the women. I concluded that the most likely interpretation was that the levels of practical and emotional support the women received antenatally from their partners may well have accumulated to a proportion beyond their reciprocation. I suggested that this resulted in additional stress, guilt, and the development of symptoms of postnatal depression. However, this study requires rigorous re-investigation on a larger sample to ascertain just how influential this caring deficit may be and how, in practice, this negative effect can be reduced.

Another potentially problematic effect of too much support is that it can increase the likelihood of dependency on a source/person for future help, the third influencing factor identified by Schumaker & Brownell (1984), i.e. that the resources exchanged by the recipient and source may not be efficient in the long term. This has been noted by Downe (1997, p. 43) who points out that 'If we [as midwives] are intensively involved in a woman's care, she will probably feel happy, and extremely grateful to us – and, when she finishes seeing us, she may well feel bereft'. She goes on to suggest that to protect against this the best strategy for midwives could be to 'teach a woman and her family how to tap into support systems and they'll be happy for life'. Future psychosocial intervention research might usefully investigate the effectiveness of such a strategy.

THE PREVENTION OF POSTNATAL DEPRESSION THROUGH ANTENATAL PSYCHOSOCIAL SUPPORT INTERVENTIONS

The negative influence of poor or inappropriate psychosocial support in pregnancy is preventable, or at least reducible, through antenatal intervention. As postnatal depression affects on average at least 10% of women, this is an area of research that needs to be tackled effectively and urgently. Antenatal psychosocial interventions have been developed but most of these have focused on physical rather than emotional outcomes. Only fairly recently has interest centred on the prevention of postnatal depression through antenatal interventions containing psychosocial support as a core component.

A review of 11 trials was carried out by Hodnett (1997) using the Cochrane Collaboration Pregnancy and Childbirth Database. Not one of the 11 trials looked at postnatal depression as a key outcome but all focused on obstetric risks such as low birth weight or preterm births. The psychosocial support in these trials was generally home visits from nurses, midwives or social workers offered throughout pregnancy. These visits sometimes followed a formal structure of once-fortnightly visits (Olds et al 1986), and sometimes visits provided when help was requested (Spencer et al 1989). The contents of the interventions varied from more formal health education to providing listening visits. However, as Hodnett (1997) concluded, 'Social support interventions for at-risk pregnant women have not been associated with improvements in any medical outcomes'.

Despite a bias towards obstetric outcome some researchers did include measures of emotional well-being. For example Olds and colleagues (1986) found that home visits by a nurse had a positive effect on women's own support-seeking behaviours and on the support provided by members of their social network, for instance 'their babies' fathers became more interested in their pregnancies . . . [and the women] reported talking more frequently to family members, friends and service providers about their pregnancies and personal problems' (p. 16).

Similarly, Oakley et al (1990) studied the effects of supportive home visits by research midwives on women considered to be at risk of low birth weight delivery, and a control group of equally vulnerable women who received standard antenatal care. The antenatal intervention consisted of social support provided by a research midwife in the form of 24-hour contact telephone numbers and a programme of home visits, during which the midwife provided a listening service for the women, encouraging them to discuss any topic of concern to them. The midwife also gave practical information and advice when asked, and carried out referrals to other health professionals and welfare agencies as appropriate. A variety of physical health outcomes were investigated at 6 weeks postpartum. Of particular relevance here, is Oakley and colleagues' finding that significantly fewer of the women in the intervention group felt worried about their babies than those in the control group. When this sample of women was followed up 7 years later it was found that 'the findings indicated that the initial advantage shown by the intervention group appeared to have been maintained. At 7 years, there were significant differences favouring the families in the intervention group in the health and development outcomes of the children, and the physical and psychosocial health of the mothers' (Oakley et al 1996, p. 7). More specifically, Oakley and colleagues report that 'women in the intervention group were significantly more likely than those in the control group to be very satisfied with life . . . to feel very happy about their child's health, . . . they were also less likely to say they had particular worries about their children' (p. 14).

Despite these generally positive findings neither Oakley et al (1990, 1996) nor Olds et al (1986) found any significant differences in self-reported depression. One possible reason for the failure of these interventions to reduce depression is that they were not targeted at those most at risk of depression.

One of the few trials to target women at psychosocial risk and whose primary aim was to reduce the prevalence of postnatal depression was undertaken by Elliott et al (1988). In their study of first- and second-time mothers identified as being vulnerable to postnatal depression, they hypothesized that those who received their antenatal intervention were significantly less likely to be depressed than the vulnerable women who had not received the intervention.

The main selection criterion was that women should be vulnerable to postnatal depression. Women were considered vulnerable if they screened positive on one or more of the following four psychological and social factors: 'poor marital relationship; personal psychiatric history including postnatal depression for second-time mothers; lacking a confidante; and high levels of anxiety' (Elliott et al 1988, p. 97). Therefore, three groups of women were studied, those who were not vulnerable to these factors and received no intervention, those who had identified vulnerability factors and received no intervention, and those who had identified vulnerability factors and did receive the intervention.

The intervention consisted of approximately 11 once-monthly sessions starting in about the fourth month of pregnancy and continuing through to 6 months postpartum. The groups were led by a clinical psychologist and a health visitor. Four groups completed the intervention. The average group size was 10–15 women and separate groups were run for first-time mothers and women who already had one or more children. The antenatal group meetings were structured with an educational emphasis which included open discussions about realistic expectations of motherhood, postnatal depression, possible changes in lifestyle, and appropriate information seeking from support-providing organizations. All the postnatal meetings and the last antenatal meeting had no formal agenda.

Elliott and colleagues (1988) found that fewer women (12%) in the intervention group received a diagnosis of depression in the first 2 months after childbirth than did women in the control group (33%). Although findings were less clear cut at 3 months postpartum, the study does suggest that antenatal intervention in the form of a set of classes may provide an important and perhaps more cost-effective alternative to home visits by a nurse or midwife. However, Elliott and colleagues point out the low attendance by second-time mothers, which suggests that such an intervention may be less appropriate for women who already have children, and as such this strategy would appear to be limited for multigravidas. Nevertheless, they concluded that 'the program was clearly successful in engaging first-time mothers and in reducing the prevalence of depression in new mothers' (p. 107). Stamp et al (1995) ran a similar, but less intensive, intervention program consisting of two antenatal support groups and one postnatal support group. However, attendance was low, which the authors speculate may have been as a result of using groups separate from the standard antenatal classes. Stamp and colleagues (1995) also found that their 'intervention did not reduce postnatal depression' (p. 138). This would imply that the practical issues of running an antenatal intervention are integral to its potential success in preventing postnatal depression, and that particular care should be taken when considering the intervention's design for suitability and generalizability to the general population or targeted subsamples of the population.

Replication of such a study, focusing on first-time mothers at psychosocial risk, may be of value, as an intervention of this kind may well have long-term positive effects that could carry over into the next pregnancy. An antenatal intervention, intended to operate within the NHS, is currently being investigated for both short-term and long-term effects on first-time mothers' emotional well-being by the postnatal depression research team in Leicester.

All women expecting their first child, booking in to Leicester General

Hospital, who are 16 or more years old, are asked to complete a questionnaire regarding the stresses and strains they may encounter at this time in their life. This initial contact is made by a research psychologist at 20 weeks' gestation in the antenatal clinic. Those women who screen positive on one of the six depression items included in the initial questionnaire are then visited at home for a baseline assessment, about 4 weeks later, by another research psychologist. It is then explained that they are being given the opportunity to attend a set of classes to help prepare them for parenthood (the antenatal intervention). The intervention consists of a package which challenges the coping styles, problem-solving skills, and psychosocial support-seeking behaviours (amongst other factors) of the pregnant women. It aims to then empower the women with information relevant to them at this time in their lives and for their future, to increase their awareness of their capabilities and potential as a parent, and to reduce the prevalence of postnatal depression, all of which is outlined to the participants at this baseline stage.

A period of 24–48 hours is then left open to the woman to reflect on the choice of whether to agree to have the opportunity of attending the 'Preparing for Parenthood' intervention classes. The same research psychologist then contacts the women, and upon confirming their agreement to continue with the research, the participating women are then randomized either to the intervention or control groups. The intervention consists of once-weekly classes of approximately 10 women per class meeting antenatally for 6 consecutive weeks. Five out of the six sessions are held during the day with only the pregnant women attending. One session is held in the evening and the women's partners/mothers/best friends are invited to attend when the topic of identification and prevention of postnatal depression is discussed.

Each of the six classes is run by two female trained course leaders selected from a core of eight occupational therapists and community psychiatric nurses – all of whom were chosen because of their experience of working in a group setting. For the evening session a third male course leader joins the groups to maintain the gender balance in the group. After the six sessions have ended the women meet for one postnatal reunion session, about 6–8 weeks after the birth, where they are invited to bring along their baby. This final class is more informal than the antenatal classes. The classes are a mixture of information provision following a specific package (covering the topics previously mentioned) and general discussion of related issues raised by the women.

Women in both the intervention and control groups are followed up at 3 months postpartum for an outcome assessment consisting of a repetition of the baseline assessment with an additional clinical psychiatric interview measure (SCAN – Wing et al 1990) by the research psychologist trained in its use. A second outcome assessment is carried out when the child is 12 months old. At this assessment all previous maternal assessments are undertaken and are complemented by child health and developmental assessments carried out by a third research psychologist.

Over 1200 women are expected to take part in the screening, with 1 in 4 (300) expected to screen positive, and it is anticipated that at least 200 of these women will give informed consent to be randomized. Owing to the lengthy period of follow-up, the earliest short-term or immediate effects of the intervention will not be available until mid-1998.

This study will have real world research value as it has been run interlinking all those areas of practice which have expertise and knowledge in this field, and it has fitted in with services already provided in the maternity care system. This will allow cost projections to be made taking into account its impact on postnatal depression.

One important conclusion from this overview of antenatal psychosocial interventions is that there is no evidence that psychosocial interventions during pregnancy have any detrimental effects whatsoever. Therefore the addition of a core psychosocial element to antenatal care may well have an important beneficial effect on women's emotional health.

Key points for caregivers

- Theoretical knowledge about the nature and effects of psychosocial support in pregnancy can help caregivers when they are considering the psychosocial needs of their clients.
- It may be helpful for caregivers to identify the social networks of the women they are caring for, to see whether support may be lacking, and where additional support is needed.
- There appears to be an optimum level of support for each individual. Too little support can lead to depression, but too much support can also be problematic, as it may lead to dependency or a caring deficit.
- Antenatal psychosocial interventions appear to be able to reduce postnatal depression, but need to be carefully planned, and targeted at the appropriate group of women.
- Clinical research spanning the past 20 years has yet to find an antenatal psychosocial intervention that has produced a single negative effect on either women's physical or emotional health. Caregivers might usefully examine the evidence on the effectiveness of antenatal supportive interventions and consider how such interventions might be part of *standard* maternity care.

REFERENCES

Arieti A, Bemporad J 1978 Severe and mild depression: the psychotherapeutic approach. Tavistock, London
Ball J A 1987 Reactions to motherhood: the role of postnatal care. Cambridge University Press, Cambridge
Brown G W, Harris T 1978 Social origins of depression: a study of psychiatric disorders in women. Tavistock, London
Brugha T S, Stuart E, Maccarty B, Potter J, Wykes T, Bebbington P E 1987 The interview measure of social relationships: the description and evaluation of a survey instrument for assessing personal social resources. Social Psychiatry 22: 123–128
Champion L A, Goodall G M 1994 Social support and mental health: positive and negative aspects. In: Tantam D, Birchwood M (eds) Seminars in psychology and social science. Gaskell Press, London

Cobb S 1976 Social support as a moderator of life stress. Psychosomatic Medicine 38: 300–312
Cohen S, Wills T A 1985 Stress, social support and the buffering hypothesis. Psychological Bulletin 98(2): 310–357
Culpepper L, Jack B 1993 Psychosocial issues in pregnancy. Primary Care 20(3): 599–619
Downe S 1997 The less we do, the more we give. British Journal of Midwifery 5(1): 43
Elliott S A 1989 Psychological strategies in the prevention and treatment of postnatal depression. Bailliere's Clinical Obstetrics and Gynaecology 3(4): 879–903
Elliott S A, Sanjack M, Leverton T J 1988 Parents' groups in pregnancy: a preventive intervention for postnatal depression? In: Gottlieb B J (ed) Marshalling social support formats, processes, and effects. Sage, California, ch 3, p 87
Hodnett E D 1997 Support from caregivers during at risk pregnancy. In: Neilson J P, Crowther C A, Hodnett E D, Hoffmeyr G J, Keirse M J N C (eds) Pregnancy and childbirth module of the Cochrane database of systematic reviews. Update Software, Oxford
May K A 1982a Factors contributing to first-time fathers' readiness for fatherhood: an exploratory study. Family Relations 31: 353–361
May K A 1982b The father as observer. The American Journal of Maternal Child Nursing 7: 319–322
May K A 1982c Three phases of father involvement in pregnancy. Nursing Research 31(6): 337–342
Oakley A 1992 Measuring the effectiveness of psychosocial interventions in pregnancy. International Journal of Technology Assessment in Health Care 8(1): 129–138
Oakley A, Rajan L, Grant A 1990 Social support and pregnancy outcome. British Journal of Obstetrics and Gynaecology 97: 155–162
Oakley A, Hickey D, Rajan L, Rigby A S 1996 Social support in pregnancy: does it have long-term effects? Journal of Reproductive and Infant Psychology 14: 7–22
Olds D L, Henderson C R, Tatelbaum R, Chamberlain R 1986 Improving the delivery of prenatal care and outcomes of pregnancy: a randomised trial of nurse home visitation. Paediatrics 77(1): 16–28
Palkovitz R 1992 Changes in father–infant bonding beliefs across couples' first transition to parenthood. Maternal–Child Nursing Journal 20(3/4): 141–154
Palm G F, Palkovitz R 1988 The challenge of working with new fathers: implications for support providers. Marriage and Family Review 12: 357–376
Power M J, Champion L A, Aris S J 1988 The development of a measure of social support: the significant others (SOS) scale. British Journal of Clinical Psychology 27: 349–358
Rankin E A D, Campbell N D, Soeken K L 1985 Adaptation to parenthood: differing expectations of social supports for mothers versus fathers. Journal of Primary Prevention 5: 145–153
Schumaker S A, Brownell A 1984 Toward a theory of social support: closing conceptual gaps. Journal of Social Issues 40(4): 11–36
Spencer B, Thomas H, Morris J 1989 A randomised controlled trial of the provision of a social support service during pregnancy: the South Manchester Family Worker Project. British Journal of Obstetrics and Gynaecology 96: 281–288
Stamp G E, Williams A S, Crowther C A 1995 Evaluation of antenatal and postnatal support to overcome postnatal depression: a randomised, controlled trial. Birth 22(3): 138–143
Wing J K, Babor T, Brugha T et al 1990 SCAN: schedules for clinical assessment in neuropsychiatry. Archives of General Psychiatry 47: 589–593

FURTHER READING

Brugha T S (ed) 1995 Social support and psychiatric disorder: research findings and guidelines for clinical practice. Cambridge University Press, Cambridge
Champion L A, Goodall G M 1993 Social support and mental health: positive and negative aspects. In: Tantum D, Birchwood M (eds) Seminars in psychology and social science. Gaskell Press, London
Cohen S, Wills T A 1985 Stress, social support and the buffering hypothesis. Psychological Bulletin 98(2): 310–357
Elliott S A 1989 Psychological strategies in the prevention and treatment of postnatal depression. Bailliere's Clinical Obstetrics and Gynaecology 3(4): 879–903
Oakley A 1992 Social support and motherhood. Blackwell, Oxford

4

Continuity of carer: the experiences of midwives

Natalie Fenwick

INTRODUCTION

Continuity of care and continuity of carer are much used terms in both maternity services and health care generally. In maternity services, continuity of care is a broad term which suggests that a woman receives consistent care, advice and information from midwives and doctors who are familiar with her history and who are aware of her needs and preferences during pregnancy, for the birth and postnatally. Continuity of carer has a more specific definition and implies the provision of care to a woman during pregnancy, childbirth and postnatally by a midwife whom she has got to know and with whom she has built a relationship.

This chapter begins by examining the changing emphasis on continuity of care and carer in maternity services in the UK throughout this century, and the resulting impact on the work and status of midwives. A review of schemes designed to improve continuity of care and carer follows. The main section of the chapter focuses on the implications for individual midwives of working in a system aimed at providing continuity of carer for women, with particular emphasis on the resulting impact on their job satisfaction. In addition, consideration is given to implications for the midwifery profession as a whole of moving towards a maternity service aimed at increasing continuity of carer.

CONTINUITY OF CARER: THE CYCLE OF CHANGE

This century has seen dramatic changes to the role of the midwife and in the care received by the women they serve. This has involved a shift from community-based midwifery care to hospital care with greater involvement of medical staff, followed by a recent return to more autonomous midwifery practice.

Historical context

Early this century, midwives and general practitioners provided a full maternity service in the community where midwives enjoyed the professional status which comes from autonomous practice. Continuity of carer was an integral part of a holistic and personal service; women were looked after during pregnancy, childbirth and postnatally by their GP and midwife. The provision of continuity of carer allowed midwives to use all their skills and to practice independently, taking full responsibility for the care of pregnant women. In 1946, prior to the introduction of the National Health Service, 50% of pregnant women in the UK received full maternity care from their general practitioner and district or hospital midwife (Smith 1990) and only 54% of births took place in hospital (Campbell & Macfarlane 1987).

The domiciliary midwifery service declined rapidly over the next 20 years. Deliveries instead began to take place in hospital or small GP-run maternity units in either cottage hospitals or attached to district general hospitals. By 1985, the number of hospital births had risen dramatically, with less than 1% of babies born at home. This shift from community- to hospital-based care resulted in increased intervention during labour and delivery (Cartwright 1979). With the rise of hospital-based care, greater emphasis was placed on the involvement of medical staff and restrictions were imposed on the type of care midwives could provide (Robinson 1989). This caused a hierarchy to develop within the professions as care of the pregnant woman became based around a 'medical model'. Obstetricians increased their role and influence in the maternity services. The change in emphasis was to have far-reaching implications for the role of midwives, changing the type of care they could provide.

Whereas previously midwives had been able to provide comprehensive care to women and their families, they found that the shift to a hospital-based service caused their role to be eroded and fragmented. Advances in technology, new interventions and the central role of the obstetricians required midwives to adapt, learn new skills and change their pattern of work. They began to specialize in certain areas such as the antenatal clinic, labour ward, the postnatal ward or the special care baby unit. Community midwives remained able to provide greater continuity than their hospital counterparts owing to less specialization. However, even they found that they were no longer able to provide intrapartum care for all their women. This was due to two factors: a greater workload at antenatal clinics in health centres (an attempt to reduce the burden on hospital clinics); and an increase in the number of postnatal visits they were expected to do as a result of the early discharge of postnatal women from hospital.

Fragmentation of care

The specialization of care by midwives led to fragmentation of care for women. Instead of a personalized experience of maternity care, women began to see different midwives and doctors during pregnancy, for labour and for their postnatal follow-up. Continuity of carer and the reassurance gained from a familiar face were lost. Care became focused on the task in hand: 'we have become assembly line workers with each midwife doing a little bit to each woman who passes by' (Thomson 1980). For some midwives, this resulted in a loss of skills and confidence (Garcia et al 1990) and reduced job satisfaction. Combined with an increase in the control afforded to doctors as decision-makers in the care of women, the role of the midwife began to lose its autonomy, responsibility and thereby its professional status.

The 1970s and 1980s saw morale among the midwifery profession at a low, and recruitment and retention of midwives a problem for health authorities. Midwives felt that their professional status was being undermined and that they were destined to be 'assistants' in a hierarchy headed by the obstetrician. Against this dispirited background, however, ways to increase job satisfaction and to provide better care for women were being discussed and piloted. In addition, midwives were not alone in voicing their dissatisfaction with the way in which maternity services were developing. Many women receiving care were unhappy, and there were criticisms of the lack of choice and control afforded to women, the dominance of the medical profession in decision-making and the high levels of intervention common to hospital-based care.

In 1982 the Maternity Services Advisory Committee was set up to investigate maternity and neonatal services. Their report 'Maternity Care in Action' was produced in three parts and set down recommendations to improve standards of care (Maternity Services Advisory Committee 1982, 1984, 1985). Continuity of care was identified as an important issue and has been the focus of much work and research since then. The reports also emphasized the importance of promoting the recognition and use of valuable skills of midwives and GPs, recommending that more antenatal care should be provided in the community.

A shift in policy

The 1980s saw a number of innovative schemes set up with the aim of increasing continuity of care and carer. The experience of the majority of women, however, remained unchanged and criticisms of a 'conveyor belt system' of maternity care were common. An inquiry by the Health Committee (House of Commons 1992) provided hope for women and exciting possibilities for midwives. The report, published in 1992, emphasized the importance of continuity of care, citing evidence that it was what women were demanding of maternity services, and linking it to quality care: 'the importance of continuity of care needs underlining very heavily for the professionals who are involved in delivering the maternity services of the NHS. Many still demonstrate an insufficient awareness of its prominence among the criteria which women use to judge the quality of care they have received.'

The report also identified midwives as the group best placed and equipped to provide continuity of care throughout pregnancy and childbirth. Perhaps more importantly, however, the report concluded that a 'medical model' of care should no longer drive the service. Maternity services were heading for far-reaching changes.

Responding to the report, the government announced that it was to set up an expert committee to review policy on NHS maternity care, particularly during childbirth, and to make recommendations. This culminated in 'Changing Childbirth' (DoH 1993). Central to the theme of the report was the assertion that maternity care should be 'woman centred', with its focus on choice, continuity and control. It set down a number of targets which purchasers and providers were encouraged to try to meet within the 5 years following publication. Two of the 10 'indicators of success' were directly related to continuity of care and carer:

Every woman should know one midwife who ensures continuity of her midwifery care – the named midwife.

At least 75% of women should know the person who cares for them during their delivery.

Continuity of care and carer had finally been recognized as an essential part of new government policy. As in the first half of the century, personalized and continuous care for women became an important priority. Making it a reality, however, involved radical changes to the ways in which midwives were working. Perceived benefits to midwives included increased job satisfaction, broader skill use and increased autonomy from the medical profession.

While the benefits to both midwives and women seemed great, 'Changing Childbirth' acknowledged that changes would not always be greeted with wholehearted enthusiasm and that some midwives might not be ready for changes with such a far-reaching impact on their practice: 'Making continuity of carer a reality will require a substantial degree of flexibility from midwives and their managers. Some midwives will welcome the opportunity to develop their skills more fully, and will be able to adjust their personal lives so that they can be available when a woman needs them. For other midwives this will not be the case.' (DoH 1993).

The following section of this chapter examines some of the models of care which midwives have developed with the aim of increasing continuity of care and carer for the women they look after.

TEAM MIDWIFERY AND CONTINUITY OF CARER

The term 'team midwifery' first entered the midwifery literature in 1980 when it was suggested as a means of providing continuity of care for women within the hospital setting (Thomson 1980). It was proposed that women would 'book' with a team of midwives in hospital (as opposed to the tradition of booking with a team of obstetricians) who would then be responsible for care during normal labour, referring to medical colleagues when necessary. Claims were made that creating teams would not only improve the standard of care received by women and their families, but would give 'meaning' and a 'recognizable job identity' to midwives.

The convergence of the needs of women and the needs of midwives provided an environment in which change was to be welcomed. Despite providing an enormous challenge, it was hoped that a focus on the provision of continuity of care and carer would reduce consumer dissatisfaction and increase morale and job satisfaction among midwives.

Continuity of care and carer in practice

In 1983 the 'Know Your Midwife' (KYM) scheme was set up and evaluated as a randomized controlled trial at St George's Hospital in London (Flint et al 1989). The trial aimed to assess the feasibility of a team of four midwives providing total care to 250 women of low obstetric risk per year and to determine whether this type of provision would provide greater 'continuity of care' and would be acceptable to women.

At their first antenatal visit women were assessed against a set of criteria in order to exclude those deemed to be of high risk of developing complications. Provided they met the criteria they were viewed to be of low obstetric risk and were randomly allocated to either the KYM scheme or 'normal' hospital care. If enrolled into the KYM scheme, women were looked after antenatally, during labour and delivery, and postnatally both on the postnatal ward and at home by the KYM midwives. Unless referred by the midwives, women were seen only once routinely by the consultant obstetrician at 36 weeks.

The team approach, such as that adopted by the KYM midwives, is a practical compromise which attempts to provide both continuity of care and continuity of carer. Continuity of care, in the sense of consistent advice and care from a small group of professionals, was to be provided during pregnancy by the four midwives. It was also hoped, however, that the scheme would provide continuity of carer with women being looked after for labour and delivery by a midwife who they had got to know and with whom they had developed a relationship during the antenatal period.

The study indicated that women enrolled in the KYM scheme did indeed see fewer caregivers during pregnancy and labour than women in the control group who received standard hospital care. Of the KYM women, 79% saw fewer than eight caregivers during pregnancy whereas the figure was 49% for the control group. Similarly, 69% saw fewer than three midwives during labour as opposed to 48% in the control group. More noticeably, however, KYM women experienced greater antenatal–intrapartum continuity of carer. They were much more likely to have had with them during labour a midwife who had looked after them antenatally (98% compared with 20%). Most importantly, the women themselves were happier with their care than those in the control group. They found it easier to discuss their anxieties, were more likely to feel that they had been well prepared for labour, felt more in control during labour and those women who had a normal delivery were more satisfied with pain relief. Furthermore, the KYM women were more likely than those receiving standard hospital care to have felt able to discuss things postnatally and to have felt prepared for child care.

In addition to being acceptable to women, the scheme proved to be of benefit to the midwives involved. They felt better able to use every aspect of their skills, and felt more confident doing so (Neil 1985). Flint (1991) also acknowledged, however, that the KYM scheme demanded extra responsibility from midwives than was usual at that time and that the change in practice was stressful for the midwives involved.

The KYM scheme was considered a success and the findings well publicized in midwifery literature. An influential piece of research, it firmly established continuity of care and carer as realistic goals of maternity care.

Since the KYM initiative, a number of schemes have been set up and evaluation has produced similar findings to those of Flint and her colleagues (Fleissig & Kroll 1996). Concern has been expressed, however, that midwifery-led care and reduced obstetrician input may put mothers and babies at greater risk. A recent study compared midwife-managed and traditional 'shared care' provided by GPs, midwives and obstetricians in terms of clinical outcomes and women's satisfaction (Turnbull et al 1996). They found that women in the midwife-managed group were less likely to have induction of labour or an episiotomy, and were more likely to have an intact perineum with no difference in perineal tears. There were no significant differences for any fetal or neonatal intervention or outcome. Furthermore, women in the midwife-managed group expressed greater satisfaction with their care in relation to choice, information, decision-making and individualized care. The authors concluded that midwife-managed care was clinically effective and enhanced a woman's satisfaction with her care.

Expansion of team midwifery

Throughout the late 1980s and early 1990s a number of health authorities set up teams of midwives with the explicit aim of improving continuity of care and carer by reducing the number of midwives and other health professionals with whom each woman comes in contact and in some cases increasing the chances of her knowing her labour midwife. The term 'team midwifery' became commonplace although it was subject to a variety of interpretations and the models of care developed differed widely.

In 1993 the Institute of Manpower Studies (IMS), funded by the Department of Health, conducted a survey of all midwifery units in England and Wales (IMS 1993). It was the first major study of team midwifery to be conducted. Of the midwifery managers they surveyed, 37% (representing 100 midwifery units) claimed to have established team schemes. Of those, 86% stated that one of the aims of the new approach was to improve continuity of care. 46% stated that they aimed to improve the job satisfaction of midwives. The IMS found that while many of the aims of teams remained constant, with continuity of care as the main priority, team schemes varied considerably in practical approach, from the size of the team to the case mix of women included for care. They identified three main models of team midwifery:

- teams of midwives providing hospital care only
- teams of midwives providing community care only
- teams of midwives providing care in both hospital and community.

Different models of care lead to different levels of continuity at different stages through the pregnancy, birth and postnatally. Surprisingly, however, the IMS found there to be few data describing these differences. In their survey they found that only one-third of units with teams could identify the proportion of women who receive care in labour from a midwife who is known to them. This figure, in the majority of cases, was over 60%. Even fewer of the units without team schemes could identify this statistic (20% of the total number of units without team schemes), and of those 40% stated that fewer than one in three deliveries was by a known midwife.

In the early 1990s team midwifery was viewed as being the way forward for maternity services. It was acknowledged, however, that in order to improve continuity of care and carer, teams would have to be restricted to a certain size. 'Changing Childbirth' further endorsed this view, 'Continuity of care will probably best be provided by small teams of midwives with their own caseloads, working between hospital and the community and linked with primary health care teams.' (DoH 1993).

A number of innovative midwifery schemes aimed at increasing continuity and putting women and midwives back in control of maternity care have developed from the team midwifery model. One-to-One midwifery practice was developed by the Hammersmith Hospitals NHS Trust. One-to-One midwives are community based and have their own individual caseload of women who they look after antenatally, during labour and postnatally. Each midwife has a partner who is available to provide on-call cover for her caseload at certain times. Partnerships are organized into group practices providing further support. McCourt & Page (1996) found that One-to-One midwifery provided good antenatal and postnatal continuity, with most care being given by the woman's named midwife, and over 80% of women being looked after in labour by a midwife they knew from their antenatal care.

Midwifery group practices are another recent development aimed at improving continuity of care and carer. A midwifery group practice is characterized by a small group, usually of between six and eight midwives, who provide 'total' care to a defined caseload of women. They work in both the community and hospital, giving antenatal, intrapartum and postnatal care.

The following section of this chapter examines data from our study of midwifery group practices and illustrates the implications for both midwives and the midwifery profession of striving to provide continuity of carer for women.

CONTINUITY OF CARER: THE IMPLICATIONS FOR MIDWIVES

Ensuring that women receive continuity of carer antenatally or postnatally for routine care requires planning and careful management. Providing a woman during labour with a midwife who she has come to know antenatally, however, is a challenge for maternity services and has the greatest potential implications for midwives themselves. First and foremost it requires midwives to work an on-call rota so that between them, the midwives are available for all deliveries. The result is a need to alter their work patterns dramatically and to adapt and work flexibly in a way which is very different from the structured shift system common to the experience of most hospital midwives.

Research about midwives' experiences

Research into the impact on midwives of schemes aimed at increasing continuity of care and carer has highlighted a number of benefits. McCourt & Page (1996) reported that One-to-One midwives highly rated their job satisfaction, and gained particular satisfaction from the different relationships they formed with women and work colleagues. Furthermore, they suggested that providing continuity of care created a rich learning environment which allowed them to assess their advice or treatment. Drawbacks, however, were also reported particularly in the beginning when midwives felt the work heavily disrupted their social lives. Stock & Wraight (1993) found on-call work to be the greatest difficulty for midwives. Increased stress and feelings of 'burnout' experienced by midwives have both been linked to the provision of continuity of carer. These have created concerns about the sustainability of such schemes (Sandall 1997). Many of the schemes which form the basis of published research recruited self-selected midwives who were committed to the principles of the schemes. Little is known about how the general population of midwives feel about working in this way.

THE MIDWIFERY GROUP PRACTICE STUDY

In our study, we looked at two community-based midwifery group practices which were set up in south London. As mentioned previously, midwifery group practices stem from the development of team midwifery. Interestingly, the midwives often referred to themselves as working in 'teams' and there was overlap in their use of the terms 'group practice' and 'team'.

The six midwives in each group practice worked as autonomous professionals providing care for a caseload of approximately 250 women per year. They looked after women antenatally, taught parentcraft classes, cared for women during labour and delivery and provided postnatal care for a minimum of 10 days. High-risk women were referred to obstetricians in the normal manner, but remained within the care of the midwifery group practice. The midwives carried pagers allowing them to provide 24-hour cover both in the community and on the labour ward.

Both group practices were a response by senior management to the recommendations of 'Changing Childbirth'. Both practices were set up at the same time, within the same trust and with common aims. They have evolved, however, in very different ways and with different emphases on continuity of carer. Table 4.1 provides a brief summary of their organization.

As illustrated in the table, one practice focused on the provision of antenatal continuity of carer while the other emphasized antenatal–intrapartum continuity of carer. Despite these differences, the implications for the working practice of the midwives in each group practice have been very similar since they all care for women from their first antenatal visit through to postnatal discharge, and provide on-call cover. The two group practice leaders recruited to join the teams were both experienced community midwives. All the other midwives, however, had previously worked in a hospital setting and were used to a structured shift system. Apart from community attachments as students, this was also their first experience of community midwifery.

Working in a group practice was a radical change for all the midwives involved. As well as adjusting to working an on-call rota, they had to adapt to working in all areas of midwifery, using their range of skills, liaising with GPs, obstetricians, and health visitors, and taking greater responsibility for the care of pregnant women. It was hoped that in addition to providing greater continuity for women, these changes would improve the working environment of the midwives concerned and hence increase their job satisfaction.

Table 4.1 Characteristics of the midwifery group practices included in the study

Group practice A	Group practice B
GP attached – caseload based on referrals from three GP practices who refer all their women to group practice care	Geographically based – caseload based on referrals from over 20 GPs who refer only a proportion of their women to group practice care (based on a variety of factors, e.g. woman's choice, geographical area)
Antenatal clinics based at the three GP surgeries – two midwives (same pair each week) provide antenatal care at their surgeries	Antenatal clinics based at a health centre – all six midwives provide antenatal care (different midwives from the team each week)
Strong emphasis on continuity of carer antenatally – woman given a named midwife, most antenatal care provided by her	Less emphasis on continuity of carer antenatally – no named midwife, antenatal care provided by the team, women encouraged to see all six midwives for antenatal checks
Antenatal – intrapartum continuity of carer encouraged – women invited to 'Meet Your Midwife' sessions	Strong emphasis on antenatal – intrapartum continuity of carer – most women should have met the midwife who delivers them through their antenatal care

What influences job satisfaction?

Literature from occupational, organizational and social psychology shows that job satisfaction is linked to a number of different factors, for example pay levels, promotion prospects, security and status (Argyle 1989). Individual differences are also an important and acknowledged factor. An influential cause of job satisfaction, however, are the characteristics of the job itself.

Hackman et al (1978) identified five core characteristics which they felt to be predictors of job satisfaction. These were:

1. autonomy – the degree to which the job provides freedom and independence
2. skill variety – the degree to which a job requires different activities and therefore different skills and talents of the employee
3. feedback – the extent to which the employee is able to obtain information about the effectiveness of his or her performance
4. task identity – the degree to which a job requires completion of an identifiable piece of work
5. task significance – the extent to which the job has an impact on others. They studied the effects of changes in the above characteristics on clerical workers whose jobs were redesigned owing to innovations in technology. They found that those people doing jobs which were felt to be 'enriched' by the changes became stronger on the above characteristics, in other words increased their job satisfaction. The opposite was true for those whose jobs scored lower on the job characteristics.

A substantial amount of research has examined the relationship between job characteristics and job satisfaction (Loher et al 1985) and identified similar themes across different occupational groups and work situations. For example, among women managers, jobs felt to be limited in responsibility, variety and autonomy were linked to low job satisfaction and a greater intention to leave work (Rosin & Korabik 1991). In the health field, Shoham-Yakubovich et al (1989) reported that increased autonomy improves job satisfaction and professional self-image among primary care nurses. Williamson (1993) found that only a minority of the neonatal nurses in her study felt fully able to use their nursing skills and resented this under-usage. Changes in these aspects of work are thus identified as important means of 'enriching' jobs to improve employee performance and satisfaction.

The midwives in our study all experienced a radical change in the way they were working. Semi-structured interviews were held with the 12 midwives working in the group practices to examine the implications for them of working in a system developed to provide continuity of carer. The data reported below come from these interviews.

The benefits to midwives of working in a midwifery group practice

The five job characteristics identified by Hackman as predictors of job satisfaction provide a useful model for looking at the impact on midwives of their new role.

Autonomy

Hackman's model identified autonomy, the degree to which a job provides freedom and independence to make decisions and determine how they will be carried out, as an important predictor of job satisfaction. By having minimal contact with the hospital environment and medical hierarchy, the midwives in the group practices in our study were able to achieve greater autonomy and take on greater responsibility than they had experienced previously. From Hackman's point of view, therefore, their new role should have brought with it increased job satisfaction.

The midwives in our study were aware of the change in their role and valued their new-found freedom:

I'm my own practitioner. You don't have to keep on asking someone. It's expected of you to use your initiative and your brains. (Midwife, group practice B)

Coming out in the team is a little bit different because you've got to make more decisions, you've got to stop and say 'right this is what has to be done'. In hospital, although you've still got that leeway, you still think 'oh well, the doctor is here, get the doctor to see this person'. (Midwife, group practice B)

There's nobody breathing down your neck. You haven't got someone hanging over you. You are just left to do it. (Midwife, group practice A)

Some also felt that their professional status among medical colleagues had increased and they were regarded on a more equal footing:

I think the relationship with the GPs has changed. I would say it has improved because we have a much higher profile. We're on much more of an equal standing . . . and we also have a much better role within the hospital in that we can now refer directly to such places as X-ray and scan and physiotherapy, which used to have to be done through either the obstetrician or GP. (Midwife, group practice A)

Confirming Hackman's prediction, autonomy and job satisfaction have been found to be closely linked in the midwifery profession. In their longitudinal study of midwives' careers, Robinson & Owen (1994) found that midwives preferred it when they were responsible for decisions themselves, and were least satisfied when decisions were made by medical staff. Hundley et al (1995) examined job satisfaction in a midwife-managed delivery unit. They found that the most important factor in predicting midwife satisfaction was the responsibility of the midwife for all management decisions in labour. Like those in previous studies, the midwives we interviewed were aware that their autonomy had increased. While recognizing this was a challenge, it was one which they welcomed and felt was to the benefit of their midwifery practice and the profession as a whole.

Skill variety and feedback

Skill variety, the degree to which a job requires a variety of activities using a number of different skills and talents, is another characteristic in Hackman's model which is very relevant to the work of group practice midwives and is a predictor of job satisfaction. Working in a midwifery group practice allows midwives to gain confidence in and use all their skills. One midwife in our study had applied to work in a group practice because she felt she was not able to use the skills in which she had been trained, and was missing out on the experience of midwifery:

I wanted to be able to give complete midwifery care which I wasn't getting the chance to do . . . and I was hearing other midwives talk, and the experience they were getting I just wasn't. I was really frustrated. (Midwife, group practice A)

Other midwives felt that working in a group practice had extended their skill use and enabled them to develop professionally, to the benefit of their midwifery skills:

It gives you more knowledge and that actually improves your service because you are doing everything, not just stuck on one line. (Midwife, group practice A)

In addition to broadening and improving their skills, midwives in a group practice are able to follow their work through and see the results of their advice or practice. Hackman identified this characteristic as feedback, the degree to which a job results in the individual obtaining information about the effectiveness of her performance. In our study, some midwives felt that by providing continuity of carer and following women through to the postnatal period they could assess the results of their work, for example sutures for an episiotomy, which was of educational benefit and improved the quality of their care.

Task identity

Hackman described task identity as the degree to which a job requires completion of a 'whole' and identifiable piece of work, in other words doing a job from beginning to end. By providing continuity of carer, midwives in a group practice are able to provide total care and look after women from initial booking to postnatal discharge. The midwives enjoyed this aspect of their work and felt that they were involved in 'complete' midwifery care:

There are so many things that we never realized happened in the community . . . that's really good because otherwise if you are stuck in the hospital you are not actually sure what is happening, you haven't completed the job. (Midwife, group practice B)

Task significance

The final one of Hackman's characteristics, task significance, is described as the degree to which a job has substantial impact on the lives or work of other people. Intrinsically, midwifery is a profession which would score very highly on this particular characteristic. However, by providing continuity of carer, and therefore a personalized and holistic service, group practice midwives experience an improved relationship with the women they look after and therefore have a more personal impact on them. The midwives found that getting to know the women in their caseload was gratifying, and a real advantage of group practice care. In some cases the women became more like personal friends:

An advantage is getting to know the women. I really enjoy that, seeing them all the way through. (Midwife, group practice A)

I think it's a deeper relationship you have with some people. (Midwife, group practice B)

You actually get to know them, their likes and dislikes, and they can tell you anything . . . even their partners. They just build up a rapport with you. (Midwife, group practice B)

. . . to have them, not so much as 'you are a patient, I am a midwife' but you have that closer relationship with the mothers. You are more like friends. (Midwife, group practice B)

In addition to building a closer relationship with women, being able to provide antenatal–intrapartum continuity of carer was extremely important for some of the group practice midwives. When asked whether being able to deliver women they had got to know made a difference to their own job satisfaction, the answer in the majority of cases was an overwhelming 'yes':

Oh yes to me it does definitely [make a difference] . . . it really gives me so much joy and satisfaction to deliver a woman who I've participated in her antenatal care. (Midwife, group practice B)

I love it . . . when I've got the pager if I am on call [I say] 'oh gosh it's Maria from my clinic', and the excitement when she sees me 'oh it's you, I'm glad you are on'. I love it. (Midwife, group practice B)

It's really nice when you are there for the delivery as well, it really does make the job worthwhile. (Midwife, group practice A)

Previous studies have also found a link between the ability to provide continuity of carer and satisfaction. Hundley et al (1995) found continuity of carer within the delivery suite, i.e. throughout labour, an important factor in midwife satisfaction. The number of other midwives involved in a woman's care was the second best predictor of satisfaction, the first being responsibility for decisions. A higher number of other midwives involved in a woman's care led to reduced satisfaction.

Limitations of midwifery group practices

In addition to identifying areas where they felt their role had improved, the midwives in our study identified a number of limitations of group practice work and expressed their concerns for the future.

The pressures of on-call

Providing continuity of carer requires midwives to work an on-call rota covering all nights. The two group practices in our study developed different patterns of shifts. Group practice B preferred to work nights in blocks of five at a time with the day off following each night on-call. Group practice A, however, split nights so that midwives would work on average three nights each week (but not consecutively). If they were not called out during the night they were expected to work the following day; however, if they were called out they were only expected to work the following afternoon. This allowed them to keep their antenatal clinic commitments. Both group practices required two midwives to work the weekend – one covering the days, and one covering the nights. Each midwife was therefore expected to work one weekend in three.

Whatever the rota, the result is a need to be extremely flexible in working patterns and to be prepared to work long shifts, particularly at the weekends when staffing is lowest. This was the most common source of dissatisfaction among the midwives in our study. Tiredness, having to work long hours and the unpredictability of being on-call were all mentioned as disadvantages of the group practice set-up:

It can be very tiring. I find the on-calls very tiring. (Midwife, group practice A)

Even though you are not called you are on duty mentally . . . you can't switch off. (Midwife, group practice B)

At times you just don't stop, it's exhausting. I just get utterly drained because you miss out on meals and drinks and all sorts of things. (Midwife, group practice B)

These pressures had a significant impact on midwives' personal lives, which in some cases were felt to suffer from their work. There is evidence that schemes requiring an on-call commitment lead to an increase in stress experienced by midwives and feelings of 'burnout' (Watson 1990). Burnout is an excessive stress reaction to the work environment which is manifested by emotional and physical exhaustion coupled with a sense of frustration and failure. In her study of three types of community-based maternity care, Sandall (1997) reported that nine of the 48 midwives she interviewed identified themselves as experiencing burnout. Disillusionment resulting from an inability to provide continuity of carer in a system designed for team care was identified as a major source of this. None of the midwives in our study, however, reported feelings of 'burnout' although they did have some concerns for the future.

Concerns for the future

Some of the midwives in our study, while enjoying their current work, worried that they could not keep working in such a way forever. Interestingly, the midwives who had opted for or been asked to work in the group practices either had no children themselves or had children who were grown up and were no longer dependent. Among the younger midwives, there were concerns that it would be impossible to combine group practice work with a young family:

It's not something that I can see myself doing for the rest of my life. Much as I enjoy it now, I find the burden of on-call too much really. I love it and it's far better [than what I was doing before] but it's just very tiring. And I would like to have children and I just couldn't ever imagine doing this. (Midwife, group practice A)

The majority of midwives we interviewed agreed that part-time work in a group practice would be difficult and might lead to a decrease in continuity of carer for women, which was identified as one of the main aims of the group practice set-up. Job sharing was suggested as a possibility, but only for one post within the team.

Although not an implication of providing continuity of carer per se, there was a real concern among the midwives in our study that their pay levels did not reflect the commitment and responsibility of their new role. The group practice leaders were graded G, but the other team members were all graded F. The interviews revealed a strong dissatisfaction with the grading and feelings that they were being undervalued and exploited. For some midwives, these concerns were strong enough to make them look for work elsewhere:

I don't like the fact we are doing a G grade job [but are paid as F grades] . . . we've actually been exploited in our grade extremely. That annoys me immensely . . . people will leave to get G grades. I don't know why they can't see that. (Midwife, group practice A)

The final section of this chapter takes a further look at the issues for midwives of working in a system aimed at improving antenatal–intrapartum continuity of carer for women, and considers implications for future practice in midwifery.

THE WAY FORWARD

It is evident from our research that the provision of continuity of carer allows midwives the chance to take on a role with many positive characteristics which are linked to high job satisfaction. These, however, are present alongside a number of limitations, some of which have serious implications for midwifery in the future.

Issues for midwives

For midwives, the provision of continuity of carer both solves and creates problems. These are illustrated in Figure 4.1. On the one hand, many of the concerns of the midwifery profession in the 1970s and 1980s are addressed. By providing continuity midwives enjoy the professional status which comes from autonomous practice. At the forefront of decision-making, they are able to use all their midwifery skills and no longer have to experience a 'conveyor belt' style of working where they see women for only one episode in their maternity care. Their relationship with women is more personal as they are able to provide holistic care catered to individual needs. All these factors are important contributors to job satisfaction.

On the other hand, schemes such as midwifery group practices demand more of midwives than previously expected. The midwives in our study felt that their new role and responsibilities were not reflected in the grading structure, and they resented being undervalued and underpaid for their work. By taking on the challenge to provide complete care, midwives need to provide on-call cover, work flexibly and adapt to the demands of their caseload. For some midwives this has had a negative impact on their personal life. In their case studies of midwifery, Stock & Wraight (1993) found that although some midwives felt that their work intruded into their personal lives

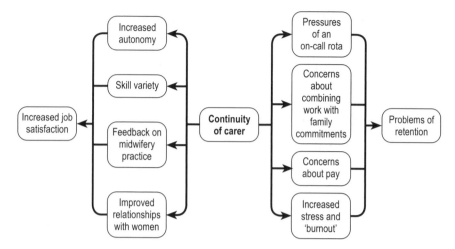

Fig. 4.1   Continuity of carer – the implications for midwives.

and required them to be flexible about hours, this was compensated for by greater autonomy and independence. Some midwives, however, may not be prepared to make this sacrifice and our study showed that there were real concerns about the problems of combining on-call work with family life. These concerns are an important finding. Robinson & Owen's (1994) study of midwife retention showed that increased flexibility to allow for family commitments was viewed as more important in encouraging midwives to stay in or return to midwifery than less involvement of medical staff in decision-making and increased opportunities for the provision of continuity of care.

The development of schemes such as midwifery teams and group practices has led to fears that midwives with family responsibilities might be excluded from working in such schemes (Robinson 1993). The result of potentially excluding this sizeable proportion of the workforce may be that the profession becomes divided (Sandall 1995). In a two-tiered system those able to commit themselves flexibly and full time to midwifery would enjoy the satisfaction and status which comes from autonomous practice, while those unable to do so may be relegated to the periphery of the workforce and limited to shifts and part-time work in potentially less rewarding areas.

What is important in terms of continuity of carer?

'Changing Childbirth' set as one of its targets the goal of at least 75% of women knowing the person who cares for them during their delivery. This is perhaps the aspect of continuity of carer which has been given most prominence in recent literature. It is widely accepted that women knowing their delivery midwife is a good thing, although the extent to which it is essential to good quality care is a source of discussion (Lee 1994). For the midwives in our study, delivering women they had got to know was a significant contributor to job satisfaction and there is evidence to suggest that it is what women want (Garcia 1995). Some midwives, however, did not consider it to be essential to either their own job satisfaction or the satisfaction of women themselves.

Further debate is needed about the importance of women 'knowing' their delivery midwife. With increased attempts to ensure that women are not looked after during childbirth by midwives they have never met, wide variations exist in the extent to which women actually 'know' their delivery midwife. This varies from a familiar face to a good friend, and it is important that we determine the resulting implications for women and midwives of these different relationships. Research is needed to explore these issues further.

As illustrated in our study, one group practice focused on antenatal-intrapartum continuity of carer while the other placed its emphasis on continuity of carer throughout the antenatal period. There is a potential difference in the impact on midwives of working in schemes with differing emphases on continuity of carer. Because of the unpredictability of when labour will occur, schemes aimed to increase antenatal–intrapartum continuity will always require an on-call commitment and flexibility from the midwives working in them. In schemes whose focus is continuity of carer in the antenatal or postnatal period, however, there is less potential disruption for the midwives themselves and some of the limitations identified in this chapter may be avoided.

The extension of schemes such as the midwifery group practices in our study will have a significant impact on both individual midwives and the midwifery profession. While many midwives may welcome the opportunity to provide continuity of carer, it is important for midwifery managers to recognize that not all midwives will be able to make the commitment which antenatal–intrapartum continuity of carer demands. It is essential that these midwives are not excluded from the service and the benefits which autonomy, varied skill use and other characteristics associated with high job satisfaction can bring. It is important, therefore, that other aspects of continuity of carer and differing models of delivery are explored to determine their implications for both midwives and women.

Key points for caregivers

- The ability to provide continuity of carer increases the job satisfaction of midwives. It gives them greater autonomy, varies their skill use and enables them to develop a closer relationship with the women they look after.

Key points for caregivers *(Cont'd)*

- Providing continuity of carer is demanding. Midwives need good preparation for the change in their role, and realistic expectations of what it will be like. Additional support in the early stages will be important when midwives will be trying to adapt to a very new style of work.
- Continuity of carer requires midwives to take on greater responsibility. The grading structure and pay levels should reflect this to prevent midwives from feeling undervalued and exploited in their work.
- The potential stress and tiredness of working an on-call rota need to be recognized and adequate support provided to prevent the possibility of burnout. The importance of protected time off should also be acknowledged.
- Caseloads should be kept at a realistic size and carefully monitored. This will ensure that continuity is maintained and prevent midwives from becoming overstretched.
- Midwifery managers need to recognize that continuity of carer requires a degree of commitment not all midwives will feel able to make. Midwives should be able to choose whether they work in this way. It is important that those unable to work an on-call rota are not excluded from this potentially rewarding style of work.

ACKNOWLEDGEMENTS

I am grateful to Myfanwy Morgan and Charles Wolfe for their comments on this chapter and to the King's Fund for supporting our evaluation of midwifery group practices.

REFERENCES

Argyle M 1989 The social psychology of work, 2nd edn. Penguin Books, London
Campbell R, Macfarlane A 1987 Where to be born? The debate and the evidence. National Perinatal Epidemiology Unit, Oxford
Cartwright A 1979 The dignity of labour. Tavistock Publications, London
Department of Health 1993 Changing childbirth: report of the Expert Maternity Group. (Cumberlege Report) HMSO, London
Fleissig A, Kroll D 1996 Evaluation of community-led maternity care in South Camden, London. University College London Medical School, London
Flint C 1991 Continuity of care provided by a team of midwives: the Know Your Midwife scheme. In: Robinson S, Thomson A (eds) Midwives, research and childbirth. Chapman & Hall, London, vol 2
Flint C, Poulengeris P, Grant A 1989 The Know Your Midwife scheme: a randomised trial of continuity of care by a team of midwives. Midwifery 5(1): 11–16
Garcia J 1995 Continuity of carer in context: what matters to women? In: Page L (ed) Effective group practice in midwifery: working with women. Blackwell Science, Oxford
Garcia J, Kilpatrick R, Richards M 1990 The politics of maternity care. Oxford University Press, Oxford, ch 4
Hackman J R, Pearce J L, Wolfe J C 1978 Effects of changes in job characteristics on work attitudes and behaviours: a naturally occurring quasi-experiment. Organisational Behaviour and Human Performance 21: 289–304
House of Commons 1992 Health committee second report: maternity services. (Winterton Report) HMSO, London, vol 1
Hundley A et al 1995 Satisfaction and continuity of care: staff views of care in a midwife-managed delivery unit. Midwifery 11: 163–173
Institute of Manpower Studies 1993 Mapping team midwifery: a report for the Department of Health. Institute of Manpower Studies, Brighton
Lee G 1994 A reassuring familiar face? Nursing Times 90(17): 66–67

Loher B T, Noe R A, Moeller N L, Fitzgerald M P 1985 A meta-analysis of the relation of job characteristics to job satisfaction. Journal of Applied Psychology 70: 280–289

McCourt C, Page L 1996 Report on the evaluation of one-to-one midwifery practice. Wolfson School of Health Sciences, Thames Valley University, London

Maternity Services Advisory Committee 1982 Maternity care in action Part 1: antenatal care. HMSO, London

Maternity Services Advisory Committee 1984 Maternity care in action Part 2: care during childbirth. HMSO, London

Maternity Services Advisory Committee 1985 Maternity care in action Part 3: care of the mother and baby. HMSO, London

Neil C 1985 Delivering the goods. Nursing Times 81(5): 19

Robinson S 1989 The role of the midwife: opportunities and constraints. In: Chalmers I, Enkin M, Keirse M J N C (eds) Effective care in pregnancy and childbirth. Oxford University Press, Oxford, vol 1

Robinson S 1993 Combining work with caring for children: findings from a longitudinal study of midwives' careers. Midwifery 9(4): 183–196

Robinson S, Owen H 1994 Retention in midwifery: findings from a longitudinal study of midwives' careers. In: Robinson S, Thomson A (eds) Midwives, research and childbirth. Chapman & Hall, London, vol 3

Rosin H, Korabik K 1991 Workplace variables, affective responses and intention to leave among women managers. Journal of Occupational Psychology 64(4): 317–330

Sandall J 1995 Choice, continuity and control: changing midwifery towards a sociological perspective. Midwifery 11: 201–209

Sandall J 1997 Midwives' burnout and continuity of care. British Journal of Midwifery 5(2): 106–111

Shoham-Yakubovich I, Carmel S, Zwanger L, Zaltcman T 1989 Autonomy, job satisfaction and professional self image among nurses in the context of a physician strike. Social Science and Medicine 28(12): 1315–1320

Smith L 1990 Is there a future for GPOs? Association for GP Maternity Care Newsletter August: 2–3

Stock J, Wraight A 1993 Developing continuity of care in maternity services: the implications for midwives. Institute of Manpower Studies, University of Sussex

Thomson A 1980 Planned or unplanned? Are midwives ready for the 1980s? Midwives Chronicle 93(1106): 68–71

Turnbull D, Holmes A, Shields N et al 1996 Randomised control trial of efficacy of midwife-managed care. Lancet 348(9022): 213–218

Watson P 1990 Report on the Kidlington midwifery scheme. Institute of Nursing, Radcliffe Infirmary, Oxford

Williamson S 1993 Job satisfaction and dissatisfaction amongst neonatal nurses. Midwifery 9: 85–95

FURTHER READING

Page L (ed) 1995 Effective group practice in midwifery: working with women. Blackwell Science, Oxford

Robinson S 1989 The role of the midwife: opportunities and constraints. In: Chalmers I, Enkin M, Keirse M J N C (eds) Effective care in pregnancy and childbirth. Oxford University Press, Oxford, vol 1

Sandall J 1995 Choice, continuity and control: changing midwifery towards a sociological perspective. Midwifery 11: 201–209

Stock J, Wraight A 1993 Developing continuity of care in maternity services: the implications for midwives. Institute of Manpower Studies, University of Sussex

5

Choice, control and decision-making in labour

Jane Weaver

INTRODUCTION

This chapter is intended to help those who care for women during childbirth to think about their practice in relation to choice, control and decision-making, and to challenge any assumptions they might be making about their clients.

The chapter begins with discussion about the concept of control. The format of the remainder of the chapter consists of a series of statements about choice, control and decision-making during childbirth. Each statement is followed by an account of some of the research which helps to support it. The statements are also supported, in many places, by quotations from a piece of research which I am currently undertaking. This is a study of women's thoughts and feelings about control during childbirth. It is referred to throughout this chapter as the 'Control in Childbirth Study'.

THE CONTROL IN CHILDBIRTH STUDY

This research consists of a series of three semi-structured interviews with 15 women having their first baby. The interviews took place at 36 weeks antenatally, and at 1 week and 16 weeks postnatally. The areas covered in the interviews were determined from pilot interviews with women 1 year after the birth of their first child. Antenatally the 15 women were asked about themselves and their experiences of control in their lives generally, as well as their expectations for childbirth. Postnatally they were asked to talk about their perception of what had happened during labour and their feelings about the experience. The midwives who cared for the women during delivery were also interviewed. All the interviews were tape recorded and transcribed, then analysed using a thematic analysis (Plummer 1995). Owing to the theoretical knowledge base behind this type of research, these women's comments cannot, by themselves, be used to make assumptions about the requirements of all childbearing women. Moreover the sample is small, and although the women came from a wide range of social backgrounds and a fairly wide age range (19–34 years), they were all Caucasian and mainly gave birth at the same maternity unit. They are therefore not representative of women generally. For these reasons the quotations, using false names, are used illustratively, and the statements made are intended to be thought provoking rather than to make unequivocal claims which cannot be challenged.

THE CONCEPT OF CONTROL

Although choice, control and decision-making in labour are topical issues, they are not new ones. History shows that childbearing women's concerns and requirements have changed over time (Lewis 1990). However Lewis points out that what has remained constant, until recently, is the tendency for these requirements to be viewed as unimportant and in conflict with the priorities of the medical profession. The recent moves to give childbearing women choice and control, and to respect their wishes, can only be commended. This does not mean, however, that giving women control is easy.

It is useful, as a starting point, to look at existing psychological research into the concept of control. Although it has long been recognized by psychologists as an important issue in everyday life, control is a notion which is still not well understood when applied to a highly complex situation like childbirth.

Psychologists have developed several theories in their attempts to conceptualize control. Two of the most central and long-standing concepts are locus of control (Rotter 1966) and self-efficacy theory (Bandura 1977). However, both define control in very narrow terms. For example, locus of control is described as a person's belief about whether his or her behaviour can determine a certain outcome or not. Internal locus of control is the belief that one's own behaviour can control what happens, whilst external locus of control is the belief that the outcome is determined by chance or by powerful others. As such, locus of control says little about belief in what one should do (Wallston et al 1987). Neither does it address beliefs about what the individual might want to do. It also does not take into account such issues as the value of the outcome to the individual, the psychological situation and the choices of alternative behaviour available in that situation (Rotter 1975).

Locus of control has been adapted by one researcher to address the specific domain of control in childbirth (Schroeder 1985). Schroeder set out to develop and test a questionnaire which could be used to assess women's expectations and experiences of control during labour and birth. This measure focused specifically on three areas: the control of pain; control of the emotions; and the control of interpersonal relationships with staff. Although the Schroeder Labour Locus of Control Scale is a useful measure of women's expectations of control, because of the narrow nature of the locus of control concept, it is of only limited use in understanding childbirth control in a broader sense. It is such a broad understanding that is required if those who care for women during labour and birth are to be able to apply it to their practice.

Similar criticisms can be made about self-efficacy theory. Self-efficacy can be described as a person's belief that he or she will be able to successfully execute a particular behaviour. Manning & Wright (1983) point out that self-efficacy theory is limited unless outcome expectancy is also taken into account; that is, the belief that the particular behaviour can actually result in a desired outcome. Manning & Wright used self-efficacy theory to explore women's control of pain during labour and birth. They asked first-time mothers to make self-efficacy judgments of pain control both before and during labour. Post-delivery the women were asked about the amount of medication they had required. It was found that self-efficacy expectancies of pain control predicted actual pain control better than other predictors, such as locus of control and the importance to the woman of having a medication-free labour and delivery. Again this is interesting research, but because of its specificity it is limited in its practical applications for those giving care during labour and birth.

A different contribution to psychological concepts of control is made from a psychoanalytic perspective. Raphael-Leff (1991) describes two types of woman in terms of their orientation towards pregnancy, birth and motherhood. Each orientation is closely bound up with issues of control. The facilitator is a woman who is absorbed by the process of pregnancy and birth. She wants nature to be allowed to take its course as far as possible throughout. She is therefore keen to have a natural childbirth and is anxious that she may not be allowed to do this. Conversely, the regulator resents the invasion of her body by the fetus, and fears that the pain of labour may overwhelm her. She is determined to use everything available to ensure minimum discomfort, and maximum self-possession throughout labour. In their own ways both types of woman require control during childbirth. The facilitator wants to be able to control and prevent unnecessary intervention, whilst the regulator wants to be able to control the pain and her own reactions to it. Raphael-Leff points out that there are few women who fit either of these models perfectly. However, she claims that most women gravitate towards one type or the other. She suggests that it is important for professionals to recognize each type of woman so that they can understand the issues of importance to them. Thus carers should be able to foresee, and ameliorate the effects of, situations in which women may feel they have failed. Although such an approach has uses, no system of categorization can replace getting to know an individual woman, with her unique set of fears and hopes.

There is therefore a need to move beyond narrow constructs of control, to understand the issues in broader terms and to relate them to the choices which are, or should be, available to childbearing women. There is existing research which addresses these issues, although it appears in a variety of places, not just psychology and midwifery texts. This chapter will focus on such research. It will elicit some of the important psychological aspects of control that have to be considered before caregivers and childbearing women can begin to give and to take control.

CHOICE, CONTROL AND DECISION-MAKING ARE OFTEN, BUT NOT ALWAYS, RELATED

In this chapter choice and control will often be discussed as if they are synonymous. However Wallston and colleagues (1987) point out that choice alone will not always increase a person's level of perceived control. The nature of the choices must also be considered. Two negative alternatives may not necessarily even be perceived as choice. Therefore, if the woman who wants to give birth at home is given the choice between delivery in a large maternity unit or a small GP unit, she may not perceive herself to have really had any choice or control over her place of birth. Richards (1982) observes that the concept of choice in childbirth assumes that there is a full set of options and that the chooser can freely exercise choice in an informed way. Even then, this may not always mean that the woman perceives herself to be in control. Green and colleagues (1988) comment on the fact that, although control is achieved in part through active participation in decision-making, and an absence of choice implies an absence of control, choice can also decrease a woman's sense of control by increasing her anxiety levels. This can happen in at least two ways: some women may feel threatened by the responsibility of having to make a choice; whilst others might feel swamped by all the options. Theresa, one of the participants in the Control in Childbirth Study, illustrates this last point:

Theresa: And she was telling you all the different methods of pain relief during childbirth. And there was loads and loads of different things. And she was like going on and on and on and on. And then the next week when we went back, she was sort of asking us loads of questions and I couldn't even remember one of them. And I thought, 'Oh my God, I must be really thick or something'.

Moreover, it is possible to have control without choice. Green and colleagues observe that a woman may be given her own notes to look after, thus having control of them. However, she may not be given the choice as to whether she wants to do this. Giving women control during childbirth is therefore not as simple as giving them a catalogue of choices. Neither will women necessarily feel empowered if they are made to take control when they do not want to. This last point will be discussed in more detail later.

CHOICE, CONTROL AND DECISION-MAKING ARE ISSUES FOR BOTH CHILDBEARING WOMEN AND THEIR CARERS

Hall (1993) describes how obstetricians, senior midwifery staff or hospital managers can feel constrained by such factors as the budget they are given or fear of litigation. This causes them to limit the autonomy of more junior midwives and doctors, who in turn are therefore unable to allow their clients to take control. In other words those whose own control is limited will find it difficult, if not impossible, to give others full control. Control giving is therefore a political issue, a question of power relations, and the resolution of political problems is seldom easy. Good communication between hospital staff at all levels is essential for solving such problems, and is therefore often the first step in giving childbearing women control.

Control and power are two members of a closely linked triad. The third member is knowledge (Rosenthal et al 1980). Information represents power. Therefore it is not surprising that midwives, who are usually recognized as knowledgeable by the women they care for, are also seen as powerful. Many of the women in the Control in Childbirth Study acknowledged antenatally that, however much they wanted some control, they would probably, when the time came, bow to the expert knowledge of the midwife:

Theresa: If they say to me, you know, 'Would you like an epidural?' If I feel that I don't need one, I'm going to say, 'No'. But if then they say, 'We think it might be a good idea if you had one', I'd probably say, 'Oh, go on then', you know? Because in the long run they're the experts, you know.

However, it is important for caregivers to remember that childbearing women also have a great deal of knowledge of their own. Although a woman may not attend antenatal classes, she is still likely to make a specific quest to find out about childbirth, from family and friends, books, magazines and television (Lovell 1996). All the women in the Control in Childbirth Study had obtained information from one or more of these sources, although they had not all attended classes. The problem, however, when knowledge is acquired from very informal sources such as friends, is that the woman may gain an understanding of what she would like, but not gain the language to express these wishes clearly. Carers have therefore to learn to listen carefully and patiently, and not to belittle the woman who has not been to classes and who does not know the correct terminology.

Even if a woman were to make no attempt whatsoever to acquire knowledge about the childbirth process, she would still arrive at the delivery ward with another form of knowledge. This is the knowledge of her own body, what it has been doing during the time leading up to her arrival, and of at least some of its capabilities. Moreover, the woman will develop this understanding of herself throughout her labour as she discovers what she can and cannot achieve. Although the antenatal women in the Control in Childbirth Study recognized the midwife's expertise, they still anticipated that their knowledge of themselves would be taken into account:

Barbara: Even though you know, I know I have the final say, because at the end of the day, it's still my body.

Hunt & Symonds (1995) demonstrate graphically the disempowering effect for childbearing women when caregivers fail to acknowledge their clients' expertise about their own bodies: when, for example, a woman is told that the contractions which she describes as strong, are really quite weak.

These two forms of knowledge which childbearing women bring into the situation should be recognized as powerful and this power should only be challenged if the caregiver feels that it is absolutely necessary. Caregivers also have a responsibility to give women unbiased information during labour, to increase their knowledge and thus enable them to make decisions.

LABOURING WOMEN ARE A COMPOSITE OF THEIR PAST EXPERIENCES

Kumar (1982) mentions that childbirth has a different significance for different women. This is a reasonable statement as women do not come to childbirth as a blank slate. Each woman brings with her a plethora of past experiences, not only from her impressions of pregnancy and any past labours, but also from her life more generally. Many of these experiences will colour her anticipation of childbirth, and will have an effect on the way she perceives labour and delivery. Some examples of this arose in the Control in Childbirth Study. For example, antenatally, Alice described the importance to her of not being overwhelmed with too much attention when she was in labour. She traced this attitude back to the way in which she had been brought up:

Alice: I suppose I'm not an attention person. I don't like too much attention. And I think that's what midwives can give you all too much of. Do you know what I mean? I mean that's one thing I'm hoping not to get, like, you know, when I go into hospital is like too much attention. I mean perhaps when the baby's born, when it's been born, yeah, fine. But if it's at the really early stages, I'd rather be just left on me own with a magazine, or something like that, and just get on with it in my own way ... And I don't know whether that's got anything perhaps to do with Mum. 'Cos

Mum's not a panicky person. I mean if one of us fell off our bikes and cut our knees, I mean we'd be screaming. And she'd be the one going, 'Now shut up, it's nothing to scream about', you know.

Postnatally, Alice was pleased that she had, as she had hoped, been left alone for much of the earlier part of her labour:

Alice: I really wanted just to be left in the room, sort of like in the early stages, just to be left alone for a little while. Which did happen. I was just like left alone to get on with it like. So it weren't until, like, later stages of labour that they actually came in and started fussing. But that was quite nice to be able to be, like, left alone to get (laughs) on with it.

Other women expressed fears which were very likely to affect the way they would behave when they were admitted in labour:

Wendy: It's the thought more than anything else of actually going in to hospital. 'Cos I can't stand hospitals.

The midwife who admitted Wendy in labour picked up on this anxiety, although she interpreted it as a fear of labour itself:

Midwife Fay: She was extremely anxious about the whole process. I would say very, you know, highly anxious. And was clearly not relishing going through labour at all.

If childbearing women are affected by a variety of past life experiences it seems reasonable to suggest two things. The first is that each woman's exact expectations and desires for control will be complex. She is likely to want more control over some things than others. For example Alice, described above, felt very strongly about the amount of attention she received, but had much less decisive views about the various interventions she might experience. It is therefore too simplistic to talk about women who want high levels or low levels of control. In fact when, in another phase of the Control in Childbirth Study, midwives were asked to define women in this way, they found it extremely difficult to do so. The second suggestion is that each woman's exact needs will be unique. Thus formulae, for example, looking to see if a woman has been to classes, to assess her desire for control, will be of limited use. In fact it is quite possible for women to attend classes and to obtain very little information from them, as did Theresa:

Theresa: She's a lovely woman, the lady who used to take the classes. And she used to waffle on, all these facts and figures and everything like that. And if you didn't sort of have a notebook there with you, there was no point, 'cos by the time you'd got out the room you'd forgotten everything she'd said. So they didn't benefit me at all. I can safely say that. (laughs) I might as well have just got a video out or something about it and watched it. And it might have sunk in a bit better then.

Another formula that is sometimes used by caregivers to assess how much control a woman is going to want during childbirth, is the employment of stereotypes. For example, it has been argued that working class women want a pain-free and rapid labour, whilst it is middle-class women who favour a sense of control over the process, and who prefer to avoid technological intervention (Nelson 1983). However, Green and colleagues (1988) found that the relationship between expectations of control and social status was much more complicated than this. Again, if women are considered as individuals with a variety of experiences which may affect their desires for control, it is easy to understand why this may be the case.

In the extreme case a woman's past experiences may have included her being the victim of sexual abuse. This can have strong effects upon her attitude towards control, either making her totally pliable, or giving her an overriding need to be in command (Tidy 1996). For this reason alone, caregivers must treat each woman as an individual and always bear in mind that a woman's expectations of control come from somewhere. If these expectations seem unrealistic or unreasonable, there may well be a good explanation.

It is important to recognize that carers also approach each case with an expertise which is coloured by past experience, both good and bad. Those who care for women during labour and birth need to reflect upon their own practice as well as the attitudes of their clients.

THE ISSUE OF CONTROL IS IMPORTANT TO CHILDBEARING WOMEN, AND THE MEMORY LINGERS LONG

Green and colleagues (1988) found that various aspects of control during labour were associated with a sense of satisfaction, fulfilment and emotional well-being at 6 weeks postnatally. Although this demonstrates the psychological importance of control to childbearing women, it could be argued that if these effects are only short term, they are of limited importance. However, Simkin (1991) found that the psychological effects of control in childbirth can be very long lasting. Women who had a sense of control over what happened to themselves and over decisions about their care during labour were more likely to express long-term satisfaction over the whole experience 20 years later. Moreover, it is not just positive memories of childbirth which have long-term effects. Kitzinger (1992) describes women who, 50 or 60 years after the event, were still trying to deal with memories of horrific childbirth experiences over which they had little or no control.

To deprive a woman of control during childbirth is therefore no small matter, and it seems unlikely that her memory of the event will be obliterated by either the pleasure of a healthy baby or by the passage of time. However, it was found that women in the Control in Childbirth Study who objectively had very little control, could still feel satisfied with the experience if they understood why things had happened as they did, and if they had felt involved in the experience. Take Anna, who had two failed attempts at a ventouse delivery before a successful forceps delivery, talking about her experience a year afterwards:

Anna: We still felt we were involved in every stage. I mean, it sounds weird, but I felt positive about the birth afterwards. I felt I was involved and treated properly all the time. And it's just that's what it took to get Liam born really. I don't think we could have changed it anyway.

Conversely, Tanya was not allowed to feel involved in her ventouse delivery, since her obstetrician did not, apparently, speak to her directly. Tanya felt responsible for her failure to achieve the natural childbirth which she had wanted:

Tanya: He (the consultant) ignored me to be honest. He didn't talk to me, he talked to my husband . . . And my husband said one minute I was being treated really well by Diane (midwife), and the next minute it was just like I was being treated like a piece of meat. Suddenly my legs were stuck up in stirrups and it was just a medical procedure that they were doing. There was no bedside manner, if you know what I mean. They were just concerned about getting the baby out and cutting me open and pulling it out sort of thing. There was no bedside manner by any of the doctors that came in . . . And I did feel as if I'd failed in a way. 'Cos I'd heard all these stories about these natural births. And I thought, 'Well if they can do it, I'm sure I can'. And I couldn't do it. When I was down after the birth, I did really feel as if I'd not done very well at all.

Simkin (1992) suggests that sometimes the initial euphoria after giving birth will minimize less positive aspects of the experience, and that it is only with time that women realize the full extent of any negative psychological effects.

CONTROL HAS MORE TO DO WITH INDIVIDUAL RELATIONSHIPS THAN WITH UNIT POLICIES OR WHAT HAPPENS TO THE WOMAN

A woman's feelings of control over what is done to her during labour are more closely related to her perceptions of the individuals who care for her than they are to either the unit in which she gives birth or her sense of having an active part in decision-making (Green et al 1988, Green et al 1994). This, according to Hunt & Symonds (1995), is because communication is the underlying issue in both control and choice during childbirth.

Several other writers also highlight the relationship between communication and control. Ralston (1994) describes the language of consent, the way in which compliance is frequently gained from women by instilling fear, or by using technical terms, or most commonly of all by such techniques as tacking an 'OK' on to the end of a statement of intent (i.e. 'I'll just examine you and then break your waters, OK?'). The midwife perceives that she is giving the woman the option to say 'no', but from the woman's point of view this is simply a statement of what the midwife intends to do.

Coercive language is not the only problem, however. Kirkham (1989) describes the ways in which women who request information during labour can be controlled by blocking of the conversation, as the midwife changes the subject or denies the woman's worry or concern. Sometimes apparent reassurance is used as a powerful block. The words, 'You must not worry' to a woman who is obviously very concerned function to deny her apprehension. To the midwife the woman has been reassured, but the woman can take it to mean that she is doing something wrong, and after this she is unlikely to raise those concerns again.

Once the importance of communication is acknowledged it is easier to see why someone like Anna, described earlier, could experience a highly interventionist delivery and still feel involved and positive about it in the long term. Anna felt that her midwife took notice of what she said and responded appropriately:

Anna: And I said, 'Well, could we try ventouse first?'. And she said, 'Well, we can', but she said, 'I think it probably won't work, but we will try'.

The possibility that good communication might ameliorate the disempowering effects of obstetric interventions has also been suggested in the literature. Green and colleagues (1988) showed that, in most cases, it is not the interventions themselves which are associated with women's postnatal emotional well-being, but the woman's perception of the appropriateness of the intervention. This sense of appropriateness is only likely to be gained if the communication between the woman and her carers is good, so that she is helped to understand why the intervention is necessary.

Most women talk about control as a joint effort with their midwife, and often with their partner as well. In other words there is a balance between the woman's control, and the midwife's and the partner's support (Walker et al 1995). Caroline and her husband Steve are one example:

Caroline: I mean I certainly felt that I had Steve's support throughout, and that any decisions that I'd made, if he didn't feel happy about them, he would have said something. Because all the discussions were with both of us . . . And I was actually very impressed by the way they [the staff] did discuss everything with me.

The women in the Control in Childbirth Study did not want total control or to be totally controlled. They desired this interaction, to be given advice and to be able to decide which to take. They wanted a midwife that they could trust. They also expected their midwife to be knowledgeable, able to listen properly and reassure.

JW: Given, you know, the perfect world, what sort of qualities would you want in the midwife who delivers your baby?

Andrea: That she knows what she's doing.

JW: Right. Yes. (laughs)

Andrea: (laughs) And that she listens. That she gives the information that's wanted, and has the time to explain things really. So that you feel that, one that she's interested in your delivery, and that she has some understanding of what you need.

Although a woman may have more anxieties about the unknown when she is awaiting her first labour, the need for a midwife with whom she can communicate is never likely to become less important, however many labours she has, because childbirth is always a momentous experience in which a woman needs to feel secure (Flint 1986).

CHOICE AND CONTROL CANNOT BE GIVEN PURELY BY INSTITUTING A SET OF FORMULAE

There is a tendency for obstetric units to institute sets of procedures which are meant to ensure that childbearing women are allowed control. For example all women may be given the opportunity to complete a birth plan, or it may be policy that anyone wishing to enter a labour room must knock first. However, birth plans are of no use if they are simply ignored when a woman is admitted in labour, or if they are adhered to rigidly despite the woman's changing view of her situation (Garforth & Garcia 1987, Nelson & McGough 1983). Neither must it be assumed that because a woman has not written a birth plan, she wants no control. Not all women feel comfortable with the written word (Green et al 1994, Lovell 1996). A caregiver must therefore find out what the woman wants when she is in labour as well as antenatally. This is reassuring for both the woman and her partner:

Caroline's husband: The thing they did do that I thought was interesting and I quite approved of was when we first went in. And the first midwife that was put in charge of us chatted in a very friendly way about, in general terms, what kind of birth Caroline wanted and so on. And took note right at the beginning.

Knocking before entering the labour room is of no use if the person requesting entry then walks in without waiting for a response (Flint 1986), or if the woman's views about who should be present are ignored. Knocking and waiting to be allowed in is more than a nicety. Women are far more likely to feel relaxed if they have a sense of privacy when they are in labour (Beaton & Gupton 1990). For some women concerns about the lack of privacy in labour, and the fear of exposure obliterate all their other anxieties:

Barbara: This is one thing I'm dreading about childbirth, is privacy . . . In one way that is more of a worry than the pain.

Therefore formulae to give women control do not work if they are not applied thoughtfully. Again the issue is the individuality of every woman and the uniqueness of her requirements, combined with the need for her carers to give her the opportunity to express those requirements, and to respond to them appropriately.

CONTROL IS MANY FACETED

Midwives often talk about a woman being in control or out of control without thinking fully about what they mean. However, control is complicated. It can be subdivided in many different ways. Green and colleagues (1988) make broad subdivisions between 'internal' control, that is a woman's control over her own behaviour, and 'external' control, that is her control over her environment and what is done to her. In the Control in Childbirth Study many women did talk about wanting control over their behaviour:

Barbara: So I hope I shall cope appropriately.

JW: So how do you define appropriate behaviour then?

Barbara: (sighs) Not too much screaming, not too much shouting and very few obscenities if you can get (laughs) away with it.

However, others were also aware of another type of internal control, the control (or lack of control) over what their body did in labour:

Caroline: There are two different kinds of control, one is mental control about what you expect, or want other people to do for you to help the situation. And the other is whether or not you have any control over what your body actually does. And in fact you have very little control over what your body does . . . In fact you have very little control over the physical aspect of it. But you can have a certain amount of control over how it's managed.

According to Green and colleagues (1988), internal control might include feeling in control during contractions or in control of one's behaviour. However, interestingly, they found that making a noise in labour was not particularly relevant to women's sense of internal control and was less related to the psychological outcome measures than other aspects of internal control. In other words, although not making a noise was important to Barbara, quoted above, some women can make a lot of noise in labour and still feel in control. The converse must also be considered. It is likely that not all women who are quiet during labour feel in control. Slade and colleagues (1993) found that control of panic during childbirth was more important than control of labour pain in promoting personal satisfaction postnatally, and it seems reasonable to assume that not all women who make a noise are panicking, whilst some women might panic quietly.

Another distinction made by Green and colleagues (1988) is the difference between expected control and wanted control. Although they found a significant relationship between antenatal wants and expectations of different aspects of control, fewer women in their sample expected control than wanted it. Green and colleagues also comment on the difference between an objective estimate of control and a perception of control. It has already been shown here that a woman can have a delivery in which the objective possibility of her having had any control seems low, but if she has experienced good support and communication, she may perceive that she was highly involved.

Green and colleagues (1988) also suggested that it might be a sense of potential for control that mattered to the women in their study as much as any actual control. This was also apparent with women in the Control in Childbirth Study:

Alice: So I just went along with whatever they decided. I mean I suppose if they'd have sort of like said anything really earth shattering, then I might have said something. But there was nothing like completely unexpected or anything like that.

In other words, Alice did not objectively take control, but it was important to her that she felt she could if she had wanted to.

Control of the situation is more than the woman getting what she wants. It is also concerned with whether she does not get what she does not want (Lovell 1996). This was clearly expressed by Lisa and Tim, her partner, who spoke antenatally about the need for carers to be flexible with them over their birth plan.

Tim: If it gets to the stage where she feels like she doesn't want to go in the pool, she's going to say, 'Well look I don't want to go in the pool'.

Lisa: Changed my mind. (laughs)

Tim: If somebody at the hospital says something that she's got written in her birthing plan, and she doesn't want to do it, are they going to push it, or are they going to leave it? And if they don't take any notice of Lisa then they're going to have to take notice of me. Because I shall be there as well.

These subdivisions of control emphasize again the tenor of this whole chapter, the fact that control is not a simple issue and that it is easy for carers to talk about giving childbearing women control, but that it is much more difficult in practice. However, an awareness of this complexity, and that it is the woman's feelings which must be taken into consideration as well as the objective features of her labour and delivery, will help to give midwives and doctors the insight and careful practice necessary to help childbearing women achieve the control that they want.

CONTROL AND DECISION-MAKING ARE NOT STATIC ENTITIES

Folkman (1984) observes that people and their environment have a dynamic relationship which changes continuously. This is a two-way relationship with the person and the environment each able to act upon the other. This can be seen during labour and delivery when there is the potential for the woman to affect what goes on around her, by her demeanour or her requests, but where the environment will also have a strong effect upon her. What is more, the direction of effect, that is whether the woman is having a greater consequence upon her environment or the other way around, will shift back and forth over time. Folkman observes that when the person–environment relationship is stressful, then appraisals of personal control will change as the relationship shifts. It can therefore be expected that a woman's perception of control and thus her willingness to make decisions will ebb and flow throughout her labour. Walker and colleagues (1995) did in fact observe in their study that the balance between the women's need for control and support shifted over time.

Another reason for a shift in the desire for control during labour may be due to the fact that women's expectations and desires for control are often different in emergency and non-emergency situations (Green et al 1988). This was well illustrated by the comments of some of the women in the Control in Childbirth Study:

Diana: I mean with things like pain relief and that sort of thing, then yes I'd want quite a large amount of say, what I have and what I don't have. But if any problems or complications arise then I'd want to be told what was going to be done, and why it was going to be done. But if it was for the benefit and the health of my baby, then that's paramount to me.

Because control and the desire to make decisions are not static entities, but dynamic processes which ebb and flow throughout labour and birth, carers have to beware of labelling the women they care for, either to themselves or when they hand over their care to somebody else. All childbearing women should be allowed the space to go with the flow of their labour whether it be totally natural or high in interventions.

ALL WOMEN WANT A HEALTHY BABY

In the past there has been a tendency to label childbearing women who wanted control as troublemakers who put their own emotional experience before the well-being of their baby. However, several authors have pointed out that every pregnant woman wants her child to be healthy above everything else (Martin 1989, Walton & Hamilton 1995). The comments of Diana, recorded in the previous section are typical of the remarks of the women in the Control in Childbirth Study when talking about this issue.

This means that childbearing women are unlikely to demand control in such a way that it might put themselves or their baby at risk, as long as they can be helped to understand the situation as it really is. However, this poses a danger: it makes it very easy for carers to use the issue of the baby's safety coercively, for example as an excuse for the unavailability of something the woman requests (Richards 1982). Such coercion must be avoided at all costs. At the least it strips the woman of her rightful control. However, at the worst it leads to a loss of credibility for those who care for women during labour and birth, and can eventually lead to women demanding the unsafe because they no longer believe what they are told.

REAL CONTROL INCLUDES META-CONTROL – CONTROL OF WHEN AND WHERE YOU TAKE CONTROL

Caregivers have a clear responsibility to advise a woman if, during labour, she chooses options which are unsafe. However, if a childbearing woman is to have full control, she must still be able to choose things which, although safe, might be considered 'wrong'. It has sometimes been assumed that all women who want choice will want natural childbirth, alternative delivery positions, and home birth, for example. However, real control also includes allowing women to have elective caesarean sections, elective episiotomies and epidurals, when this is an informed decision based on full evidence of the risks and benefits. Most importantly of all, the woman must be allowed to have control over the areas in which she takes control. Mander (1993) claims that, although carers do offer childbearing women choice, they still retain the ultimate sanction by virtue of the fact that they choose which choices the woman is allowed to make. The same can be said of control. Women are often only given limited areas of control, which are chosen for them. For example, in the 'Control in Childbirth' pilot study, Freya was acutely aware that the hospital where she was sent for her first antenatal visit were trying to control her place of delivery:

Freya: I waited for them to finish, you know, asking if my great grandmother had diabetes. And then at the end they just booked me in at the hospital. And I said, 'Actually, I don't want to come to the hospital', and it was, 'Oh! Oh, right. Oh right, well we do have a home birth unit'. But they weren't going to say, 'These are your options, what would you like to do?'

When childbearing women are not allowed to have control over the areas where they can take control, this suggests a hidden agenda. Kohler-Riessman (1983) points out that reforms aimed at minor issues are often in danger of silencing more important concerns. For example, attempts to make the birth environment more congenial to women in the USA in the early 1980s, by making labour rooms look more like bedrooms, distracted attention from the fact that birth was still treated as a pathological event, under the control of the medical profession.

If a childbearing woman is to take control in the widest sense, she must not only be able to control the areas where she takes control, but also when she takes control. In other words, she needs the freedom to relinquish control exactly when she wants to, and to take it back when she feels ready. This is very different, however, from the situation where control is wrested from her. In her first postnatal interview, Caroline described just such a voluntary relinquishment:

Caroline: So I was quite happy to hand over control to her. And I didn't feel that I was abdicating control, which I think is important. It was just a case of, not so much handing over control, but allowing her to take control, because she knew what she was doing in the circumstances. And I needed to be told what to do.

Midwives and doctors must think carefully if the things a client is requesting are contrary to their own beliefs. They must ask themselves upon what these beliefs are based. If it is reliable research data, then they should share this information with the woman, in a way which is respectful of her level of understanding. If it is simply their own opinion, then they need to be honest about this, with the woman and with themselves. Controlled choice and control are not really choice and control at all.

SOME OF THE PROCEDURES OF CHILDBIRTH ARE DISEMPOWERING IN THEMSELVES

However concerned a carer is with giving the client a sense of control, some of the procedures the woman may encounter can, in themselves, make her feel vulnerable and powerless. Examples of such procedures are vaginal examinations, the use of lithotomy poles, forceps delivery, suturing and episiotomy (Crompton 1996). Crompton points out that a procedure which is deemed highly traumatic by the woman may not be perceived as such by her carer. It was worrying, in the Control in Childbirth Study, to find that two women had episiotomies and were not told about them until the next day. When they were told they needed to be sutured they assumed, in the absence of any other information, that they had torn. One can only speculate as to why this information was considered unimportant enough to be overlooked.

Crompton (1996) advises carers to remember, not only that the childbearing woman is entitled to control, but also that she is entitled to respect, and under all reasonable circumstances she should never be touched until her permission has been obtained.

CONTROL AND CHOICE IN CHILDBIRTH ARE PART OF A MUCH LARGER WHOLE

Childbirth is an important experience, but it is one experience embedded in the larger context of a woman's life. Just as it has already been suggested that a woman's antenatal experiences can colour her desires and expectations for control during childbirth, it is not surprising that, in the Control in Childbirth Study, postnatal care also became part of the picture that women drew upon when they remembered their childbirth experiences. How they were helped and supported then was as important as whether they received support during labour:

Barbara: I felt perhaps I could have done with just a little more support. Labour ward appeared to be worried about me enough to keep me there for a considerable time after he was born. And yet when I got to the ward I was, not abandoned, but 'Well you're here now. Look after yourself', sort of thing.

It is therefore of no use to invest immense efforts in giving women choice and control during delivery if antenatal and postnatal care is dehumanizing or disempowering. To discuss choice, control and decision-making before and after labour and delivery is obviously outside the scope of this chapter. However, it is important that, in the current climate of improvement to care during childbirth, these other important areas are not overlooked or, worse still, allowed to deteriorate.

CONCLUSION

The importance of giving all women a sense of meta-control, or control over the amount of control they take during childbirth, cannot be emphasized enough. It has been shown that both highly positive and very negative childbirth experiences can have profound psychological effects on women both in the short and long term. However, it is important to remember that control is complex. Because of this, and because every carer is also subject to control, it will be impossible to always give every childbearing woman the exact amount of choice and control she desires. This does not mean that midwives and other carers should not try to achieve this, but it means that it is important for them to learn to practice reflexively, regarding what they do with critical eyes and trying to improve, whilst also treating themselves and their colleagues with respect and patience as they learn.

Key points for caregivers

- Work to improve communication between staff at all levels of obstetric care. This is the first step to giving each other the necessary autonomy that will eventually result in childbearing women receiving more choice and control.
- Recognize and respect the childbearing woman's unique knowledge of her own body, and that all women have different control requirements. Do not assume that the same practices will empower all women.
- Recognize that a woman's expectations and wishes may have a root in past, possibly traumatic, events.
- Give women unbiased, research-based information. This means keeping yourself up to date.
- Think about the way in which you communicate. Seek to improve. Do you give each woman real choice? Do you really hear what she is saying to you, believe her, and respond appropriately?
- Assume that all women want some control, even if it is just to be in control of handing the decisions over to you. Do not make a woman take control when she does not want to, or presuppose, if she does not want control in one situation, that she does not want it at all.
- Find out a woman's expectations in early labour (as well as antenatally if possible), but do not assume that these will not change over the course of labour. Find out, not only what she wants, but what she does not want.
- Respect each woman's privacy in every possible way. Appreciate how vulnerable she feels. Think before you do a vaginal examination or use lithotomy poles. Is it really necessary? Always seek and obtain a woman's explicit consent before procedures are undertaken.
- Remember that you are still accountable for your practice. Be honest if you think something is not advisable or safe, but never coerce a woman by pretending safety is an issue when it is not.
- Find out what each woman knows. Do not assume that any woman knows things. But also, do not assume that she does not. She may have read extensively on the subject and know more than you do.

ACKNOWLEDGEMENTS

My thanks go to all the mothers and midwives who have given up time to talk to me or to complete questionnaires, thus making the Control in Childbirth Study possible and also to my PhD supervisor, Dr Jane Ussher, for her help and encouragement.
The Control in Childbirth Study is funded by a Medical Research Council studentship.

REFERENCES

Bandura A 1977 Self-efficacy: towards a unifying theory of behavioural change. Psychological Review 84: 191–215
Beaton J, Gupton A 1990 Childbirth expectations: a qualitative analysis. Midwifery 6: 133–139
Crompton J 1996 Post-traumatic stress disorder and childbirth: 2. British Journal of Midwifery 4: 354–373
Flint C 1986 Sensitive midwifery. Heinemann, London
Folkman S 1984 Personal control and stress and coping processes: a theoretical analysis. Journal of Personality and Social Psychology 46: 839–852
Garforth S, Garcia J 1987 Admitting . . . a weakness or a strength? Routine admission of a woman in labour. Midwifery 3: 10–24
Green J M, Coupland V A, Kitzinger J V 1988 Great expectations: a prospective study of women's expectations and experiences of childbirth. Childcare and Development Group, University of Cambridge, Cambridge
Green J, Kitzinger J V, Coupland V A 1994 Midwives' responsibilities, medical staffing structures and women's choice in childbirth. In: Robinson S, Thomson A M (eds) Midwives, research and childbirth. Chapman & Hall, London, vol 3, pp 5–29
Hall J 1993 Power games in midwifery. Midwives 106: 375
Hunt S, Symonds A 1995 The social meaning of midwifery. Macmillan, Basingstoke
Kirkham M 1989 Midwives and information giving during labour. In: Robinson S, Thomson A M (eds) Midwives, research and childbirth. Chapman & Hall, London, vol 1, pp 117–138
Kitzinger S 1992 Birth and violence against women: generating hypotheses from women's accounts of unhappiness after childbirth. In: Roberts H (ed) Women's health matters. Routledge, London, pp 63–80
Kohler-Riessman C 1983 Women and medicalisation: a new perspective. Social Policy (Summer): 3–18
Kumar R 1982 Neurotic disorders in childbearing women. In: Brockington I F, Kumar R (eds) Motherhood and mental illness. Wright, London, pp 71–118
Lewis J 1990 Mothers and maternity policies in the twentieth century. In: Garcia J, Kilpatrick R, Richards M (eds) The politics of maternity care. Clarendon Press, Oxford, pp 15–29
Lovell A 1996 Power and choice in birthgiving: some thoughts. British Journal of Midwifery 4: 268–272
Mander R 1993 Who chooses the choices? Modern Midwife 3(1): 23–25
Manning M M, Wright T L 1983 Self-efficacy expectancies, outcome expectancies and the persistence of pain control in childbirth. Journal of Personality and Social Psychology 45: 421–431
Martin E 1989 The woman in the body. Oxford University Press, Milton Keynes
Nelson M K 1983 Working-class women, middle-class women, and models of childbirth. Social Problems 30: 284–297
Nelson M K, McGough H L 1983 The informed client: a case study in the illusion of autonomy. Symbolic Interaction 6: 35–50
Plummer K 1995 Life story research. In: Smith J A, Harré R, Van Langenhove L (eds) Rethinking methods in psychology. Sage, London, pp 50–63
Ralston R 1994 How much choice do women really have in relation to their care? British Journal of Midwifery 2: 453–456
Raphael-Leff J 1991 Psychological processes of childbearing. Chapman & Hall, London
Richards M P M 1982 The trouble with 'choice' in childbirth. Birth 9: 253–260

Rosenthal C J, Marshall V W, MacPherson A S, French S E 1980 Nurses, patients and families. Croom Helm, London
Rotter J 1966 Generalized expectancies for internal versus external control of reinforcement. Psychological Monographs 80(1): No 609
Rotter J 1975 Some problems and misconceptions related to the construct of internal versus external control of reinforcement. Journal of Consulting and Clinical Psychology 43: 56–67
Schroeder M A 1985 Development and testing of a scale to measure locus of control prior to and following childbirth. Maternal-Child Nursing Journal 14: 111–121
Simkin P T 1991 Just another day in a woman's life? Part 1: women's long-term perceptions of their first birth experience. Birth 18: 203–210
Simkin P T 1992 Just another day in a woman's life? Part 2: nature and consistency of women's long-term memories of their first birth experiences. Birth 19: 64–81
Slade P, MacPherson S A, Hume A, Maresh M 1993 Expectations, experiences and satisfaction with labour. British Journal of Clinical Psychology 32: 469–483
Tidy H 1996 Care for survivors of childhood sexual abuse. Modern Midwife 6(7): 17–19
Walker J M, Hall S, Thomas M 1995 The experience of labour: a perspective from those receiving care in a midwife-led unit. Midwifery 11: 120–129
Wallston K A, Wallston B A, Smith S, Dobbins C J 1987 Perceived control and health. Current Psychological Research and Reviews 6(1): 5–25
Walton I, Hamilton M 1995 Midwives and changing childbirth. Books for Midwives Press, Hale

FURTHER READING

Green J M, Coupland V A, Kitzinger J V 1988 Great expectations: a prospective study of women's expectations and experiences of childbirth. Childcare and Development Group, University of Cambridge, Cambridge
Hunt S, Symonds A 1995 The social meaning of midwifery. Macmillan, Basingstoke
Kirkham M 1989 Midwives and information giving during labour. In: Robinson S, Thomson A M (eds) Midwives, research and childbirth. Chapman & Hall, London, vol 1, pp 117–138
Kitzinger S 1992 Birth and violence against women: generating hypotheses from women's accounts of unhappiness after childbirth. In: Roberts H (ed) Women's health matters. Routledge, London, pp 63–80
Lovell A 1996 Power and choice in birthgiving: some thoughts. British Journal of Midwifery 4: 268–272
Mander R 1993 Who chooses the choices? Modern Midwife 3(1): 23–25
Quine L, Rutter D 1996 Birth experiences. In: Niven C A, Walker A (eds) Conception, pregnancy and birth. The psychology of reproduction 2. Butterworth Heinemann, Oxford, pp 114–119
Richards M P M 1982 The trouble with 'choice' in childbirth. Birth 9: 253–260

6

Having a homebirth: decisions, experiences and long-term consequences

Jane Ogden

INTRODUCTION

In the late 19th century, it was the prerogative of the wealthy woman to have her baby at home (Foster 1995). A homebirth supported by private health care providers was viewed as the safe and preferable alternative to hospital births with their high rates of maternal mortality and unsanitary conditions. However, throughout most of the 20th century the medical profession has been intent on reversing this position. Hospitals have been recommended increasingly as the safest place of birth and the wide range of possible medical interventions such as caesareans, forceps and induced births have been presented as central components in the safety debate. However, the 1990s have seen a shift in perspective and homebirths have begun to make a reappearance. Following a thorough examination of the research into the safety of home and hospital births, Tew (1990) argued that changes in infant and maternal morbidity and mortality were in response to nutrition and general health rather than the use of medical interventions or increased hospitalization. Furthermore, the Winterton Report (DoH 1992) argued that the 'policy of encouraging all women to give birth in hospitals cannot be justified on the grounds of safety'. In response to the recommendations from this report the Expert Maternity Group was established by the Government in 1992 and produced the Cumberlege Report 'Changing Childbirth' (DoH 1993). This report also questioned the policy of systematically recommending hospital births. In particular, the 'Changing Childbirth' document called for the development of a woman-centred service which met the needs of the individual and proposed that women should 'be able to choose where they would like their baby to be born'. Therefore, the potential benefits of having a homebirth are now being given serious consideration. However, although the document provides guidance as to where information about the place of birth can be accessed, most of the cited sources are experts such as midwives, GPs and obstetricians. In effect, this means that women's own experiences remain a neglected source of information. What do the women themselves think about homebirths? Is the experts' increasing enthusiasm reflected by those women who have actually been through the process? At a time of a consumer-led health service the views of women who have had a homebirth remain an untapped source of information. This chapter draws upon the results from the Memories of Homebirth Study, which I carried out with my colleagues Adrienne Shaw and Luke Zander (Ogden et al 1997a,b,c). The Memories of Homebirth Study was designed to examine women's experiences of having a homebirth and aimed to address the three questions outlined below.

When hospital birth is the norm, what processes are involved in choosing to go against this norm?

The 'Changing Childbirth' document argues that a woman's choice about the place of birth should be 'respected and every practical effort made to achieve the outcome that the woman believes is best for her baby and herself' (DoH 1993, p. 25). The document also states that 'women should receive clear, unbiased advice' in order to facilitate their decision. This desire for choice is reflected in the results of a MORI survey of women who had recently given birth, with 72% saying that they would have liked the option of a different system of care; of these, 44% wanted a midwife-led domino delivery and 22% would have liked the choice of a homebirth (DoH 1993, p. 23). This emphasis on the need for choice is also reflected in publications aimed at both the professional and lay person (e.g. Kitzinger 1987, Kitzinger 1989, Moorhead 1996). However, the great majority of women still have their babies in hospital and therefore choosing to have a homebirth involves going against the norm. Further, because of unresolved issues surrounding the safety of homebirths, the literature on this issue remains open to alternative interpretations (Dowswell et al 1996, RCOG 1992). Therefore, in parallel with other health-related decisions (Ogden 1996) deciding to have a baby at home is a complicated process. The popular literature on maternity issues has provided some insights into the factors involved in deciding upon the place of birth. For example, Wesson (1990) details her own personal reasons for choosing to have her fourth baby at home and provides a range of factors involved in the decision-making process based upon interviews with women in the UK. Reasons such as the belief that a homebirth would be more relaxed and less stressful, that going into hospital can slow labour down, the need for privacy and previous experiences of hospital births are presented in her book as a source of information for women considering the place to give birth. Likewise, Mosse (1993) provides insights into the often contradictory feelings women have about both home and hospital as the right place to have their baby. For example, she describes how women describe the home as comfortable and yet are worried about the mess and how hospitals are seen as both safe and lacking privacy. The first part of the Memories of Homebirth Study was concerned with the factors involved in deciding to have a homebirth.

What is it like to have a homebirth and can these experiences be used to inform women in the future?

'Changing Childbirth' (DoH 1993) indicated that 'professionals cannot quantify the enriching experience which some women feel when they have their baby in a place of their choice' (p. 23). Research has used both quantitative and qualitative approaches to explore the childbirth experience and the role of the place of birth on the women's satisfaction with this experience. Further, this research has been presented in both the academic and popular press. In a recent systematic review of the use of home-like birth settings, Hodnett examined the results from studies exploring women's experiences (Hodnett 1996a,b). She reported that women preferred to have their baby in a home-like setting rather than within a traditional hospital ward and further stated that the continuous presence of a trained individual increased the women's satisfaction with their experience and was associated with decreased interventions such as operative vaginal delivery and caesarean delivery, and decreased the duration of labour (Hodnett 1996a,b). Research has also examined the experiences of women who have planned to have a homebirth but have been referred to hospital either before or during labour (Davies et al 1996). The authors of this study concluded that even though these women ended up having a hospital birth they stated that they valued the chance to have part of their labour at home. Studies have also attempted to define the kinds of factors which predict satisfaction with the birth experience. Drew et al (1989) explored the correlates of satisfaction with hospital births in the UK and concluded that explanation of the procedures, patient involvement with administering and choosing these procedures, the presence of the partner and qualified staff and the physical comfort of the ward were important. Similar components were also reported by Seguin et al (1989) following their study in Canada, and Brown & Lumley (1994) following a study in Australia. In line with this, the popular literature has also examined women's experiences of birth. In her review for the National Childbirth Trust, Moorhead (1996) reported many accounts from different women describing their experiences of having a birth either in hospital or at home. These accounts provide insights into the birth process, any interventions and the involvement of supportive (or less supportive) others. However, the accounts are fairly brief and are provided by self-selected women. Therefore, although they provide a source of information for others their value as research data is limited. A more detailed selection of accounts is provided by Clement (1995) in her book exploring women's experiences of having a caesarean section. The literature has also examined women's experiences of a range of births over different time periods and within different countries. For example, Oakley (1986) provided detailed descriptions of women's experiences of having hospital births in the 1970s in the UK and highlights factors such as the clash between expectations and reality, the question of control and the problem of recognition (is this labour?) as central to this experience. Isaacs Ashford (1984) examined not only the mothers' but also the fathers' and grandmothers' accounts of their birth experiences over a 70-year period and explored changes in this experience over this time and compared the experience from different perspectives. Wesson's (1990) book is one of the few to focus on exploring the experience of having a homebirth and uses the experience of women as the basis to provide information for others considering home as the place for the birth of their baby. The Memories of Homebirth Study also aimed to provide detailed accounts about women's experiences of having a homebirth.

Does choosing to have a homebirth have an impact upon the mother beyond that of the actual birth?

Over recent years there has been an increasing interest in the possible longer-term effects of childbirth. Simkin (1992) examined women's long-term memories of their birth experiences and concluded that women's memories are strikingly vivid. Kitzinger (1992) analysed women's accounts of their birth experiences and suggested that the stress of the experience and feelings of being invaded and violence may be associated with long-term distress. Moorhead (1996) emphasized the emotional content of birth and introduces her book with the statement 'childbirth isn't just something that women go through. It's something that changes them as individuals, something that shows them their vulnerability and their strength, something that teaches them about themselves' thus emphasizing childbirth as having an impact beyond the confines of the birth itself. Some research has examined the possible impact of the birth experience on postnatal depression. A recent prospective study of 303 women in the Netherlands examined the effect of place of birth on the occurrence of the blues and depression 4 weeks postpartum (Pop et al 1995). The authors reported no differences between those who had had their baby at home and those who had given birth in hospital. However, little research to date has explored women's own beliefs about the longer-term impact of having a homebirth. Therefore, our study also aimed to explore the consequences of having a homebirth in the broadest sense from the woman's perspective.

THE MEMORIES OF HOMEBIRTH STUDY

Four GPs and one independent midwife in Lambeth, Southwark and Lewisham, South London who provide care to women having homebirths were asked to select 25 women (five women each) who had had a homebirth between 3 and 5 years ago and who varied in terms of age, length of time since birth, number of previous births, number of subsequent births, and experiences of hospital births. They were asked to contact the women by letter or telephone to request their permission to be interviewed and then to supply the women's names and addresses to the interviewer.

The interviewer contacted each woman and arranged for an interview. The interviewer was a research nurse (SRN, RMN) who has received interview training and is experienced in interviewing individuals in both a clinical and non-clinical context. Each interview took place in the interviewee's own home, were audiotaped and lasted for between 1 and $1\frac{1}{2}$ hours. The interviews were in depth and were designed to encourage free recall from the interviewee. Each interview was designed to cover the following aspects of the birth:

1. *The decision to have a homebirth*, consisting of the open-ended question: 'Can you tell me about why you decided to have your baby at home and what led up to that decision?' The women were also asked to reflect on their decision.

2. *The experience of the homebirth*, consisting of the open-ended question: 'Could you tell me as much as you can about what happened during the birth and how you felt about it?' The following prompt questions were then added if the interviewee did not cover them in depth: 'What role do you feel other people played during the birth?', 'What is your memory of pain during the birth?' and 'Did you feel in control during the birth?'

3. *The subsequent effects of the homebirth*, consisting of the open-ended question: 'Can you tell me what effect you feel the birth has had on your life?'

The interviews were transcribed and analysed by examining the transcripts for themes and categories. The analysis aimed to explore the range of views expressed by the different women and to provide quotes to illustrate the kinds of comments that were made. The results are not quantified and the numbers of women who made comments belonging to any particular theme are not provided as the sample size and methodology does not render such a quantitative approach appropriate. All names are changed throughout.

RESULTS

All the women contacted by the interviewer were very positive about the study. During the interviews many women became quite emotional. Some women were tearful and several expressed an enthusiasm for being able to talk in depth about their experiences. None of the interviewees expressed regrets about having chosen to have a homebirth and when asked to reflect on their decision made comments such as 'One of the best things I have ever done. It was really the best decision I could have made, that's all I can say', 'One hundred percent . . . the right thing' and 'I feel good. I think it was the best decision I made'. When asked about the consequences of having a homebirth, most were clear that the birth had had a generally very positive impact on their lives. One woman said 'I think it is one of the nicest things that ever happened to me . . . it is a nice experience that you can remember for the rest of your life'.

The results will be presented in terms of three components of the homebirth experience.

Making the decision

Most women could explain the decision-making processes in detail and talked about their choice to have a homebirth in terms of the following themes and categories.

Being at home

Women stressed the importance of maintaining the routines of normal life, particularly those involving their other children:

There were lots of children and some of them wanted to be there . . . I just didn't want to leave them, so I just thought it would be nice as a family if we could just all be here together.

Several women felt it was important to bring the baby directly into the home. One woman said:

It has something to do with actually me not going away and not leaving him and coming back with a new baby.

The women described their decision in terms of the simple benefits of being at home:

I felt it would be nice to be at home, surrounded by the immediate family, not to have to travel in labour, which is really uncomfortable.

Not being in hospital

Several women described their decision as a reaction to not wanting a hospital birth. For example one woman said, 'I hated the idea of being in hospital. That was almost a negative decision'. Another described how she changed her decision to have a homebirth at 36 weeks after going to hospital for antenatal care and:

not seeing the same midwife and answering the same questions and nobody actually reading the notes and you go and one doctor would say 'come back in 4 or 2 weeks' and you would get back there and they would say 'why have you come back so soon'.

The women described their negative feelings about the general hospital atmosphere. One woman who was initially planning to have her baby in hospital described her feelings when she first went to the hospital:

I was about 33 weeks when I went to the hospital. I looked around and said 'No, it is not for me'. We could hear people, all sort of impersonal. We could hear other people having babies. I think it is quite frightening because when you come in you are not at that stage and you hear people screaming their heads off – it puts you off.

Some women described their previous experiences of hospital births in terms of the medical interventions:

Because I had had such an awful time having Rebecca. I just felt it was very high tech and they jabbed me when I didn't want to and I don't even remember the birth I was so blotto.

Women also described the way in which their treatment was carried out. In particular this related to feeling out of control in hospital, being treated like a child and feeling 'I was one of a number' and that 'it was so impersonal'.

When I became pregnant with my second one, I thought I couldn't cope being somewhere where everybody was telling me that I was doing it wrong and I wasn't fitting in and I was causing trouble and I thought I want to have this next one at home.

The role of others

Some of the women described their decision as a very personal process involving no-one else. One woman said that she went to her GP and said, 'Look, I want a homebirth'. Another said, 'I was quite determined I wanted a homebirth. It is just what suited me, what suited my lifestyle . . . It feels like an achievement that I have done . . . it's standing up for a choice'. However, many women described the decision-making process in the context of discussions with several other people. Sometimes other people were perceived as being supportive and facilitative and sometimes they were described as being obstructive.

Several women described the role of their GP and the midwives. For many, the involvement of these professionals was a positive experience:

My doctor at the time had given me so much confidence and support with this, because she had said that the decision was entirely mine and if I wanted a homebirth it was fine . . . She just gave me the confidence to go ahead with it.

I felt I was supported by the community midwives who knew that I was serious about what I wanted to do.'

However, others described negative experiences with the professionals:

Well she [GP] said basically their practice don't do them full stop for whatever reason . . . well, one of the reasons we wouldn't want to have the responsibility for a baby's death or something like that.

The women described a range of positive and negative lay views about their decision, offered by their partners, parents and friends.

Some partners were reported as being positive, with one woman saying that her main reason for having a homebirth was:

to have John involved. He, my husband, is a very shy person and in hospital . . . he didn't really feel he could take much part in what was going on and he was just an onlooker really. Whereas at home, he'd have felt more comfortable. All in all that is what we hoped for.

Several women had to convince their partners that the homebirth was a good idea:

When my husband heard, he was a little bit shocked. He is very worried about change but when he sees that it is good he is all for it. And of course once he realized that, well yes, there is a potential here to have a successful birth at home he was all for it.

However, not all partners could be convinced:

My husband was not overenthusiastic about me having a baby indoors. He is not one of those fathers who will be there at the birth . . . he was a bit panicked that he would be involved if it was a homebirth. That was his only fear, if I had a baby at home would I ask for help. I said no I did not need his help, I knew I could cope on my own.

The women also described the views of their parents. Some mothers were positive:

My own mother had two babies in hospital and two at home and for her there was absolutely no comparison. Home was the place to be, so she was very supportive.

Other parents were not so positive:

My mum was a bit worried because she only lives across the road. She didn't want to be in the house at the time, and she didn't want to be in here. She thought you should go to hospital and if anything goes wrong then you are there.

Many women indicated that their friends had been supportive and encouraging:

I had quite a few women friends who had had babies at home . . . I think because when you have got one child you tend to get to know people who are having babies around the same time and there were certainly a few people who had had wonderful experiences of having their babies at home . . . So you know you heard about their birth experiences and they were all very positive about it.

One woman suggested that she started to select friends who were positive about her decision:

I just mixed with people who could be positive and supportive and I didn't really want to spend that much time with people who were not very supportive.

Others indicated that their friends were surprised by their wish for a homebirth:

My friends weren't keen . . . because they were thinking predominantly about my health and the health of the baby and they thought that in hospital if anything goes wrong I would be completely supported by modern technology.

The women also described how they dealt with the more negative views:

I think that in that situation I knew what I wanted for me, in the way that I wanted to do it and it is not for other people.

Another stated that she explained to both her own parents and her partner's parents that 'I can understand what your feelings are but we have chosen to do this and I felt confident enough not to be put off, and they did support me'.

Several women also described other sources of information they had used either to come to their own decision or to convince others:

The midwife kept giving me, telling me bits of information to tell him . . . to have the baby at home, because they said there was . . . less chance of the baby catching any sort of infections if it is born at home.

Risk and safety

The women also described their decision to have a homebirth in terms of risk and safety and the implication for responsibility and blame.

Several women described their belief that the home was a safer place to have a baby:

I think you can get more infections being born in hospital than you can at home.

Birthwise I have always thought that it was a very safe option. You have a very skilled midwife, or probably two skilled midwives, possibly a student midwife as well at the birth, possibly a GP. For many births that take place in hospital, you don't have that skilled attendance. The house was easily accessible for emergency services and not very far from the hospital.

Several women felt that hospital may be safer:

Oh God am I making a risky choice . . . I don't know whether I would feel different if I lived in the middle of the countryside, you know, quite a long way from hospital . . . but it is so close . . . I sort of felt that if anything was going to go wrong, I would be bailed out . . . that was a security in my mind.

The women also discussed the issue of responsibility. In particular, they indicated that although they wanted to feel in control they did not want the feeling of responsibility if something went wrong:

I didn't really want to go into hospital. I have heard a few scary stories which have put me off . . . but having said that I didn't want to put my baby's life at risk. If anything happened with me not going into hospital, I know I would never have forgiven myself.

Others believed that there would be sufficient support in case of an emergency:

I knew some people who had haemorrhages and things and had been whipped in and it all ended quite safely in the end so I wasn't too alarmed about anything that went wrong.

Deciding to have a homebirth involves going against the norm. Therefore the choice to have a baby at home is a complex process involving the weighing up of the pros and cons, listening to and sometimes ignoring the views of others and planning how to deal with issues of responsibility.

The homebirth experience

The women talked about their experiences of having a homebirth in terms of the following themes and categories.

Normality

Many emphasized the normality of having their baby at home:

It just seemed to be the right and normal thing to do and I put it down to having been born at home actually myself and it seeming a perfectly natural and normal thing to do.

Women used terms such as 'normal', 'comfortable', 'warm', 'cuddly' and 'peaceful' and described this normality in terms of physical comfort, carrying on as usual and their partner being able to carry on as usual. This comfort was important during the birth:

I felt it made all the difference you know, being at home, being able to walk around my own living room, my bedroom and go to the bathroom and have a bath and stay there as long as I wanted to.

And after the birth:

I remember it being wonderful, giving me a bath afterwards, feeling like the queen and then I got back into my own clean bed with clean sheets and everything and I couldn't believe it. I mean now, years later I can remember it so well. It was such a wonderful feeling.

Many women commented that having a homebirth enabled them to carry on as usual, keep themselves occupied in labour by such things as making tea, cooking pasta and pottering around:

It just felt as if I was getting on with my life and it was just a natural part of life. I think that I could just keep all the routines going.

The next day after I had had Simon I was up. I believe I did a load of washing. I remember cooking, it was only simple but I did cook dinner . . . I did just get back into the routine of life very quickly.

Many women also commented that being at home gave their partner a role to play:

He was making some lunch, it is just life went on really, it was much easier to slip her into our ordinary life.

The atmosphere

The women talked about the general atmosphere of the birth in terms of feeling relaxed, peaceful and quiet:

I was in my own room and I was being loved and trusted and with everyone around me and people that I loved and trusted.

The role of professionals

The women discussed the role of health professionals in their birth experience, and the midwives in particular appeared to play a prominent role. The professionals were described as either being involved or being separate. This is summed up by one woman who said:

It was all happening but it wasn't intrusive. So I just felt it was just nice, people were there but they weren't there . . . they played a really nice role in my birth, as being there but not being there and not interfering really.

In terms of being involved, many women commented that the midwives were friendly, chatty and fun. In addition, they described them coming in and out of the room and being available and keeping them informed:

She was very very responsive to what I wanted to do and really very calm and would have been quite willing to sit there all through the night. Considering that they had been at work all day and there was no hurrying, no getting irritable with me or anything.

Women also commented on how the midwives gave them space and were not intrusive:

They left us to it quite a lot. They just left myself and my partner in the bathroom . . . So yes they were very relaxed and that made me feel confident in their ability and I had absolute faith in the midwives.

Pain

Pain featured frequently in the women's memory. It was often described in conflicting ways using terms as varied as 'intense', 'severe', 'shock', 'irritating', 'wonderful' and 'lovely'. In particular, pain was described in terms of its function:

you never get more pain than you can manage . . . each contraction is one step nearer to giving birth.

Some women described how the experience of pain was offset by positive aspects of the birth:

It was jolly painful. Because it is such a positive experience, it is not uppermost in my mind, it is not the pain I remember. It is all the nice things, all the lovely things.

Pain was also described in terms of the effect of being at home:

I think having the freedom to walk about and be where I wanted to be is probably quite significant and I felt you know how I was in control of where I wanted to be or have who I wanted to have, to rub my back or rub my stomach for me or whatever really, so yes, I think being here helped in my perception of the pain probably.

Pain was also discussed in terms of the impact of being at home on the use of medication.

One woman, who had a difficult birth and whose baby was born with its cord around its neck commented that having a homebirth was the right decision and said:

I knew that there wasn't anything else anyone could do, we had to get her out, so I think perhaps we worked harder then and we did get her out.

One woman commented that she had less analgesia than she would have liked because she was at home:

I just wanted her to do something . . . And I think if I had been in hospital, you know it would have been a round of pain killers and I would have accepted it quite readily but here she didn't have time to go out, you know, and she said afterwards that she felt that by the time she went to the car which was just outside and came back, that I would be at the next stage.

Control

A sense of control played an important part in the women's memories of their homebirths, with women using phrases such as 'I was in control because I was in my own home'.

The women described the role of control in the actual birth. Sometimes this was in terms of feeling in control over factors such as their position, control over medication and control over timing:

I certainly felt I was absolutely and utterly in control of the whole, the whole thing . . . the fact that it is in your home is very important, because it is your environment and the people who are there come into your home so they are not in control.

Many women described how, although they were in control of the birth, it was important for them to know that the midwives were there for them:

It was mainly in the hands of the midwives, which I was pleased about. Because I feel really they are the ones who, unless there is anything going wrong, they are the ones in the business of delivering babies.

Several women also described some degree of conflict of control:

She said, I think, I can't see enough with you down there on the floor, will you get up on the bed and I thought, Oh God no, this isn't what I envisaged being in my own house, you know I was very happy down there on the floor . . . I said I didn't want to do that and she said I think you are ready to push. I think in the end we had to reach a compromise.

Such conflict may have appeared greater because the women were in their own home and therefore expected to have more control.

Several women described how they felt in control over what was happening because things were explained to them and they were asked what they wanted to do:

I was listening to the midwives and taking advice about things, but in the end it always felt like everything was my decision and the power remained with me.

Not in hospital

Many women described their homebirth in comparison to their experiences of hospital births and remembered aspects of the birth simply as not being in hospital. Sometimes this comparison was in terms of risk and safety:

I've spent a lot of time in hospital, but I know that they can be quite dirty places and I know that infection can be rife and things like that . . . I was worried really and I knew a lot of people that had complications from a birth in hospital and had infections or I know I was just happy to be at home really, happy with our own germs.

Sometimes homebirths were described as being more natural:

It is so intimidating being in a delivery suite . . . even midwives and doctors in a situation just let science take over whereas maybe nature might have got me further on.

Sometimes they described the inhibitions created by being in a large institution:

If you go into hospital its much harder to feel that you can question when there is this huge organization and they are all obviously supporting each other.

The women appeared to accept hospital births as the norm and experienced their own homebirth in comparison to this norm.

Sharing

Many women emphasized the importance of sharing the birth experience with many different groups of people.

Women described sharing the birth with their partner:

And John's role was he had something to do which I think he needed, you know he had a role to play . . . so he had to make sure that I drank and that I weed and so he had that to do.

And sharing with their family and other children:

I wanted the baby to be sort of integrated into the family right from the word go. And she was and that is how it happened and that is really nice, Jane really remembers that too. She says 'I was one of the first to hold you'.

Women also described the importance of having the family together immediately after the birth:

The most wonderful thing, that I couldn't have predicted, which was absolutely wonderful, was that 2 hours after I'd given birth, everybody had gone. The place was cleared up and Peter and I just went to bed together, in our own bed with our baby in between us and it was just wonderful.

Many women also commented on a sense of sharing with other women in general:

it felt quite a woman-centred experience . . . It just felt like, you know, you were in a world of your own, and doing a job women do.

They also described sharing with their own mothers:

I think we have become a lot closer since that experience . . . It's levelled us out quite a bit because we are both women who have given birth to children. We are both mothers and we have both got our family responsibilities.

The women therefore described the homebirth experience in terms of factors such as normality, control, pain and the role of others.

The longer-term impact of having a homebirth

The women described the impact of their homebirth in terms of the following themes and categories.

Perceptions of self as a woman

The women described the impact of the homebirth in terms of coming to terms with and fulfilling their role as women:

I would say I felt very exhilarated by it all really. It was so nice to know my body worked properly and I had managed to do that.

One woman who had had difficult births in the past said:

I felt very confident in my body as a mother . . . It sounds strange . . . but the way the birth went, I think previously I'd thought from the hospital-managed birth as if it had all been taken away from me . . . but the second birth really put that right for me, really gave me the confidence that, oh yes, I do function all right really.

The women also described the impact of having a homebirth in terms of changes in their emotional state:

It made us feel more confident, peaceful and able to do things. I definitely do feel a lot more comfortable with myself . . . so I think it has made me feel, I am definitely . . . not so scared of life.

One woman discussed the possible relationship between homebirths and postnatal depression:

I never had any slight bit of postnatal depression, who knows whether that is my personality, what happened to me or whether it is connected, but I have a strong feeling that having had such a good birth experience and being at home and the breast-feeding went well, could be connected.

Previous experiences

The women described the impact of the homebirth in terms of how they made sense of their previous births. For example, one woman who had had two difficult births before said:

I didn't get any stitches and I wasn't induced and I didn't have a caesarean or anything like that . . . I felt, yes. I had achieved something really good, that birth doesn't have to be horrible.

Another woman who had had one difficult birth said:

The first time I had a child I really felt I needed to talk about it and if anybody was talking about pregnancy or birth I had to get in with my little comments. But now I don't. It's as if having Gregory was like a healing for what happened the first time.

The women also described the effect of the homebirth on how they identified with their surroundings at the time of the birth including the specific room, the house and the general area:

'It was a very positive experience and particularly for this house, because actually a few years earlier I nursed my father here while he died, he actually died here while he was at home and it felt good to have a sort of counterbalancing experience for this house – sort of one out and one in.

Future experiences

For many women their experiences had encouraged them to have other homebirths. One woman said:

After my second child I was very negative but Simon being such a nice calm experience . . . If I was to get pregnant this would make me do it again.

Another said that her experiences had resulted in her having more children:

One of the jokes I have made which may have some truth in it is that I may not have ended up with three if it hadn't been so good. That is a pretty lasting implication.

However, one woman who had had a difficult birth said:

It did make me nervous about having Amy. I decided that I would have Amy in hospital.

The women also described the impact of the homebirth on their relationships with the child who had been born at home:

The relationship with your child starts right at the beginning, the birth and then the breast-feeding. My bond was there instantly.

Also, they described their relationship with their other children:

We are lucky enough to have it on video and the children love to see it so we talk about it and discuss it.

In particular, some women discussed how the birth may have influenced the child's behaviour. For example one woman said:

I felt it made all the difference, you know, being at home, being able to walk around in my own living room . . . I was thinking it made a difference to them as well. I don't know maybe it was just me and that's the way they are . . . the way they are calm and they were really calm . . . The mother and child are relaxed, the baby is happy and not so traumatized.

The women also described the effect of the homebirth on their future relationships with their children:

It has certainly given me positive experiences to look back on and . . . no fears to pass on to my children about the whole event.

Many women described the consequences of the homebirth in terms of their relationships with their mothers. For many, the homebirth was seen as something which had brought them closer to their mother:

It's levelled us quite a bit because we are both women who have given birth to children. We are both mothers and we have both got our family responsibilities and I am no longer her little girl.

However, for some the homebirth had highlighted some of the problems with this relationship:

I couldn't have spoken to my mother about it she just can't cope with anything like that . . . there wasn't anybody that I felt that, that had the right to know everything I felt, you know, so I didn't discuss it an awful lot.

And at times the homebirth was seen by women as a way to move on from a problematic relationship with their mother:

I haven't got a very good relationship with my mother and particularly for me it has been very positive in a way to break the shackles of that kind of relationship.

The women also described the effect of the homebirth on their relationships with other women. In the main the women described the network of women friends which had resulted from the homebirth experience:

They are all personal friends now, but at the same time they were just all in the same boat at the same time and this time I had a really good network.

The women also described the homebirth in terms of its influence on their environment. For example one woman said:

Where I had Matthew has become Matthew's bedroom, we were decorating the bedroom differently and he is really really chuffed and now after, because he was born in that room and now he's back in that room I think he was pleased, I think it makes more sense to him.

The women therefore described the impact of the homebirth in terms of their role as women, and its impact on their understanding of both past and future experiences.

DISCUSSION

This chapter aimed to explore women's experiences of having a homebirth and indicates that even up to 5 years after the birth the women's memories remain rich and evocative.

In terms of the processes involved in choosing to have a homebirth, the results suggest that some women are clear from the beginning of their pregnancy that they want a homebirth and are determined to stand by their choice whatever the obstacles. However, for the majority, the decision to have a homebirth involved balancing up a range of sometimes conflicting factors which both helped and hindered their decision, some of which are in line with those indicated within the popular literature (Mosse 1993, Wesson 1990). The facilitative factors which the women considered included the benefits of being in their own home, the perceived negative aspects of being in a hospital, and the relative safety of their home environment. In particular, although hospitals were regarded as safer in the case of an emergency, the women believed that hospitals were associated with illness and disease and therefore in certain ways more dangerous than their own home. The women reported being exposed to a range of both professional and lay views which had supported their decision and indicated that the views of their GP, midwives, partners, friends and families had helped them to decide on a homebirth and carry this decision through to fruition. The women, however, also reported several obstacles which had hindered their homebirth. Some GPs and midwives were reported as being obstructive and partners, families and friends were sometimes seen as unenthusiastic, worried and concerned for the woman's health or anxious about their own potential involvement. The women indicated a variety of ways of dealing with these obstacles ranging from using information to change the minds of these people, deciding to persist with their intention in spite of their reduced support or choosing to avoid people with negative attitudes and mix only with those who were like minded. Even though faced with such obstacles, the women in the study ended up having a homebirth. But there may be many others, who considered the possibility of a homebirth, but ended up opting for a hospital birth when exposed to such opposition.

When discussing their experiences of actually having a homebirth, the women described a range of factors relating to their environment such as the importance of normality, the peaceful atmosphere and the role of other people around them. They also described the impact of this environment in terms of factors such as feeling in control, their pain and being able to share their experiences with others important to them. Many of their experiences of the actual birth were related directly to the birth being in their own home. For example, the familiarity of the environment helped them to integrate the time leading up to the birth into their normal life with other family members. It increased their sense of control as they felt a sense of ownership over the birth and it also provided a role for the partner. Further, it appeared to influence how they experienced pain. Being at home was also directly linked to their memories of the postnatal period in terms of remaining with their partner and other children, being able to accommodate the new baby into normal life immediately and being able to bathe in their own bath and sleep in their own bed. In line with this, the women expressed beliefs that being at home had improved the birth experience for them. Further, this perception was illustrated through their enthusiasm to discuss the experience and their use of positive language. Many of the experiences reported by the women are in line with those described in previous literature. In particular, issues of control, the possibility of a role for their partner and the physical comfort of a familiar environment have been highlighted as central to satisfaction with the birth experience (Drew et al 1989, Oakley 1986, Seguin et al 1989). The results from the present study suggest that homebirths may be experienced in such a positive way because the very factors which are associated with a positive birth experience are more likely to occur if the birth happens at home.

In terms of the potential longer-term impact of choosing to have a homebirth, many women described the impact of their homebirth on their feelings about themselves as women and indicated that their ability to have a baby at home had made them feel more confident about themselves and subsequently better equipped to deal with their children. Further, they described feeling reassured that their bodies functioned properly. The women also described the impact of the homebirth in terms of their reappraisal of past events and their interpretation of future ones. The homebirth appeared to help some women put negative past events such as death and difficult births into a more positive framework. Further, the homebirth appeared to have a lasting positive influence on their interpretation of future relationships with a range of individuals.

Overall, the results from this study present a positive picture of the experience of having a homebirth and indicate that having a baby at home may make a rewarding experience into an event which not only changes the individual but colours the way she understands both her past and future lives. However, choosing to have a homebirth is not a simple process as it involves going against the norm and dealing with both explicit and implicit obstacles. The 'Changing Childbirth' document argues that women should be provided with sufficient information in order to make an informed choice about their place of the birth. Accordingly, the women's memories described in this chapter provide information from the service user's perspective which may contribute to future informed decisions about the place of birth. Further, the document states that women's choices about the place of birth should be respected. The results from this study indicate that perhaps the emphasis should not only be on respecting women's choices once made, but also on providing a suitable forum for women to discuss their beliefs in an informative and non-directive way whilst still engaged in the decision-making process. Further, 'Changing Childbirth' and other literature for lay readers (Kitzinger 1987, Moorhead 1996) stresses that childbirth is an enriching experience. The results from the present study support these suggestions.

CONCLUSION

The home as the preferred place of birth in the 19th century was usurped by the hospital in the 20th. However, at a time when health care professionals are beginning to question the 'hospital is best' policy of the maternity services and when patients are viewed as valued consumers whose voice should be heard, perhaps the 21st century will see a return to homebirths as an acceptable option. The voices of the women who were interviewed in our study suggest that this should be the case. Perhaps the next few years will see the option of a homebirth offered to all women. Further, women may be encouraged to make their choice about the place of birth on the basis of personal preference and an informed weighing up of the pros and cons. However, as long as women have to resort to going against the norm in order to experience the normality of a homebirth, the homebirth option may not be completely realized.

Key points for caregivers

- Some women may be determined from the start of their pregnancy to have their baby at home. However, the majority of women will be unsure as to the best place to have their baby. Such women should be encouraged to discuss their concerns and worries about both hospital and home births, be given any relevant information and be given time to come to a decision about the place of birth which best meets their own personal needs.
- Women should be encouraged to talk to other women about their own birth experiences to gain insights beyond those of the professionals.
- Many women may welcome the chance to take control of their own birth. Such responsibility is empowering if everything goes to plan. However, personal responsibility can lead to both victim blaming and self-blame if problems arise. When discussing the possibility of a homebirth with pregnant women, caregivers should emphasize that although the place of birth is her choice, professionals will be there to deal with the responsibility of any problems.

> **Key points for caregivers**
>
> - Many women may choose to have a homebirth because they wish to be in control over both their environment and the actual birth process. Further, many women may also want access to all information and to be involved in all decisions. Accordingly, caregivers should respond by providing detailed and clear information and by encouraging such women to take an active role in decisions about the birth. However, other women may welcome the opportunity at times to hand over control to their caregivers. Health professionals should match their provision of information and the opportunity for choice to the specific needs of the individual. Both too much and too little control can result in feelings of panic and powerlessness.
> - Having a baby at home appears to improve an already positive experience. This may be in the main due to environmental factors such as comfort, normality and the presence of familiar family members which cannot be replicated in a hospital setting. However, it may also be related to factors such as the calm atmosphere, the presence of familiar professionals and an involvement in decisions, all of which could be transferred, to some degree, to the hospital. Caregivers should attempt to replicate their own behaviour exhibited when managing a homebirth when within the more hectic and managed hospital environment.

ACKNOWLEDGEMENTS

The author would like to thank Adrienne Shaw and Luke Zander for their contributions to the original study and to the women for agreeing to be interviewed and speaking so honestly and openly.

REFERENCES

Brown S, Lumley J 1994 Satisfaction with care in labour and birth: a survey of 790 Australian women. Birth 21: 4–13
Clement S 1995 The caesarean experience, 2nd edn. Pandora Press, London
Davies J, Hey E, Reid W, Young G 1996 Prospective regional study of planned home births. British Medical Journal 313: 1302–1306
Department of Health 1992 Maternity services. Health Committee second report, session 1991–1992 (Winterton report). HMSO, London
Department of Health 1993 Changing childbirth: report of the Expert Maternity Group. (Cumberlege Report) HMSO, London
Dowswell T, Thornton J G, Hewison J, Lilford R J L 1996 Should there be a trial of home versus hospital delivery in the United Kingdom? British Medical Journal 312: 753
Drew N C, Salmon P, Webb L 1989 Mothers, midwives and obstetricians views on the features of obstetric care which influence satisfaction with childbirth. British Journal of Obstetrics and Gynaecology 96: 1084–1088
Foster P 1995 Women and the health care industry. Routledge, London
Hodnett E D 1996a Alternative versus conventional delivery settings. In: Enkin M W, Keirse M J N C, Renfrew M J, Nielson J P (eds) Pregnancy and childbirth module of the Cochrane database of systematic reviews. The Cochrane Library. Update Software, Oxford
Hodnett E D 1996b Support from caregivers during childbirth. In: Enkin M W, Keirse M J N C, Renfrew M J, Nielson JP (eds) Pregnancy and childbirth module of the Cochrane database of systematic reviews. The Cochrane Library. Update Software, Oxford
Isaacs Ashford J 1984 Birth stories: the experience remembered. The Crossing Press, New York
Kitzinger S 1987 Pregnancy and childbirth. Penguin, London
Kitzinger S 1989 The new pregnancy and childbirth. Penguin, London

Kitzinger S 1992 Birth and violence against women: generating hypotheses from women's accounts of unhappiness after childbirth. In: Roberts H (ed) Women's health matters. Routledge, London, pp 63–80

Moorhead J 1996 New generations: 40 years of birth in Britain. National Childbirth Publishing Trust, HMSO, London

Mosse K 1993 Becoming a mother. Virago, London

Oakley A 1986 From here to maternity. Pelican, Middlesex

Ogden J 1996 Health psychology: a textbook. Open University Press, Buckingham

Ogden J, Shaw A, Zander L 1997a The homebirth experience: women's memories 3 to 5 years on. British Journal of Midwifery 5: 208–211

Ogden J, Shaw A, Zander L 1997b Deciding to have a home birth: women's memories of help and hindrances 3–5 years on. British Journal of Midwifery 5: 212–215

Ogden J, Shaw A, Zander L 1997c Women's homebirth memories: a decision with a lasting effect? British Journal of Midwifery 5: 216–218

Pop V J, Wijnen H A, van Montfort M, Essed G G, de Geus C A, van Son M M, Komproe I H 1995 Blues and depression during early puerperium: home versus hospital deliveries. British Journal of Obstetrics and Gynaecology 102: 701–706

Royal College of Obstetricians and Gynaecologists 1992 Response to the report of the House of Commons Health Committee on Maternity Services. RCOG, London

Seguin L, Therrien R, Champagne F, Larouche D 1989 The components of women's satisfaction with maternity care. Birth 16: 109–113

Simkin P 1992 Just another day in a woman's life? Part 2: nature and consistence of women's long term memories of their first birth experiences. Birth 19: 64–81

Tew M 1990 Safer childbirth? A critical history of maternity care. Chapman & Hall, London

Wesson N 1990 Homebirth: a practical guide. Optima, London

FURTHER READING

Ackermann-Liebrich U, Voegeli T, Guenter-Witt K, Kunz I, Zuellig M, Schindler C, Maurer M, Zurich Study Team 1996 Home versus hospital deliveries: follow up of matched pairs for procedure and outcome. British Medical Journal 313: 1313–1318

Bastian H 1993 Personal beliefs and alternative childbirth choices: a survey of 552 women who planned to give birth at home. Birth 20: 186–192

Chamberlain G, Wraight A, Crowley P 1997 Home births. Parthenon, London

Tew M 1990 Safer childbirth? A critical history of maternity care. Chapman & Hall, London

Wesson N 1990 Homebirth: a practical guide. Optima, London

7

Post-traumatic stress disorder following childbirth: causes, prevention and treatment

Suzanne Lyons

WHAT IS POST-TRAUMATIC STRESS DISORDER?

Post-traumatic stress disorder (PTSD) refers to an extreme psychological distress reaction following exposure to a traumatic and threatening experience. PTSD was first defined as a diagnosis in the *Diagnostic and Statistical Manual of Mental Disorders* (DSM III) in 1980 (American Psychiatric Association 1980), although symptoms of PTSD had been observed for years. Much of our understanding of PTSD has been derived from observations made of people who participated in wars of this century. More recently there has been research into PTSD as a sequel to a multitude of different traumatic experiences, including natural disasters, bombings, train crashes, kidnapping and sexual assault.

Previously it was debatable whether a traumatic experience of childbirth fitted the DSM III-R criterion of being 'a psychologically distressing event that is outside the range of usual human experience'. Perhaps for this reason there has been a reluctance by health professionals to acknowledge that PTSD can occur following childbirth, and women have not been offered appropriate treatment (Moleman et al 1992, Ralph & Alexander 1994). However, in the revised manual DSM IV (American Psychiatric Association 1994) the diagnostic criterion is subtly different. This states that:

The person has been exposed to a traumatic event in which both of the following were present:
1. the person experienced, witnessed, or was confronted with an event or events that involved or threatened death or serious injury, or a threat to the physical integrity of self or others
2. the person's response involved intense fear, helplessness, or horror.

Classic symptoms of PTSD are: intrusive thoughts and images, nightmares, hypervigilance, avoidance and increased arousal. These are frequently accompanied or complicated by depressive symptoms. The DSM IV criteria are that symptoms must be present for more than 1 month, and the disturbance must cause clinically significant distress or impairment in social, occupational, or other important areas of functioning.

Only a small percentage of women are likely to experience a level of post-traumatic stress (PTS) symptoms following childbirth which would fulfil the DSM IV criteria for PTSD. The DSM IV criteria are useful for research purposes, but generally it is more pragmatic to think in terms of a 'clinical' level of symptoms, i.e. when a woman is experiencing PTS symptoms which are distressing to the extent that they are disruptive to her and her family. Various assessments are available to categorize and measure the frequency of PTS symptoms, such as the Impact of Event Scale (IES) devised by Horowitz et al (1979). The IES is a 15-item scale with two subscales which record the number of PTS intrusion symptoms (e.g. 'I had trouble falling asleep or staying asleep, because of pictures or thoughts about it that came into my mind') and PTS avoidance symptoms (e.g. 'I stayed away from reminders of it'). As it only takes a few minutes to complete, it is ideal to use with mothers. Although there is no strict cut-off for the IES scores, a common classification is 0–8 low distress, 9–19 medium distress and 20+ high distress, for each subscale (Church & Vincent 1996).

Oakley & Rajan (1990) commented on the trend historically to frame postnatal distress and adjustment in terms of mental illness. With this in mind it may be more useful to view the term 'PTSD' as describing a type of psychological symptom rather than using it to label mothers as suffering from a psychiatric condition.

EVIDENCE OF PTSD FOLLOWING CHILDBIRTH

Case studies and qualitative research have provided evidence that some women do experience PTSD following childbirth. Beech & Robinson (1985) drew attention to reports by mothers of prolonged nightmares following childbirth. Moleman et al (1992) described three women who had symptoms of PTSD following childbirth. Ryding (1993) in a Swedish study found that 28 mothers who had previously had a traumatic childbirth showed PTS symptoms. Ballard et al (1995) presented four case studies of women who showed symptoms fitting the DSM III-R criteria of PTSD.

Kitzinger (1992) proposed that there are similarities between traumatic obstetric experience and the experience of sexual assault: 'in childbirth as in rape, a woman may be stripped, forcibly exposed, her legs splayed and tethered, and her sexual organs put on display to all comers . . . Rape and birth trauma survivors are both at first shocked, numb and emotionally anaesthetized. Their dominant feeling is that they have survived'. Kitzinger's material came from 345 letters from women concerning their birth experiences. Using discourse analysis as a framework for studying these, one major theme to emerge was the women's use of the words 'rape', 'abuse', 'assault' or 'violence' to describe their feelings, during and after childbirth. PTSD is a recognized outcome of sexual assault; factors which have been found to influence the onset of this are related to experiences which are perceived as painful, humiliating, mutilating, and occurring in an unsympathetic environment and in which the woman feels powerless to resist (Bownes et al 1991). Menage (1993) in a study of 30 women who had experienced PTSD following obstetric or gynaecological procedures, also found that women used descriptors denoting sexual assault to describe their experiences and some of the women's scores for PTSD were of a similar magnitude to those obtained from a study of Vietnam war veterans.

There are few published studies on the incidence of PTS symptoms following childbirth. Lyons (in press) in a prospective study of 42 first-time mothers found 3 (7%) mothers scored in the medium distress range on the IES and 1 (2%) in the high distress range, 1 month after childbirth. The participants in this study were older than average, mainly from socio-economic groups I, II and IIIN, and English was their first language; additionally the maternity unit where they were delivered appeared to have higher standards of psychosocial care than were found in some other studies (e.g. Fleissig 1993). Taking this into consideration, the incidence of women experiencing a level of PTS symptoms of a magnitude which is distressing and disruptive, could possibly be greater in the general population following childbirth.

THE EFFECTS OF PTSD

Research has shown that PTS symptoms and the consequential problems can have far-reaching effects both for the women concerned and for other family members. These are some of the identified problems.

Fear of childbirth

PTS reactions can lead women to avoid pregnancy or to fear the process of giving birth. Menage (1993) found examples of women avoiding pregnancy following PTS related to obstetric or gynaecological procedures. Niven (1988) in a study of 33 women 3–4 years after childbirth, found three mothers who did not have another child because their fears relating to labour had 'put them off'. Ryding (1993) found that 10 women elected to be delivered by caesarean section because of their previous traumatic experiences of childbirth. In a qualitative study of 20 mothers who had rated their labours as having been extremely distressing 10 months post-delivery, eight mothers reported a clinical level of PTS symptoms (i.e. scores over 40); of these, six said they would not have any more children because of the experience and the remaining two would only do so with elective caesarean sections (Allen 1996).

Psychosexual and relationship problems

O'Driscoll (1994), writing about sexual problems following childbirth, cites examples which are indicative of cases of PTSD. One woman had been unable to make love since the birth of her daughter, 18 months previously, without 'mentally re-living the pain (of labour), disapproval and distaste of the sexual act, and the fear of pregnancy'. Stewart (1982), in a study of mothers showing psychiatric symptoms following unsuccessful attempts to have an intervention-free childbirth, reported that some became miserable, depressed and suicidal, and lost interest in sex and in their marriage.

Mother–child relationship

Affonso (1987) found that mothers' difficulties in adaptation following childbirth are associated with negative feelings towards their infants. One woman wrote to Kitzinger 1 year after a very traumatic birth experience, 'I was very depressed about everything, kept reliving the birth and thinking, "What did I do wrong?" I felt nothing for the baby, just looked after her through a sense of duty. It was as though I'd been given some other woman's child to look after.' She said she was starting to love her child, but still had nightmares about the birth. Ballard et al (1995) reported four cases of PTSD following childbirth: initially each mother showed problems responding to her baby and these problems continued for two of them. Problems included disowning and not wanting to care for the infant, feelings of hatred towards the baby and avoiding emotional interaction with the baby because it triggered vivid memories of the traumatic delivery.

WHAT CAUSES PTSD?

Recently researchers have argued that it is not just the nature of the traumatic event but the individual's response to and interpretation of it which determine the development and severity of a post-traumatic reaction. Feinstein & Dolan's (1991) findings from a study of individuals exposed to physical trauma suggest that the greatest influence in determining outcome is the way an individual initially assimilates and deals with a traumatic event. The traumatic event serves as an important trigger for PTSD rather than being the sole cause.

Rachman (1980) in his theory of emotional processing proposed that stressors (i.e. agents of causation) include sudden, uncontrollable, dangerous and unpredictable events. Lindy et al (1987) suggested that sudden onset, lack of preparation, threat to life and traumatic loss are core components for the development of PTSD.

Although PTSD following childbirth is a relatively unresearched area, there is a growing literature on the development of PTSD following medical procedures. Shalev et al (1993) in a study of individuals' reactions to medical procedures found commonalties between typical stressors of PTSD and some medical events. These stressors included a sense of lack of control and a perceived threat to life. This research may also be applicable to childbirth as medical procedures and interventions are common in hospital deliveries.

Psychological theories of the development of PTSD

There are several psychological theories which attempt to describe the development of PTSD and the effect of influencing variables. Outlined below are information processing and cognitive approaches, and an interactive model of PTSD.

The information processing model of PTSD describes how an individual initially reacts to the events or trauma which triggers the PTSD response. Hollon & Garber (1988) suggest that when an individual encounters new information which is inconsistent with pre-existing experience, understanding or view of the world, self or others, either assimilation or accommodation takes place. Assimilation is a process of fitting information into an existing framework of understanding. Accommodation involves changing the existing framework in order to incorporate new incompatible information.

The ability to process information during emotional distress is frequently impaired; in addition, as traumas tend to be one-off events an individual is unlikely to be able to process the experience using existing framework and concepts. Therefore new information will be remembered in detail along with the emotions which accompanied it until the individual is able to process the information. These memories, which may be experienced as intrusive recollections, flashbacks and nightmares, are likely to be associated with emotional distress. In order to avoid these unpleasant feelings an individual may try to avoid any reminders of the traumatic event; this can lead to symptoms of hypervigilance and extreme anxiety. Avoiding the 'new' information slows down the processes of assimilation and accommodation so maintaining a PTS response because the information remains too intense and threatening to be mentally processed.

The cognitive model helps to explain why some people are more likely to develop PTSD than others. This model holds that the manner in which a person thinks will determine what they focus on during an event and how this in turn is interpreted. For example a person who believes that bad things happen because of his or her actions is more likely to view events in this light and in so doing reinforce this belief and consequentially experience higher levels of distress.

Foy (1992) suggested an interactive model of PTSD which combines environmental and individual factors to further explain why some individuals are more likely to develop a PTSD response than others. The development of PTSD is seen as being influenced by three types of mediating variables which may increase or decrease the risk of PTSD developing. The first type of mediating variable does not have a direct effect in that it does not produce distress of itself but its presence interacts with the effects of a traumatic experience to increase the likelihood of a PTSD response. A review of the literature indicates that this type of mediating variable for PTSD following childbirth could be: personality, social support, socio-economic group, antenatal preparation and subsequent expectations.

The second type of variable is independently capable of producing distress. Resulting distress is increased in a contributing or additive fashion. In the case of childbirth, examples of these may be: a difficult pregnancy, obstetric interventions, and a worse experience of childbirth than expected.

The third type of variable interacts with the traumatic event or trigger to heighten the PTSD reaction beyond the simple additive effects of the two, for example memories of previous childbirth traumas, miscarriage, death of a child, sexual abuse or assault may be retriggered by childbirth. Crompton (1996) gives an example of a 17-year-old mother who experienced flashbacks of sexual abuse during delivery. Qualitative research by Parratt (1994) concerning the experience of childbirth for survivors of incest, graphically illustrates how, in particular, pain, touch, not feeling in control and lack of privacy may trigger flashbacks and associated distress during childbirth.

POTENTIAL TRIGGERS FOR THE DEVELOPMENT OF PTSD

Current research suggests that it is not possible to determine whether a traumatic event or experience will trigger a post-traumatic response for a given individual. However, the literature does suggest that there are a few common triggers which include: fear of death or permanent damage to self or baby, severe pain, and feelings of not being in control. In Ryding's (1993) study of 28 Swedish mothers the following factors were identified as causing acute distress during delivery:

- feelings of helplessness, particularly where their pain could not be alleviated

- longer or shorter periods of feeling close to death, believing that they were either dying of pain or wishing for death to end the pain
- fear of losing control following brief moments of profound loss of control during a late stage of delivery.

Memories of loss of control were terrifying and contained a fear of dying and insanity.

Fear of death or permanent damage

Fear of losing a baby was the most powerful trigger for PTS reactions among the mothers in Ryding's study. Ten women had experienced complicated deliveries, five babies had been ill afterwards and, of these, two children had died, one had very severe permanent brain damage, and although the other two had not been seriously ill their mothers believed that they had been saved at the last moment.

Research by Lyons (in press) into the occurrence of mothers' concerns for the well-being of themselves and their babies during labour, and the significance of this for the development of PTS, suggests that these fears are not uncommon. Of the 42 participating mothers, 24 (57%) felt there had been complications during their delivery, 14 (33%) said they felt that their baby had been distressed, 6 (14%) women had feared that their baby might die and 4 (10%) women had feared their own death. These results indicate that these fears are perhaps more prevalent than is generally recognized. Two mothers who said that they had experienced these fears subsequently reported a level of PTS symptoms indicative of medium and high distress (see below). The intensity and duration of these fears during labour may be a crucial factor in the development of PTS. Their two accounts also emphasize the importance of the subjective experiences or attribution associated with specific events for development of a post-traumatic stress reaction.

Mother A said that she had had an 'awful' pregnancy. During labour there had been initial examinations which she had not expected and she felt that she had not been prepared antenatally for things going wrong, which had reduced her ability to cope. There had been a discontinuity of staff during her labour which she had been unhappy about and found detrimental to subsequent communication. She felt that choice and control had been taken away from her. She had memories of the baby being distressed during the final stages of labour and of her blood pressure rising. When her baby was finally born, after an emergency caesarean section, he had a physical abnormality. At 1 month post-delivery she was 'terrified' of having another child, partly because of concern that her next child would also have an abnormality and due in part to her experience of childbirth.

Mother B had developed pre-eclampsia. She was induced early and during labour she experienced intense pain in her head and was concerned that her baby may have been harmed. At this point she thought she was going to die. Her baby was delivered by emergency caesarean under general anaesthetic. The medical staff confirmed that this mother and baby had been in a critical situation. 1 month following her delivery she said that she would not have another child because of the trauma caused by the experience and the likelihood of the condition re-occurring. An important additional factor was the fact that her husband's first wife and baby had died following childbirth.

Pain

Acute pain has been shown to be a potential trigger for PTSD: the prevalence of PTSD amongst injured survivors of stressful events has been found to be higher than that of survivors without physical injury. Schreiber & Galai-Gat (1993) showed that uncontrolled pain following physical injury can even be the core trauma in PTSD. Melzack (1993) compared labour pain with other forms of pain and found that the average intensity scores for childbirth were higher than those for back pain and cancer. During obstetric interventions there is the potential for women to experience surgically induced pain and for anaesthetics to be inadequate or to fail. Ballard et al (1995) describe how for one mother an epidural was not fully effective and 'she experienced excruciating pain during an operation which took 10 minutes. She was screaming, shouting and struggling to get off the operating table during the procedure, and was held down by the attendants.' Not surprisingly this woman developed a severe PTSD reaction which included recurrent intrusive images of the experience, nightmares, and in addition she experienced suicidal thoughts and negative feelings towards her baby.

There are other accounts of women experiencing PTSD following painful deliveries (e.g. Moleman et al 1992). Ryding (1993) found women in her study feared the intractable and excruciating labour pain which they could recall as vividly months after the birth as immediately after delivery. However, it is not possible to predict whether or not a mother will develop symptoms of PTS on the basis of pain intensity alone. Lyons (in press) found that mothers' reported pain intensity ratings of labour, using the Present Pain Intensity scale of the McGill Pain Questionnaire (Melzack 1975), did not show a statistically significant association with the number and frequency of reported PTS symptoms 1 month after delivery. This suggests that, although for some women pain is the factor which leads to the development of PTS, there is not necessarily a direct causal effect and that there are interactive factors, e.g. a woman's interpretation of pain and the context in which it occurs.

However, the mothers' selection of particular pain descriptors ('fearful', 'frightful', 'terrifying', 'punishing', 'cruel', 'vicious', 'killing', and 'torturing') when recalling their delivery 1 month later, did show a statistically significant association with a higher number of reported PTS symptoms. Interestingly, women's selection of these pain descriptors a few days after delivery was not found to be predictive of the number of PTS symptoms. This suggests that mothers who have negative feelings about their baby's birth shortly afterwards will not necessarily continue to feel these 1 month later, but for some women there is an influencing factor or process in the intervening month after delivery which maintains their negative view of their experiences which leads to an increase in reported PTS symptoms.

Feelings of not being in control

The importance of control as a trigger for the development of PTSD has already been mentioned. PTSD research and postnatal case studies have found a lack or loss of 'control' to be a salient trigger for a PTS response. Lyons (in press) found that women's subjective feelings of not being in control during labour showed a statistically significant correlation with a higher number of reported PTS symptoms at 1 month following delivery. 'Being in control' means different things to each mother, some are concerned about becoming disinhibited, others may find the level of pain they experience to be beyond their control, and for some, perceptions of staff competence and their ability to be in control may be the most important factor. Control is discussed in some detail in Chapter 5.

VULNERABILITY AND PROTECTIVE FACTORS

As mentioned above, the interactive model of PTSD holds that mediating variables may increase or reduce the risk of an individual developing symptoms of PTSD. The following are potential vulnerability factors for the development of PTSD, which of themselves may be distressing: having experienced a difficult pregnancy; obstetric interventions; and a worse experience of childbirth than expected.

Difficult pregnancy

Laizner & Jeans (1990) found antenatal depression and poor health to be important predictor variables for emotional distress following childbirth. All three of the case studies presented by Moleman et al (1992) of women with symptoms of PTSD following childbirth had complicated pregnancies. Similarly, Lyons (in press) found that women who felt they had experienced a difficult pregnancy were more likely to report symptoms of PTS and postnatal depression 1 month after delivery. One explanation for this finding is that women who have experienced a difficult pregnancy may require more potentially traumatizing medical intervention during childbirth; they may be more likely to go into premature labour or be induced for medical reasons, and consequently feel less well prepared than mothers who deliver at full term. Another possibility is that the anxiety related to a difficult pregnancy is a vulnerability factor as it affects the mother's attitude towards childbirth and predisposes her to view the experience negatively.

Obstetric variables

In a prospective study of 42 first-time mothers, mode of delivery was not found to be predictive of the reported number of PTS symptoms 1 month later; however, mothers who had had an epidural or were induced were found to report more PTS symptoms (Lyons in press). Green et al (1990) found that obstetric interventions can lead to feelings of not being in control; this was true for minor interventions such as shaves, enemas and episiotomies as well as major ones such as forceps deliveries and caesarean sections. These effects were cumulative, i.e. the more interventions a woman experienced the less she felt in control. However, it was also found that some mothers who had major obstetric interventions were still able to feel in control.

Kitzinger (1992), from her study of the letters of 345 women who had been unhappy with their childbirth experiences, found that it was not only when birth entailed surgery that a woman felt violated. Many of the births appeared to have been obstetrically straightforward and the interventions were routine practices such as artificial rupture of the membranes and episiotomy. Smith & Mitchell (1996) found that 16% of the women who chose to use a postnatal debriefing service had had 'normal' deliveries. These findings demonstrate the prime importance of a mother's psychological state and perception of an event rather than the attributes of any particular intervention.

Worse experience than expected

Crowe & Von Baeyer (1989) found that women's expectations of pain are frequently neither accurate nor realistic. In this study, women with high levels of fear before antenatal classes were less anxious during delivery, and the higher a woman's anxiety after classes the less pain she reported. From this, Crowe & Von Baeyer hypothesized that women with lower levels of anxiety experienced surprise or shock at the duration and intensity of labour pain, whereas women with higher levels of anxiety prior to delivery had recognized and dealt with their concerns earlier. Lyons (in press) found 16 (45%) mothers felt their experiences of childbirth to be worse than they had anticipated and that these mothers tended to report more PTS symptoms 1 month later. It may be that inaccurate expectations may lead to surprise or shock during childbirth which could create a predisposition for the development of PTS.

Personality

Research suggests that personality is a critical vulnerability or risk factor for the development of PTSD. McFarlane (1988) found 'Neuroticism' as measured by the Eysenck Personality Inventory (EPI) (Eysenck & Eysenck 1964) to be a significant risk factor and, in a subsequent study, 'Neuroticism' was found to be a better predictor of post-traumatic stress than the degree of exposure to trauma (McFarlane 1989).

The 'Neuroticism' scale (EPI 'N') reflects a continuum of emotionality, ranging from, for example, calm and even-tempered to having changeable moods or feeling anxious. An example of an EPI 'N' question is: 'Does your mood often go up and down?'

The 'Extraversion' (EPI 'E') is similar to an extroversion–introversion continuum. Characteristics associated with the term 'Extraversion' include: sociable, easy going, impulsive, optimistic, active and talkative. Typical features of 'Introversion' include: being introspective, reserved, quiet, careful, controlled and reliable. An example of an EPI 'E' question is: 'Do you often do things on the spur of the moment?'

The EPI 'E' and 'N' scales are independent, and therefore it is possible for people to have high scores on one or both scales. Lyons found that women with higher 'N' scores tended to report more (IES) intrusion symptoms for PTS following childbirth, in contrast to women with higher 'E' (EPI) scores who showed a trend to report (IES) avoidance symptoms. This study also indicated that at 1 month following delivery high 'N' scores (EPI) may be indicative of a vulnerability factor whilst high 'E' scores (EPI) may reflect a protective factor for PTS symptoms.

A cognitive theory explanation for why being introverted or reflective should make mothers more vulnerable to developing symptoms of PTS is that they may focus on or be sensitive to negative events, or be predisposed to remember negative events. Weiner's (1986) cognitive theory of emotions suggests that people who hold themselves responsible for events rather than attributing them to other people or environmental factors, are predisposed to feel guilty or depressed following a negative event. For example, a mother who likes to be in control or has a potentially unrealistic view of control during delivery (e.g. a belief that she should be able to tolerate pain and remain totally in control) may blame herself for 'failing' following a problematic birth; this would be likely to increase vulnerability to PTS and depression.

Personality is also likely to affect how a person subsequently copes with emotional distress. Allen (1996) found that women who used coping strategies such as active coping, planning, humour and seeking emotional and social support reported fewer PTS symptoms. Mothers' actions involving accessing practical and emotional help from more than one source of social support, and gaining information about events during labour were helpful in reducing distress following delivery. Additionally, reinterpreting a traumatic experience of labour with positive thoughts rather than dwelling on negative events was found to be advantageous.

Social support

In a time of difficulty, perception of social support is important, according to Cohen & Wills (1985); for if people perceive that they are loved, cared for and cherished, they will feel that a supportive network is available. There are several questionnaires available to measure social support, such as the Perceived Social Support Scales (PSSS) developed by Procidano & Heller (1983). The questionnaire has two subscales: one for family and the other for friends. Wade & Procidano (1988), using the PSSS, found that for first-time mothers there is a transition of the location of social support from friends to family. Interestingly, Lyons found that first-time mothers who do not perceive themselves as being well supported by their families are more likely to develop symptoms of PTS.

Joseph et al (1991) suggest from their research following the capsizing of the ferry, the *Herald of Free Enterprise*, that social support may provide consensus (or shared) information which enables a person to re-assess his or her feelings by attributing the cause of a situation more rationally. For example, many mothers find their own forms of debriefing following childbirth, through discussions with family or friends. These will provide them with a greater opportunity to re-evaluate their experiences by discovering that other people have had similar experiences or reactions. However, if a woman were to withdraw socially following childbirth, perhaps because she is emotionally distressed, she would not be in a position to benefit from this sharing of experiences.

Socio-economic group

Research by Oakley (1991) suggests that the more socially disadvantaged a woman is the less likely she is to be satisfied with her medical care. Quine et al (1993) found that mothers' satisfaction with birth was mediated by psychosocial factors including information received and social support. Women of higher socio-economic grouping were more likely to feel supported by partners, family and neighbours, to feel that they had been well prepared for labour, and to report fewer symptoms of stress and less pain than women of lower socio-economic status. Similarly, Lyons found that first-time mothers from higher socio-economic groups were less likely to report symptoms of PTS. There are many possible reasons for this but one explanation may be that women with greater access to education have more realistic expectations of childbirth.

PTSD AND DEPRESSION

People who have PTSD are often also depressed. This depression may be either pre-existing (and may intensify a PTS response) or connected with the traumatic event, or be a consequence of the symptoms of PTSD.

Lyons found a significantly high correlation between self-reported symptoms of PTS and postnatal depression (PND) 1 month after childbirth. However, there was also evidence of symptoms of PTS and PND occurring independently indicating that these are two different types of psychological state. In addition the results suggest that these were influenced differently by mediating variables including personality. Research has also detected differences in the underlying cognitive or thinking patterns of the two conditions. Muran & Motta (1993) found that people who are both depressed and show symptoms of PTSD tend to have fewer irrational beliefs about themselves and others than people who are depressed but do not have symptoms of PTSD.

PREVENTION OF PTSD
What can be done during pregnancy

Realistic information for mothers may help to reduce the risk of PTS symptoms by helping them to remain in control rather than feeling overtaken by events. It is difficult to balance providing realistic information with the need to prevent unnecessary anxiety; however, if a mother knows, for example, the rate of emergency caesarean sections at the unit where she is to have her baby, this may help her to prepare for this eventuality.

When a woman has had previous experiences of childbirth which she found traumatic, or has lost a baby, symptoms of PTS may recur during subsequent pregnancies or be triggered during delivery. Providing women with an opportunity to discuss previous experiences and for this information to be known by midwives caring for her during delivery, if the mother wishes, may help to alleviate psychological distress. However, it should be noted that people have different coping styles and that to talk about past experiences may not be welcomed by all women.

Memories of sexual and physical abuse may be triggered during childbirth. The statistics concerning the number of women who have been abused in childhood or adulthood vary considerably but suggest that this is not uncommon (Crompton 1996). This obviously has ramifications for the number of women who are likely to experience flashbacks of these events during pregnancy and childbirth. It has been argued that if a midwife does not ask about previous abuse, she may reinforce the victim's sense of shame and confirm the client's belief in the need to deny the reality of her experience. However, research (Herman et al 1986) suggests that some of these women may make a psychological recovery from childhood incestuous abuse without the help of psychotherapy. Asking questions in this case may possibly disturb distressing memories unnecessarily which might otherwise have lain dormant during childbirth.

Great caution should be exercised in the prompting of disclosure of sexual or physical abuse during pregnancy unless the mother is asking for help or her behaviour is indicative of an underlying problem. Reasons for this include the following:

• Women are frequently more emotionally vulnerable during pregnancy and consequently their reactions to disclosing abuse may be intensified. This could prove detrimental to the mother emotionally and physically and possibly affect the mother–child relationship.
• Women who were sexually abused during childhood have been found to report significantly higher rates of depression and self-harm (Sedney & Brooks 1984) and to attempt suicide (Briere & Runtz 1986).
• If a woman discloses memories of abuse to a midwife, it is possible that the mother will associate the memory of the disclosure with that particular midwife. If the midwife should then assist at the woman's delivery, her presence may actually increase the chance of the mother experiencing flashbacks of the disclosed experience.

Clearly some women do have psychological issues that need attending to prior to delivery. Other than the mother directly asking for help or a midwife's intuition that the mother requires psychological help, there may be other indications of problems such as a reticence to have an internal examination. If a pregnant woman does have psychological problems it is quite likely that it will be her midwife who has the opportunity to pick up on this and who is in a position to gain the required trust and understanding to access the most appropriate help for her. Ideally midwives should have a resource such as a clinical psychologist, with whom to consult or work, or who is able to take clinical responsibility for the mother's psychological well-being with respect to past experiences and PTS.

What can be done during labour and delivery

The complexity of a PTS response following childbirth means that it is not possible to predict which mothers are more likely to develop symptoms of PTS. Being aware of the mother's feelings of control during childbirth, providing her and her partner with information and including them in the decision-making are all important factors which have been shown to be protective for the general well-being of the mother and are therefore likely to reduce the risk of PTS symptoms.

Crompton (1996) emphasizes the importance of empowering women during childbirth by always asking permission to touch a woman, and, if a vaginal examination is necessary and the woman gives permission, providing the reassurance that it will stop the moment the mother wishes it to. This kind of practice is likely to increase women's sense of control and diminish the possibility of a woman feeling violated, which should reduce the incidence of PTS.

Being aware of a mother's fears and reassuring her where possible may help to reduce the possibility of a mother falsely interpreting a situation traumatically. Allen (1996) found that 18 of the 20 women who had rated their labours as extremely distressing had attempted but failed to access adequate practical and emotional support, including reassurance that their labour was under control. Indications that staff were panicking, of errors during interventions and ineffective pain relief were taken as evidence by the mother that the situation was not under control.

Care of women following birth

The term 'debriefing' has come to have many meanings and may be confused with the term 'critical incident stress debriefing'. Mitchell (1983) originally described four similar techniques incorporated under the term 'critical incident stress debriefing'. One of these was psychological debriefing (PD) which was described by Dyregov (1989). This was devised for use with emergency workers within 48 hours of traumatization. It allows individuals who have been exposed to the same trauma the opportunity to piece together what happened. The primary aim of psychological debriefing is to provide the person with as much information as possible to enable the person to assimilate and emotionally adjust to the traumatic event. Other aims of PD are to facilitate constructive coping strategies, to provide social support and information about PTSD.

One of the reasons for critical incident stress debriefing taking place 48 hours following an incident is that it was easier to bring people together shortly afterwards and for people to share their experiences and perceptions of an event. It may be advantageous for midwives and other medical staff to meet shortly after a traumatic delivery, perhaps following the death of a baby, but for the mother at this stage it may do more harm than good. Debriefing before an individual has become accustomed to the level of anxiety which accompanies PTS may lead to retraumatization of the experience (Busuttil 1995). In the short term the best form of care for a traumatized mother might be general support, acknowledging that she may be shocked or traumatized, and providing answers to any questions that she may have. It may be worth noting, also, that Ballard et al (1995) suggest that in cases where adverse incidents have occurred during delivery, e.g. epidural failure during a caesarean section, a prompt apology by hospital staff may reduce psychological distress which could otherwise maintain a PTS response.

The term 'debriefing' in a postnatal context is becoming increasingly common and generally refers to providing a mother with the opportunity to tell her own story of childbirth and to gain access to information about her childbirth experience (Smith & Mitchell 1996). This facilitates the mental processing of the event and allows the mother to find the 'missing bits' of her experience, or sort out confusions by asking questions, and it also provides the opportunity for midwives to help the mother to positively re-evaluate her experience. For example, a mother who had an emergency caesarean section following a difficult labour, may be left with a sense of failure; sensitivity to this and a focusing by the midwife on positive qualities shown by the mother, perhaps courage and stamina, could help to enable a mother to recognize that she had not failed. Research may show that the process of debriefing if undertaken with an empathic and knowledgeable listener may be a significant factor in preventing symptoms of PTS following childbirth. Debriefing may also act as a kind of screening process, where mothers who are found to have continuing symptoms of PTS which are causing apparent distress may be referred for clinical assessment and psychological intervention if applicable.

There are likely to be some occasions where debriefing by the midwife who was present at the birth is not advisable. For example, where a mother appears to have ambivalent feelings about her delivery or is angry or distressed about the care she received, it may be difficult for her to express her feelings openly. Brant (1972) found that mothers may be restrained in what they say to their midwife out of courtesy. In such a situation it may be better for the mother to have access to a specialist counsellor who has direct links with the maternity unit.

If a mother does have specific questions concerning her labour, often it is not until some time after she returns home that she is ready to talk about her experiences and by this time she may no longer be in contact with maternity services. To answer this need seven midwives in Winchester set up 'Birth Afterthoughts' a service for women who have unanswered questions and unresolved feelings about their birth experiences, a model which has been followed in many parts of the country. It is not a counselling service but an 'information and listening service, providing a one off meeting and not on-going support' (Charles & Curtis 1994). The service offers a mother the opportunity to meet with a midwife, either at home or in a hospital setting, to discuss her delivery. The midwives in this group felt that mothers often need a period of reflection before wishing to talk about their delivery in depth. Prior to the meeting the midwife reads the mother's notes and brings them to the meeting with the mother to share with her. In an evaluation of the service, all of the 38 mothers who completed a questionnaire felt that one visit was enough to clarify the concerns that they had at that time. This kind of service offers a first line of defence postnatally against the development and maintenance of PTS symptoms. It can also serve as an entry to other types of help and support where needed.

Other areas have also developed similar services. Allott (1996), a consultant obstetrician, describes a service called the 'post-delivery stress clinic' from which women who need further help are referred on: e.g. to a clinical psychologist, psychosexual counsellor, genetic counsellor or paediatrician. A debriefing service in Oxford, where mothers postnatally were given a telephone number they could contact and were able to be seen at home if they wished, was also found to serve as an effective quality control and risk assessment system for maternity services (Smith & Mitchell 1996). This development may in turn lead to better practice and correspondingly reduce the incidence of PTS amongst those women using the maternity service.

If financial or other constraints prevent individual debriefing being generally available, consideration could be given to providing a service for mothers identified at greatest risk of developing PTS. For example, antenatally, midwives or GPs may be aware that a woman is at greater risk of developing symptoms of PTS due to previous experience of difficult or traumatic labour, losing fetuses or babies, or through having a history of sexual assault or abuse. Postnatally another group to target might be mothers who appeared to be distressed; particularly if a mother indicated that she did not feel in control, or was concerned that her baby or herself would be permanently harmed or not live. Postnatally the Impact of Event Scale (Horowitz et al 1979) may prove an effective routine screening tool for identifying mothers who may benefit from clinical assessment and help.

As each delivery is unique, attempting to provide group debriefing for mothers on a postnatal ward may be detrimental because:

- some mothers may not feel able to express their true feelings in front of others
- emotions may be very raw and intense which could be distressing for some mothers
- a mother who is traumatized may experience group debriefing as retraumatization.

PSYCHOLOGICAL TREATMENT OF PTSD

For a mother reporting symptoms of PTS, providing information concerning PTSD would be the first step in helping her to understand what is happening to her, and may offer reassurance. Effective psychological care needs to be tailored to each woman as the cause of PTS differs for each individual; determined by past experiences, personality, coping styles, understanding of the events during delivery, subsequent home environment and level of social support.

A psychological assessment for a women with PTS would involve taking a personal history, including: the woman's perception of the cause of the PTS, the type of symptoms and the severity, frequency and duration of these, the implication of these for herself and family, her methods of coping with the symptoms and an assessment for depression.

The central components of psychological treatment for PTS would be:

- to provide the mother with information on PTSD
- to assist in the process of assimilating the traumatic experience and to develop non-avoidant strategies
- an assessment of thinking style and the development of alternative ways of thinking (e.g. changing a mother's belief that she has failed because she had a caesarean section)
- to assist in the development of coping strategies
- to attend to secondary problems occurring as a consequence of PTS, such as psychosexual difficulties, disruption of the mother–child relationship, etc.

Psychological therapy also provides a non-judgmental environment where a woman can express feelings of disappointment, loss and anger.

PROTECTING THE WELL-BEING OF THE MIDWIFE

Protecting the psychological well-being of midwives as providers of a debriefing service is an important issue to consider. Working with people following personal traumas can be very demanding and so the caregiver also needs to be supported. Palmer (1995) acknowledged the potential stress of counselling following a traumatic experience stating that 'it can prove an abusive experience for all parties'. For this reason individuals who provide psychological debriefing or treatment for PTS reactions must have good psychotherapeutic skills and supervision, i.e. support from a trained counsellor or psychotherapist who is able to help disentangle the personal issues which arise when counselling people who have encountered traumatic experiences.

A midwife who has assisted at a traumatic birth or one where the baby has physiological problems or has not survived, may need to put his or her emotions 'on hold' temporarily, in order to continue to work effectively. In this situation it would be more appropriate for the midwife to be receiving support than to be expected to assume the role of actively counselling a distressed mother or couple. One reason for this is that it is common for people who are distressed to project their anger on to others, i.e. to blame them for what has happened: this could prove devastating for a midwife who had been directly involved in a delivery.

Key points for caregivers

- A woman who has previously had a traumatic birth may delay attending to her distress or unanswered questions until she is contemplating a further pregnancy or delivery. Discussing this with her antenatally or accessing other resources could improve the mother's psychological well-being during pregnancy and prevent the risk of retraumatization.

Key points for caregivers *(Cont'd)*

- As not feeling in control during childbirth has been shown to be a central risk factor for the development of PTS, sensitivity to this and corresponding action would assist in reducing this risk. Significantly, failure to adequately obtain a mother's consent for a procedure may lead to her interpreting events in terms of violation. The following are likely to increase a mother's sense of being in control:
  - assisting a mother to have realistic expectations of labour in order to lessen feelings of being unprepared, surprised or shocked
  - communicating effectively during delivery, e.g. to establish the appropriate type and level of control for the mother, some prefer minimum input whilst others may wish for frequent information, reassurance and pain relief
  - providing adequate information and explanations of procedures during delivery thus enabling a mother to make an informed decision about an event or procedure, whenever possible.
- As fears of harm or death to self or infant are triggers for the development of PTSD and as these fears are not uncommon, sensitivity to these and appropriate reassurance, particularly where these concerns are unfounded, could help to prevent unnecessary cases of PTS.
- As intense and continuous pain has been found to be a trigger for PTSD; prompt and adequate pain relief when requested should reduce the incidence of PTS following childbirth.
- It is important to be aware that retraumatization of past experiences (e.g. sexual abuse and assault) can be triggered by childbirth and that this needs to be responded to appropriately. Since personality, past experiences and other influencing factors affect a person's perception of an event, a delivery which does not appear to be traumatic to an onlooker may still cause the mother to feel traumatized. For this reason, it is important to acknowledge and attend to a woman's distress during and following delivery whenever it is evident.
- As PTS can be severely detrimental to the mother, baby and other family members, a simple screening process (e.g. using the Impact of Event Scale) could be implemented as early as 1 month following delivery to identify those mothers needing further help.
- Midwives or specialist counsellors could offer a debriefing service for mothers, with the back-up of mental health professionals, such as clinical psychologists, who are trained to treat PTSD and other psychological problems, and who could also act as a resource and provide support.
- Resources might be targeted at groups of women who are known to be at greater risk of developing PTS. These include women who have previously lost a fetus or baby, experienced a traumatic birth or been sexually abused.

REFERENCES

Affonso D D 1987 Assessment of maternal postpartum adaptation. Public Health Nursing 4(1): 9–20

Allen S F 1996 Post traumatic stress disorder symptoms following traumatic labour: causal factors, mediating variables and consequences. Doctorate Dissertation (Clinical Psychology), Southampton University, Southampton

Allott H 1996 Picking up the pieces: the post-delivery stress clinic. British Journal of Midwifery 4(10): 534–536

American Psychiatric Association 1980 Diagnostic and statistical manual of mental disorders III. American Psychiatric Association, Washington DC

American Psychiatric Association 1994 Diagnostic and statistical manual of mental disorders IV. American Psychiatric Association, Washington DC

Ballard C G , Stanley A K, Brockington I F 1995 Post traumatic stress disorder (PTSD) after childbirth. British Journal of Psychiatry 166: 525–528

Beech A B, Robinson J 1985 Nightmares following childbirth. British Journal of Psychiatry 147: 586

Bownes I T, O'Gorman E C, Sayers A 1991 Assault characteristics and post traumatic stress disorder in rape victims. Acta Psychiatrica Scandinavica 83: 27–30

Brant M 1972 The post-delivery interview. Psychosomatic Medicine in Obstetrics and Gynaecology: Third International Congress, London 1971. Karger, Basel

Briere J, Runtz M 1986 Suicidal thoughts and behaviours in former sexual abuse victims. Canadian Journal of Behavioural Science 18: 413–423

Busuttil A 1995 Psychological debriefing. British Journal of Psychiatry 166: 676–677

Charles J, Curtis L 1994 Birth afterthoughts: a listening and information service. British Journal of Midwifery 2(7): 331–334

Church J, Vincent C 1996 Psychological consequences of medical accidents in personal litigants. British Journal of Health Psychology 1: 167–179

Cohen S, Wills T A 1985 Stress, social support and the buffering hypothesis. Psychological Bulletin 98: 310–357

Crompton J 1996 Post-traumatic stress disorder and childbirth. British Journal of Midwifery 4(6): 290–293 & 4(7): 354–356, 373

Crowe K, Von Baeyer C 1989 Predictors of a positive childbirth experience. Birth 16: 59–63

Dyregov A 1989 Caring for helpers in disaster situations: psychological debriefing. Disaster Management 2: 25–30

Eysenck H J, Eysenck S B 1964 Manual of the Eysenck Personality Inventory. London University Press, London

Feinstein A, Dolan R 1991 Predictors of post-traumatic stress disorder following physical trauma: an examination of the stressor criterion. Psychological Medicine 21: 85–91

Fleissig A 1993 Are women given enough information by staff during labour and delivery? Midwifery 9: 70–75

Foy D W 1992 Introduction and description of the disorder. In: Foy D W (ed) Treating PTSD: cognitive–behavioural strategies. Guilford Press, New York

Green J M, Coupland V A, Kitzinger J V 1990 Expectations, experiences and psychological outcomes of childbirth: a prospective study of 825 women. Birth 17: 15–24

Herman J, Russell D, Trocki K 1986 Long-term effects of incestuous abuse in childhood. American Journal of Psychiatry 143(10): 1293–1296

Hollon S D, Garber J 1988 Cognitive therapy. In: Abramson L Y (ed) Social cognition and clinical psychology: a synthesis. Guilford, New York, pp 204–253

Horowitz M, Wilner N, Alvarez W 1979 Impact of Event Scale: a measure of subjective stress. Psychosomatic Medicine 41(3): 209–218

Joseph S A, Brewin C R, Yule W, Williams R 1991 Causal attributions and psychiatric symptoms in survivors of the Herald of Free Enterprise disaster. British Journal of Psychiatry 159: 542–546

Kitzinger S 1992 Birth and violence against women: generating hypotheses from women's accounts of unhappiness after childbirth. In: Roberts H (ed) Women's health matters. Routledge, London, pp 63–80

Laizner A M, Jeans M E 1990 Identification of predictor variables of a postpartum emotional reaction. Health Care for Women International 11: 191–207

Lindy J D, Green B L, Grace M 1987 The stressor criterion and post traumatic stress disorder. Journal of Nervous and Mental Disease 175: 269–272

Lyons S J A prospective study of post-traumatic stress symptoms one month following childbirth in a group of 42 first-time mothers. Journal of Reproductive and Infant Psychology (in press)

McFarlane A C 1988 The longitudinal course of post traumatic morbidity: the range of outcomes and their predictors. Journal of Nervous Mental Disease 152: 110–121

McFarlane A C 1989 The aetiology of post traumatic morbidity; predisposing, precipitating and perpetuating factors. The British Journal of Psychiatry 154: 221–228

Melzack R 1975 The McGill Pain Questionnaire: major properties and scoring methods. Pain 1: 277–299

Melzack R 1993 Labour pain as a model of acute pain. Pain 53: 117–120

Menage J 1993 Post-traumatic stress disorder in women who have undergone obstetric and/or gynaecological procedures. Journal of Infant and Reproductive Psychology 11: 221–228

Mitchell J T 1983 When disaster strikes. The critical incident stress debriefing process. Journal of Emergency Medical Services 8: 36–39

Moleman N, Van der Hart O, Van der Kolk B A 1992 The partus stress reaction: a neglected etiological factor in post partum psychiatric disorders. Journal of Nervous and Mental Disease 180(4): 271–272

Muran E M, Motta R W 1993 Cognitive distortions and irrational beliefs in post traumatic stress, anxiety, and depressive disorders. Journal of Clinical Psychology 49(2): 166–176

Niven C 1988 Labour pain: long-term recall and consequences. Journal of Reproductive and Infant Psychology 6: 83–87

Oakley A 1991 Using medical care: the views and experiences of high risk mothers. Health Services Research 26(5): 651–669

Oakley A, Rajan L 1990 Obstetric technology and maternal emotional well-being: a further research note. Journal of Reproductive and Infant Psychology 8: 45–55

O'Driscoll M 1994 Midwives, childbirth and sexuality. British Journal of Midwifery 2(1): 39–41

Palmer I 1995 Response to treatment varies. British Medical Journal 311: 510

Parratt J 1994 The experience of childbirth for survivors of incest. Midwifery 10: 26–39

Procidano M E, Heller K 1983 Measures of perceived social support from friends and from family: three validation studies. American Journal of Community Psychology 11(1): 1–24

Quine L, Rutter D R, Gowen S 1993 Women's satisfaction with the quality of the birth experience: a prospective study of social and psychological predictors. Journal of Reproductive and Infant Psychology 11: 107–113

Rachman S 1980 Emotional processing. Behaviour Research and Therapy 18: 51–60

Ralph K, Alexander J 1994 Borne under stress. Nursing Times 90(12): 28–30

Ryding E L 1993 Investigation of 33 women who demanded a caesarean section for personal reasons. Acta Obstetrica et Gynecologica Scandinavica 72: 280–285

Schreiber S, Galai-Gat T 1993 Uncontrolled pain following physical injury as the core-trauma in post traumatic stress disorder. Pain 54: 107–110

Sedney M A, Brooks B 1984 Factors associated with a history of childhood and sexual experiences in a nonclinical female population. Journal of the American Academy of Child Psychiatry 23: 215–218

Shalev A Y, Shreiber S, Galai T, Melmed R N 1993 Post-traumatic stress disorder following medical events. British Journal of Clinical Psychology 32: 247–253

Smith J A, Mitchell S 1996 Debriefing after childbirth: a tool for effective risk management. British Journal of Midwifery 4(11): 581–586

Stewart D E 1982 Psychiatric symptoms following attempted natural childbirth. Canadian Medical Association Journal 127: 713–716

Wade L N, Procidano M E 1988 The effects of child rearing on mothers' social support. Paper presented at the annual meeting of the American Psychological Association, Washington DC

Weiner B 1986 An attribution theory of motivation and emotion. Springer-Verlag, New York

FURTHER READING

British Journal of Midwifery 1996 Positive care in childbirth supplement. British Journal of Midwifery 4(10): 527–538

British Journal of Midwifery 1996 Risk management supplement. British Journal of Midwifery 4(11): 581–586

Kitzinger S 1992 Birth and violence against women: generating hypotheses from women's accounts of unhappiness after childbirth. In: Roberts H (ed) Women's health matters. Routledge, London, pp 63–80

Ralph K, Alexander J 1994 Borne under stress. Nursing Times 90(12): 28–30

Scott M J, Stradling S G 1992 Counselling for post traumatic stress disorder. Sage, London

8

Psychological effects of stillbirth and neonatal loss

Patricia Hughes

INTRODUCTION

Stillbirth is legally defined in the UK as the birth of a dead infant after the 24th week of pregnancy. In older research papers stillbirth may mean the birth of a dead child after the earlier legal definition of 28 weeks' gestation. In practice, clinicians tend to use the parents' experience of their baby's maturity as a guide to whether the loss be considered a stillbirth or miscarriage, and recognize a loss after 20 weeks' gestation as representing a stillborn child to the parents. Neonatal loss is the death of a live-born infant up to the age of 1 month. In clinical practice staff also have to work with parents whose infants die more than 1 month after birth, but who are never discharged from the neonatal unit. For simplicity, the term *perinatal loss* will be used in this chapter to include both stillbirth after 20 weeks' gestation and neonatal loss in the first month. In England and Wales 0.6% of babies are stillborn, and 0.4% of live-born babies die within the first month (OPCS 1995).

Termination of pregnancy for fetal abnormality is another important perinatal loss that leads to significant grief and mourning. However, for reasons of space, this chapter is confined to naturally occurring perinatal losses, but the reader is directed to literature on this subject at the end of the chapter.

PERINATAL LOSS AS BEREAVEMENT

Until the early 1960s, perinatal loss and in particular pregnancy loss was not acknowledged by the medical profession as a real bereavement and one which deserved serious attention. An obstetrician writing in 1970 reported with surprise that one mother had told him that the stillbirth of her baby had upset her more than the loss of her mother (Giles 1970). Until the 1970s it was generally considered harmful for a mother to see and hold her dead baby, especially if the baby had been stillborn, or to plan and attend a funeral service (Davidson 1977). Staff were firm in their belief that to see and hold the dead child would increase the mother's upset, and that this must be avoided. Mothers were generally advised to forget what had happened, and to try to have another baby as soon as possible. Fathers were not considered to have feelings of distress; their role was to comfort the mother. It is now recognized that both parents' attachment to the child develops throughout the pregnancy, and that loss during or soon after birth is very real indeed to the parents (e.g. Condon 1986). By the early 1980s an increasing number of clinicians had come to believe that contact with the baby was an important experience for bereaved parents. Kirkley Best & VanDevere (1986) think that it is important for parents to realize that the death has occurred, to be parents even if only for a very brief time, and to say hello and goodbye to a daughter or son who will always have a place in the family.

It is now accepted practice in hospitals to acknowledge the severity of the loss, and to expect the parents to go through a period of mourning, at least for a full-term child or one who has reached the second half of the pregnancy. There are written guidelines designed to recognize the importance of the loss for parents, and to dignify the experience as a significant bereavement (e.g. SANDS 1991). This means that some of the earlier commentaries about management in hospitals would no longer hold true.

PROBLEMS OF RESEARCH INTO PERINATAL LOSS

There have been many papers looking at the effect of perinatal loss on parents. The research has had a number of problems. There is confusion in many papers about the distinction between normal grief and psychiatric illness, with a tendency to pathologize a normal, painful response to loss. In addition, many papers suffer the problem of poor sampling, as well as high rates of dropout before the study is complete. Almost no research is available on the longer-term effects of the loss on the parents or on other children in the family.

In recent years, several researchers have pointed out that the difficulty in getting a truly representative sample of the population has been a consistent weakness in all studies of perinatal loss. In some studies full research data have been available for fewer than half of all eligible parents (Bourne & Lewis 1992). In studies of parents who have suffered a loss those who have agreed to take part in the study are more middle class and more educated than those who refuse or who cannot be contacted (Zeanah et al 1995). Women from lower socio-economic groups are thus under-represented in investigations of all types of losses (Osterweis et al 1987). Women who refuse to take part are less likely to be married, are more likely to have a baby who died on the first day after birth, and are less likely to consent to post-mortem examination (Tudehope et al 1986). Those who have more dismissing responses to painful experience may also be under-represented (Zeanah et al 1995). There has been relatively little research on fathers, and when researchers have attempted to include them in a project, their rate of non-compliance is even higher than that of mothers.

This raises important questions about the extent to which research results can be generalized. Both the lack of long-term studies and the shortcomings in sampling mean that we cannot predict with certainty which parents and families will make a full recovery and which will have difficulties in the longer term. It is possible that the parents who do not take part in research studies are more vulnerable than those who agree.

BEREAVEMENT, GRIEF AND MOURNING

Bereavement, *grief*, and *mourning* are often used interchangeably. *Depression* is sometimes equated with mourning. Zeanah (1989) has suggested how we might distinguish these terms.

• *Bereavement* is the state of having lost someone or something to whom one is significantly emotionally attached.
• *Grief* refers to all the painful emotions associated with loss, including sadness, anger, guilt, shame and anxiety.
• *Mourning* refers to a complex interplay of the psychological processes that are triggered by the loss. This includes biological reactions, such as loss of appetite; behavioural reactions, such as searching and weeping; and cognitive and defensive operations related to the loss, such as preoccupation with the lost person, and sometimes idealization of him or her. Mourning is the process by which a person resolves a loss. According to Bowlby (1980) *resolution of mourning* is the person's acceptance of a change in the external world, with a reorganization and reorientation of the internal (mental) representation of the world.
• *Depression* is both a psychiatric symptom and a diagnostic category. The normal sadness of loss or bereavement should not be confused with the pathological condition of depression, although sometimes depressive illness may be precipitated by a severe loss, and may need psychiatric treatment.

Writers quoted in this chapter use both *grief* and *mourning* to describe the process following loss. Readers are invited to use their common sense to understand what is intended.

WHAT DO WE MEAN BY NORMAL MOURNING

In 1944 Lindemann published his classic study of the normal course of grief. He described the acute distress of the early weeks and months, with sadness, weeping, insomnia and often loss of appetite. The bereaved person shows little interest in social activities, and is usually preoccupied with images of the deceased.

Bowlby writing nearly 20 years later (Bowlby 1961) conceptualized mourning as taking places in stages. This work was developed further by Parkes (1965) and by Kubler Ross (1970). These clinicians described the now familiar *stages of mourning*, with numbness and shock initially, followed by yearning and searching, disorganization, and finally reorganization, when the bereaved person adjusts to a world in which he or she finally accepts that the loved person is gone.

The usual duration of mourning is generally agreed to be 6 months to 1 year (Parkes 1965, Lake et al 1983), but it is not unusual and should not in itself be considered abnormal for mourning to last 2 years before the bereaved person substantially adjusts to the loss. One study (De Frain 1990–91) found that both mothers and fathers thought that it took an average of between 2 and 3 years for them to almost fully recover after a stillbirth.

GRIEF AFTER PERINATAL LOSS

There are two kinds of research assessing the course of normal and abnormal grief. In empirical research (e.g. Forrest et al 1982, Tudehope et al 1986) assessment of the course of normal grief has generally been done using scales developed to measure clinical depression, although more recently Toedter et al (1988) devised the Perinatal Grief Scale, which includes questions specific to perinatal grief.

In clinical and descriptive studies (e.g. Condon 1986, Lewis & Page 1978) a smaller number of patients are described in detail, and symptoms are quantified by clinical evaluation rather than questionnaire. Each of these approaches has its advantages: the questionnaire method may lack depth and clinical sensitivity, but gives an overview of population patterns, whilst the clinical papers are fresh and lively, but the smaller numbers sometimes limit the generalizability of the findings.

The many studies of parental grief after perinatal death are unanimous in finding that this is a significant and intensely painful loss for parents. It is usual in the period immediately after the death for parents to be intensely sad, unable to sleep or eat, preoccupied with the dead baby, and to lose interest in normal activities.

About 20–30% of women have symptoms of depression at a level which could be diagnosed as a psychiatric case during the first year after loss. We do not know if this predicts longer-term problems.

Change in symptoms over time

Those studies which have looked at parents over time have found that the severity of disabling symptoms diminishes over the first year.

As might be expected symptoms are usually most severe in the first 3–6 months. Jensen & Zahourek (1972) found that 6 weeks after the loss, one-third of mothers had symptoms at the level of clinical depression; Harmon (1984) found that mothers rated themselves as most affected 2–4 months after the loss, and that 77% said that 'things were not going well' at 3 months. LaRoche et al (1984) found that 20% of mothers had 'inappropriate grief reactions' at 3 months. 6 months after bereavement Forrest et al (1982) found that 34% of mothers had scores in the range of psychiatric disorder, and that 49% had significant symptoms of depression or anxiety.

Towards 1 year after the death, researchers report that women are generally improved although many still suffer the effects of their loss. At 9 months, Harmon found that 32% said that things were not going well, and 74% said they had some symptoms of depression. At 1 year, Jensen & Zahourek found 20% of mothers suffering depression at case level, and at 14 months, Forrest et al reported that 23% of mothers had symptoms at the level of clinical depression.

In a retrospective study, De Frain (1990–91) found that the average time for 'almost full recovery' to pre-loss levels of happiness for both fathers and mothers was 2–3 years after stillbirth. The parents said that the time taken for full recovery was on average 8 years.

Factors which correlate with intense grief in the early weeks

A high level of symptoms of grief 2 months after perinatal loss is related to poor marital adjustment (Mekosh-Rosenbaum & Lasker 1995, Nicol et al 1986, Tudehope et al 1986), poor ego strength and poor social support (Zeanah et al 1995). For fathers, but not mothers, perceived family support is a protective factor in mitigating intensity of grief.

Age, education and social class are less useful predictors. Having other live children is a mildly protective factor for mothers, but not for fathers, in terms of intensity of grief and difficulty coping, though mothers with and without children report the same level of depressive symptoms as measured by the Beck Depression Inventory (Zeanah et al 1995).

Mothers who had poorer physical health and previous mental health symptoms are more likely to have greater difficulty coping 6 weeks after loss (Toedter et al 1988). Previous mental health problems also predict those who will have continuing symptoms of grief 1 and 2 years later. Toedter et al found that older mothers are more likely to have a high level of despair after the loss.

Factors which do not correlate with level of grief in the early weeks

Stillborn and neonatal deaths have very similar grief reactions (Peppers & Knapp 1980). The level of grief is not affected by previous pregnancy losses, nor by the gender of the baby (Zeanah et al 1995).

OUTCOME AFTER PERINATAL LOSS

Mothers' versus fathers' level of grief

Although fathers are often as attached to their children as mothers are, there is less public acceptance of the father's need to grieve after a perinatal loss (Peppers & Knapp 1980). However, studies which have investigated differences in the grieving of mothers and fathers have been bedevilled by low compliance rates in fathers.

Tudehope et al (1986) reported differences in *how* mothers and fathers grieve. 8 weeks after the loss, both mothers and fathers showed guilt, anger, hostility and social withdrawal. Mothers also had sleep disturbance, depression, anorexia and morbid preoccupation with the baby, whilst fathers were more likely to be unable to work, deny the death and misuse alcohol. Vance et al (1994) found that mothers but not fathers increased their use of sedative drugs in the 2 months after the loss. Mothers showed a greater *increase* in heavy drinking than fathers although in absolute terms fathers drank more than mothers (De Frain et al 1990–91, Vance et al 1994).

Most studies report that after perinatal loss mothers' grief exceeds that of fathers (Benfield et al 1978, Tudehope et al 1986). Two careful studies, however (Benfield et al 1978, Zeanah et al 1995), whilst confirming this average, show that in about a quarter of couples, the father's grief exceeds that of the mother. Lasker & Toedter (1991) found that although mothers' grief was more intense 2 months after loss, there was no difference between the level of grief symptoms of mothers and fathers 1 year and 2 years later.

One study (De Frain 1990-91) found that 28% of mothers and 17% of fathers 'seriously considered' suicide after the death of the baby, although no-one in his series had attempted it. The recognition that fathers may be as severely distressed as mothers has implications for planning support services.

Effect of perinatal loss on the parent's relationship

The reported effects of perinatal loss on the parent's relationship with each other vary. One study found 33% of parents having marital difficulties after the loss (Cullberg 1972); in another, half of the parents said their relationship had improved in the 6 months since the loss, and half said it was unchanged (Forrest et al 1982). However, 6% of parents in Forrest's study separated within 6 months of the death. One carefully controlled study used parents of live-born infants as controls. Marital satisfaction declined equally for both bereaved and control parents within the 2.5 years postpartum. In the 2.5 years after the loss, parents who had suffered a loss had a separation/divorce rate of 5.8% compared to 3.7% for parents whose child had lived (Mekosh-Rosenbaum & Lasker 1995).

The balance of evidence is therefore that marital satisfaction declines after perinatal loss, but no more than it does after a healthy child is born. There is some evidence that rate of separation and divorce goes up, but only slightly.

Other findings

De Frain (1990–91) found that 24% of mothers and 18% of fathers reported that they had moved house 'to escape the pain of the stillbirth'. This may be a further factor in increasing the difficulty in keeping in touch with parents for research.

Effects on existing children

The initial reaction of existing children to perinatal loss is often puzzlement and confusion about what exactly has happened. If parents do not provide an explanation, the child may fantasize active destruction or abandonment of the expected baby and may blame parents or him- or herself for what has happened. Older children may be resentful because of disappointment (Cain et al 1964). Parents may be so caught up in their own grief that the children may feel ignored or rejected (Gilson 1976).

Nightmares, bedwetting and behaviour problems may occur both in young and in school-age children after sibling loss (Phipps 1982), and a child's fear of his own death may lead to difficulty in getting to sleep and fear of illness (Mandell et al 1983).

The scapegoating of one child in the family after a sibling death (Tooley 1975) and the conscious or unconscious holding of an older child or surviving twin responsible for the death have been observed. In one case a mother believed that a surviving twin 'starved out' the twin who died (Kirkley Best & VanDevere 1986).

Cultural differences

There is almost no research on cultural differences in patterns of grieving after perinatal death. It is sometimes argued that the main stress for women from Indian families is the sense of having failed to produce a viable child for their husband. However, one study looked in some depth at nine middle-class Indian women who had suffered a perinatal death (Mammen 1995) and found evidence of substantial grieving unrelated to family blame for not producing a child.

WHAT DO WE MEAN BY PATHOLOGICAL GRIEF OR PATHOLOGICAL MOURNING

Pathological mourning differs from normal by being prolonged beyond the usual time and/or in the degree to which day-to-day behaviour and emotional state are affected (Bowlby 1980). It clinically falls into two broad categories, absent grief and prolonged mourning or grief.

Absent grief is a failure to display symptoms of grief in the first few weeks after loss. Clinicians who work with bereaved people suggest that absent grief may result in severe anniversary reactions (delayed grief), or the later development of phobic or anxiety symptoms (masked grief). (Condon 1986, Lewis & Page 1978).

Prolonged grief is also called *adjustment disorder with depression* or *unresolved mourning*. This is a grief (mourning) that initially seems normal, but which fails to resolve and continues unabated, with disabling severity beyond the 'normal' duration. The mourning time after the loss of a close and loved person is generally agreed to be 6 months to 1 year, but having some symptoms of grief continuing for up to 2 years is not unusual.

PATHOLOGICAL GRIEF REACTIONS AFTER STILLBIRTH AND NEONATAL DEATH

Most studies of pathological grief after perinatal loss define pathology in terms of psychiatric morbidity such as intense or prolonged symptoms of depression or anxiety.

Other criteria include absent grief reactions, and subsequent problems in family relationships or with children born after the loss. Lasker & Toedter (1991) distinguish what they consider to be the less severe forms of grief, namely crying and sadness, and the more severe dimensions including withdrawal and despair, with difficulty coping.

Prolonged mourning

The diagnosis of prolonged mourning is made on the basis of both the length of the mourning time and the severity of the continuing symptoms. Although this is not a hard and fast rule, most writers use 1 year as a cut-off point for defining the onset of prolonged mourning. Condon (1986) suggests that the loss should not be centre stage in the woman's emotional life after 6–9 months, and that there should be evidence of significant signs of resolution by then. It may be considered normal for a woman to feel a lot of sadness, and even weepiness 9 months after her baby's death, but a doctor or health visitor might be concerned if she is still unable to carry out her normal family or work responsibilities, or if she experiences intense anxiety around babies.

Research shows that up to a quarter of mothers meet the criteria for being classified as a psychiatric 'case' 1 year after loss. This compares to about 10% of adult women in the general population. As women from lower socio-economic groups are under-represented in most studies of perinatal loss, the true increase in morbidity is probably higher than it appears.

Mothers are much more likely than fathers to be referred for treatment because of abnormal grief after perinatal death, although frequently when the parents are interviewed it is clear that the father is equally distressed (Condon 1986). Most bereaved parents who want professional help seek it within a few months of the loss, but a few ask for treatment or are referred by another professional years later.

Psychiatric symptoms 1 year after loss

Studies variously report up to a quarter of women still have depressive symptoms at the level of psychiatric diagnosis 1 year after the loss (Forrest et al 1982, LaRoche et al 1984, Rowe et al 1978). However, an early paper by Wolff et al (1970) reported that none of their group had psychiatric symptoms 3 years after loss. They suggested that because these women had had several interviews in the immediate postpartum period, they may have been helped to express grief and that this facilitated mourning. This proposal is supported by Forrest et al (1982) who noted a sharp reduction in psychiatric symptoms at 6 months in women who had had a counselling intervention.

Absence of grief

Several writers (Cullberg 1972, Kennell et al 1970) consider that absence of grief after perinatal loss may indicate disordered mourning. Although this has been said to be a maladaptive response to loss, it is not definitively established as necessarily pathological. Systematic evaluation of depressive symptoms in the early weeks after perinatal loss shows that about a quarter of mothers and a third of fathers have a muted response to the loss in terms of the intensity of their emotional responses. They suffer less severe weepiness, less insomnia, anorexia and self-blame, and perceive themselves as coping fairly well with the loss (Zeanah et al 1995). This is clearly a common way to cope with loss and grief, and deserves more research before we can be sure that it always represents pathology.

About a quarter of a group of parents scored less than 2 on the Beck Depression Inventory (BDI) 2 months after a perinatal loss (Zeanah et al 1995). Zeanah coined the term 'minimizers' to describe them, suggesting that the 'minimizers' may either be coping well with good social support, or their responses may be defensive and they could be storing up future trouble for themselves.

In a descriptive clinical paper, Condon (1986) suggests that absent grief may be associated with later difficulty in becoming attached to the next baby. There is no systematic research to confirm this, but Field et al (1991), working with non-bereaved mothers, report that mothers who score very low on the BDI postpartum have more difficulty relating to their babies than higher scorers, perhaps indicating some insensitivity or cutting off from their own or the baby's emotional cues.

OTHER PSYCHIATRIC CONDITIONS AFTER PERINATAL LOSS

Postpartum psychosis

Stillbirth or neonatal death does *not* increase the risk of postpartum psychosis. Postpartum psychosis is a rare condition (about 1.5 per 1000 births) with an acute onset of florid symptoms including confusion, excitement, delusional beliefs and hallucinations, with onset usually within 2 weeks of delivery.

Condon (1986) notes two striking symptoms which would usually indicate severe depressive illness, but which he believes are part of the clinical picture in normal grief after perinatal loss. Firstly, the hallucination that the baby is still kicking in the womb. This corresponds to the visual and auditory hallucinations which are common after other kinds of bereavement. Secondly, an intense sense of guilt and self-denigration is common following perinatal loss. The special circumstance of the baby having been part of the mother and the mother's sense of responsibility for the fetus mean that these symptoms are not necessarily an indication of abnormal grief, but can be considered to be a normal reaction to this particular loss.

Post-traumatic stress disorder

Post-traumatic stress disorder may occur after stillbirth, and will need treatment. This is not a 'normal' reaction to perinatal loss. The symptoms are vivid nightmares of the trauma, flashbacks in which the mother feels she is going through the experience again, and sometimes feelings of panic aroused by something associated with the trauma (see Ch. 7 for further details).

PREDICTORS OF PATHOLOGICAL GRIEF REACTIONS

Research evidence is limited. Available evidence suggests that poor marital support is important in predicting pathological grief, and lack of social support and significant other stresses in pregnancy are contributing factors (Condon 1986, Forrest et al 1982, LaRoche et al 1984, Nicol et al 1986, Rowe et al 1978).

Lasker & Toedter (1991) found that pre-pregnancy mental health was the best predictor of levels of grief 2 years after the loss in both mothers and fathers. Those who had a history of depression prior to the pregnancy were most at risk of prolonged grief. The risk of a prolonged grief reaction was best predicted in their study by scores on the 'difficulty coping' and 'despair' subscales of the Perinatal Grief Inventory.

The loss of a loved person during pregnancy has been found to be a predictor of pathological mourning in mothers (Nicol et al 1986) but losses that predate the pregnancy, including perinatal losses, were unrelated to the extent of pathological mourning (Forrest et al 1982).

Social class has been reported to have no effect in predicting disordered mourning (Rowe et al 1978, LaRoche et al 1984), but neither of these papers published the figures to support these claims

Research has not explored whether personality characteristics, lack of resolution of mourning for previous losses, or the parents' own childhood experiences and relationships might be associated with pathological grief reactions.

THE NEXT PREGNANCY

There are increased fertility rates, in both developing and developed countries, following perinatal loss (Vogel & Knox 1975), and parents are more likely to have another child after a perinatal loss than after having a surviving infant with an abnormality (Rubin & Ferencz 1985).

When do women become pregnant again?

Between 50 and 60% of women become pregnant again within the year after the loss (Forrest et al 1982, LaRoche et al 1984, Rowe et al 1978). In one study, however, 20% of mothers were adamant 3 years after losing the baby that they did not want to be pregnant again, and 10% had been sterilized at their own request (Wolff et al 1970).

Anxiety and depression during the next pregnancy

It is unsurprising to find that mothers are markedly anxious during the next pregnancy after perinatal loss (Davis et al 1989). Theut and colleagues (1988) found greater anxiety in pregnant women with previous perinatal losses, as measured by the Pregnancy Outcome Inventory, specifically designed to look at anxiety in pregnancy. Fathers were not different on any measures. In our own study of 60 mothers and 60 case-matched controls, we have found a doubling of 'caseness' of depression and marked rise in anxiety using the Spielberger anxiety scale (Hughes & Turton, in preparation).

A feature of the next pregnancy which is more difficult to quantify is what has been called 'absence of involvement' (Kirkley Best & VanDevere 1986). Some mothers deliberately or unconsciously distance themselves from emotional involvement in the next pregnancy until they are sure that they will have a living child because they cannot face the pain of another loss.

Does the timing of the next pregnancy matter?

The rationale for believing that the timing of the next pregnancy matters is either that the mother may suffer more disordered mourning or that the timing may influence for better or worse her relationship with the next child. These two points may become confused in looking at studies which assess the effect which earlier or later pregnancy have on the mother.

The effect of pregnancy on symptoms of grief

There is one much-quoted study that becoming pregnant within 5 months of a perinatal loss puts the mother at risk of prolonged grieving (Rowe et al 1978). LaRoche et al (1984) on the other hand found no significant differences in the mourning of women who became pregnant under 6 months and over 6 months after perinatal loss. Some researchers (Wolff et al 1970) even take the view that the mother's willingness to embark on another pregnancy is evidence of resolution of mourning. There has been one encouraging report suggesting that a programme of support soon after the loss made a difference to depressive symptoms in women who elected to become pregnant very soon. Women who had this support and who were pregnant within 6 months of the loss had a very much lower level of depressive symptoms at 6 months than those who had not had the intervention (Forrest et al 1982).

The effect of early pregnancy on the mother's relationship with the next child

A number of clinicians have described difficulties in the mother–child relationship when the mother has suffered a previous perinatal loss. This has been postulated to be related to a failure to resolve the mourning for the dead child with a continuing preoccupation with that child, and sometimes an unconscious confusion between live and dead children. According to Lewis (1976, 1979), such difficulties will be increased if the mother becomes pregnant too soon after the loss, and before she has had time to resolve her mourning and accept the reality and finality of the baby's death. Lewis argues that the mother's focus on her new pregnancy will divert her from the necessary preoccupation with the mourning process. Her residual unconscious failure to end the relationship with the dead child will then leave her vulnerable to developing a disordered relationship with the live one.

Lewis' position is plausible, but has not been systematically investigated. There is a need for long-term follow-up looking systematically at the relationship which the mother has with the next child. At present we do not know whether delaying the next pregnancy protects against later problems in the mother–child relationship.

The child born after a perinatal loss

Green & Solnit (1964) suggest that the child born after a perinatal loss is at risk of being treated with particular anxiety, the *vulnerable child syndrome*, others (Cain & Cain 1964) have described the *replacement child*, whose needs and personal characteristics are either idealized, or denigrated as less than the lost child would have been. Akhtar & Thomson (1982) propose that the 'replacement child manoeuvre' may lead to the child being treated as very special and yet neglected because of the mother's continuing ambivalence, and suggest this may be related to later narcissistic personality disorder.

There are several single case studies describing physical illness in the child born after the death of a newborn baby, including failure to thrive in the early months (Drotar & Irving 1979) and abdominal pain in a 6-year-old related to maternal anxiety (Jolly 1976). In Forrest's group, of seven mothers who had another child by 14 months after the loss, five related well to the child, but two experienced negative feelings about their infants and seemed unresponsive to them (Forrest et al 1982).

A recent study (Heller & Zeanah, in preparation) found that 45% of 19 mothers who had suffered perinatal loss had infants who showed a disorganized pattern of attachment behaviour in the Strange Situation at 1 year. In contrast, the parents in Phipps's study (1985) thought they had no attachment difficulties to the next child, and Goldberg et al (1986) in a study of five surviving twins found that all had a secure relationship with their mothers as measured by the Strange Situation technique.

On balance there is a large amount of descriptive evidence that children born after a pregnancy loss may be more vulnerable than others to psychological and physical problems. These reports involve small numbers or are single case studies; nonetheless they are based on careful clinical assessment and cannot be lightly dismissed. These clinical reports may be telling us something important about a particular risk associated with perinatal loss, but need further research. Unfortunately, at present we have no way of knowing which parents and which children are at risk.

What advice should parents receive about the timing of the next pregnancy

Davis et al (1989) found that women did not like being advised by the doctor, whether they were advised to wait more than 6 months or encouraged to conceive immediately. Despite this observation, women are likely to continue to ask for advice from doctors, midwives and health visitors, and should be given as much information as is available when they make their decision.

There is no empirical evidence that delaying the next pregnancy confers any psychological advantage on either the parents or the subsequent child, but nor is there evidence that the pregnancy itself assists the mourning process. We can say with more confidence that the next pregnancy after a loss is stressful and the couple might want to feel reasonably emotionally and physically robust before beginning again.

Probably the best advice to parents is to recognize that they need some time to recover from a painful loss before embarking on the stress of the next pregnancy. The actual timing may vary widely. If a health professional is asked to help in the decision, he or she should encourage the parents to explore the specific issues involved for them.

GOOD PSYCHOSOCIAL PRACTICE AFTER PERINATAL LOSS

It is now usual for hospitals to have guidelines for dealing with the parents after perinatal death. This is important in promoting good practice, but carries the risk that staff may begin to apply it automatically, and without thinking about what particular parents need and can cope with (Leon 1992).

When things begin to go wrong

Parents appreciate being told in a clear and straightforward way what is going on, and what management is planned. Even in an emergency this should be done wherever possible. The information should be given by a senior person looking after the mother and baby, and other staff should know what has been said to avoid confusion.

After the baby has died or been stillborn

Parents should have privacy without being forgotten. Even in such circumstances, many people appreciate the opportunity to talk to a staff member. Parents should be asked if they want to see their baby, and have time to decide. Some will want to see the baby but not hold it.

There may be a particular difficulty when one twin has died, when the parents need acknowledgement of their loss as well as support in caring for the surviving twin.

Although most parents are grateful for the sensitive support they have had from staff after perinatal death, the main criticism has been of staff who did not acknowledge their distress, or who avoided them.

difference?

with bereaved people emphasize the
of the lost person in helping the
is why so many writers advocate that
itact with their dead baby, and why
become usual practice. There is no
and hold their baby are upset by the
s who see and hold their babies are
so; those who chose not to see and
regretting it, and others feeling that
et al 1990–91, Phipps 1982).
e baby helps parents make sense of
ned (Cohen et al 1978), and LaRoche
igher in mothers who had not seen
that some parents who had not seen
that the baby had not really died, but

an *association* between not seeing and
ems. We do not know whether seeing
. It is possible that those parents who
asons are the same parents who do

nd to hold a funeral, even for infants
ition time of 24 weeks' gestation. As
he baby, those who do have a funeral
are usually glad they did so and some say that it helps to have a ritual to deal
with the death and that it helps family and friends realize that there really
was a baby. Some parents who do not have a funeral still feel afterwards that
they made the right decision, others regret that they decided against it (De
Frain et al 1990–91).

Some hospitals hold an annual service of remembrance for babies who died
before or soon after birth. This is usually well attended and appreciated both
by parents who have suffered a recent loss, and those whose loss took place
years earlier.

Mementoes

In most hospitals mementoes are prepared by midwives. However, one
moving paper describes the pathology department's careful preparation of a
memento pack, containing photographs of the baby, clothed and unclothed, a

lock of hair, a footprint and handprint, and the bracelet label from the baby's wrist (Khong et al 1993). This hospital stores the packs for some years. 80% of parents request it and the average time of request is 8 weeks after the loss. Some parents contact the hospital several years later to ask for the memento pack.

Giving information after the death

It is usual practice for the consultant who has cared for the mother and/or baby to meet with the parents about 6 weeks after the death when as much information is available as possible.

There are four tasks at this stage:

- to give information from the post-mortem examination
- to discuss what went wrong in the pregnancy
- to talk about the risks and possibly the timing of a future pregnancy
- to assess whether either of the parents needs further specialist support.

Parents may eagerly await the result of a post-mortem examination believing that it will tell them exactly what went wrong. As many as 40% of post-mortem examinations of stillborn infants do not show any definitive reason for the stillbirth (Kirk 1984), and parents are then left dissatisfied and with their questions unanswered. In the study of De Frain and colleagues (1990–91), half the parents felt that the post-mortem was helpful, and half did not.

Specialist counselling

Many obstetric departments now have specialist counselling services. Sessions with the counsellor may be routinely offered or referral may be at the request of the parents themselves, one of the hospital staff, or the general practitioner or health visitor.

Unless counselling is routine practice, or the decision is primarily the parents', they are likely to be referred because of very intense grief reactions, difficulty coping with day-to-day activities, or inappropriate use of alcohol or drugs to help them cope. A number of papers (Defey 1995, Hopper 1991, Leon 1990) describe the issues to be dealt with after perinatal loss. Defey's summary includes:

1. addressing the damage to self-esteem because of perceived failure as a parent
2. the recognition of ambivalent feelings to the partner and the dead child
3. building up mental representations of the lost child which are realistic and rewarding
4. working through feelings of guilt about the child's death, based upon real facts as well as anxieties related to unconscious feelings

5. discussing how to allow the siblings information about what really happened
6. planning how to incorporate the dead baby as part of the family
7. avoiding the projection of guilt inappropriately on to staff
8. if planning another pregnancy, distinguishing between the dead child and the next one.

Condon (1986) adds two further issues. First, anger towards the staff because of false optimism in the delivery room or insensitivity towards the parents may predispose parents to paranoid fantasies of negligence. Secondly, he recommends that a three-generation genogram is taken from the mother. Both family history and the woman's attitude to her own femininity, fertility, and capacity to be a mother, may emerge in looking at a family genogram. Condon argues that the mother may take the stillbirth to confirm that she is non-nurturing, and that the quality of her own mothering as a child may be involved in what this pregnancy means for her.

Referral to general practitioner or to psychiatric services

This should be considered when the mother has symptoms of post-traumatic stress disorder at any stage, or if either parent is misusing alcohol or drugs beyond the early weeks. If either parent shows severe biological symptoms of depression 6 months or more after the loss (sleep disturbance, appetite disturbance and weight loss), referral is appropriate. Medical referral may be helpful even in the early weeks if sleep is a problem, as any stress is compounded by not being able to sleep, and a simple intervention may be effective.

Other support services

Some parents find parents' groups useful. A list of relevant organizations is given at the end of the chapter.

Medical needs after perinatal loss

It is important that the mother's physical needs are not ignored because of her very rapid discharge from hospital and her exclusion from child health clinics where she would have had regular contact with health visitors and her general practitioner. Suppression of lactation, contraception or infertility problems, gynaecological complications and sexual difficulties are all relevant and should be anticipated (Oglethorpe 1989). The let-down of milk, first sexual intercourse and first period may be acutely distressing (Lockwood & Lewis 1980). Good communication between the hospital team and the primary care team is essential.

Social pressures

One of the problems parents confront when they return home is the difficulty with which other people deal with their loss. Parents often need to repeatedly go over what has happened in the weeks following the loss, and may find that friends are embarrassed or impatient for them to move on. This may lead to their withdrawing from some social contacts, often around the second month (Forrest et al 1982). Parents say that what helps is having people who will listen, and who will be patient and allow them to grieve for longer than the listener feels is necessary (De Frain et al 1990–91).

Some friends and acquaintances behave as though the dead child is replaceable, in sharp contrast to the parents' feelings about the baby (Helmrath & Steinitz 1978). When one twin has died, friends may assume that parents should be grateful for the survival of one baby and overlook the death of the other twin (Wilson et al 1982).

Parents are grateful to friends and family who remember that the loss was awful for them, and who do not avoid them but who write, phone or simply ask how they are getting on. Sensitive friends also realize that the parents sometimes need to be alone (De Frain et al 1990–91).

EFFECTS OF PERINATAL DEATH ON CAREGIVERS

Health professionals have to learn to tolerate painful feelings: anxiety or guilt about our failures, fear of blame, and sadness about the suffering we are in contact with. There seems to be a particular difficulty around perinatal loss.

Bourne (1968) discovered that compared to general practitioners whose patients had had a healthy delivery, many GPs whose patients had had a stillbirth either refused to respond to his enquiries about them, or claimed that they could remember nothing about the delivery. He concluded, 'the doctor whose patient has had a stillbirth does not want to know, he does not want to notice and he does not want to remember anything about it.'

Forrest et al (1982) found that 14 months after a perinatal death, 8% of GPs refused to allow researchers to contact patients for fear of upsetting them. When we planned a follow-up study of mothers who had had a stillbirth during their next pregnancy, several professionals warned us that they were unhappy about bringing the stillbirth into the mother's mind. However, as one mother said, 'I've been thinking of it all the time since I became pregnant. How could I not?' For many years doctors considered that mothers should forget as quickly as possible, yet mothers tell us is that it is 8 years before they are fully recovered (De Frain et al 1990–91), and many remember the pain 40 years later.

Parents sometimes complain that they are avoided after perinatal loss and possibly this is a peculiarly painful area for staff. We are not immune to our own conscious and unconscious anxieties and infant death seems to be a potent trigger for these. Perhaps we should simply remember that this is an especially tricky area, and that we may be unconsciously liable to forget or ignore our patients and their distress.

SUMMARY

Stillbirth and neonatal death occur at or after about 1% of all births. Grief after the baby's death is severe, and for parents the process of mourning lasts on average 2 or 3 years. Poor marital adjustment, poor social support and previous poor physical or mental health problems are associated with more severe symptoms of depression after the loss. Fathers' grief may be as intense as mothers'. Siblings may suffer psychological and physical symptoms related to their anxieties about the death. Most parents show reduction in painful feelings of grief in the first year, and in 'normal' resolution of mourning there should be evidence of improvement in symptoms after 6 months.

Counselling after loss may reduce the duration of feelings of severe depression. Psychiatric consultation is indicated if the symptoms are very long lasting or do not diminish in intensity after some months.

The next pregnancy is an anxious time. There is no conclusive evidence that the timing of the pregnancy makes a difference to the severity or duration of grief, but the area is poorly researched. There are reports that maternal anxiety about the next child may affect the child's development, but a lack of systematic investigation.

Clear guidelines about psychosocial management are an important part of good practice. However, staff should be sensitive to the needs of a particular couple and not insist on following guidelines against the wishes of the parents. Staff should also be aware that this is a painful area for themselves, and training should include discussion of personal feelings which may interfere with good practice.

Key points for caregivers

- Parents should have clear information about what is happening when a problem arises during pregnancy or delivery, or soon after birth
- When a baby has died, parents need time together. They should have a choice about whether they want to see and hold the baby.
- Mementoes are requested by most parents and should be routinely prepared and kept for several years. They should be of good quality and not hastily put together to satisfy procedural practice.
- The consultant should see the parents a month or two after the birth to explain what went wrong and to discuss the post-mortem findings, to assess the parents' need for further support, and to answer questions about further pregnancy.
- If counselling is offered, there are a number of areas which the counsellor should expect to cover (see above).
- Parents should be warned that recovery is usually slow, and that it may be several months before they feel noticeably better.

Key points for caregivers *(Cont'd)*

- Good communication between hospital and primary care is essential for continuing support and management of the puerperium.
- Referral for psychiatric consultation should be considered if a parent shows continuing severe symptoms of depression 6 months after loss, or if there is concern about a parent's safety before that time. Severe alcohol or drug abuse or symptoms of post-traumatic stress disorder are indications for immediate referral.
- Perinatal loss is a difficult area for professional staff, and awareness of this should be part of the training of midwives, doctors and others who work with these parents.

REFERENCES

Akhtar S, Thomson J A 1982 Overview: narcissistic personality disorder. American Journal of Psychiatry 139: 12–20

Benfield D G, Lieb S A, Vollman J H 1978 Grief response of parents to neonatal death. Pediatrics 62: 171–177

Bourne S 1968 The psychological effects of stillbirths on women and their doctors. Journal of the Royal College of General Practice 16: 103–112

Bourne S, Lewis E 1992 Psychological aspects of stillbirth and neonatal death: an annotated bibliography. Tavistock Clinic, Weavers Press Publishing, London

Bowlby J 1961 Processes of mourning. International Journal of Psychoanalysis 42: 317–340

Bowlby J 1980 Attachment and loss, vol. 3. Loss: sadness and depression. Hogarth Press, London

Cain A C, Cain B S 1964 On replacing a child. Journal of the American Academy of Child Psychiatry 3: 443–455

Cain A C, Fast I, Erikson M, Vaughn R A 1964 Children's disturbed reactions to their mother's miscarriage. Psychosomatic Medicine 26: 58–66

Cohen L, Zikha S, Middleton J, O'Donohue N 1978 Perinatal mortality: assisting parental affirmation. American Journal of Orthopsychiatry 48: 727–731

Condon J T 1986 Management of established pathological grief reaction after stillbirth. American Journal of Psychiatry 143: 987–992

Cullberg J 1972 Mental reactions of women to perinatal death. In: Morris N (ed) Proceedings of the Third International Congress of Psychosomatic Medicine in Obstetrics and Gynaecology. Basel, Karger, pp 326–329

Davidson G W 1977 Death of the wished-for child: a case study. Death Education 1: 265–275

Davis D L, Stewart M, Harmon R J 1989 Postponing pregnancy after perinatal death: perspectives on doctors' advice. Journal of the Academy of Child and Adolescent Psychiatry 28: 481–487

De Frain J, Martens L, Stork J, Stork W 1990–91 The psychological effects of stillbirth on surviving family members. Omega 22(2): 81–108

Defey D 1995 Helping health care staff deal with perinatal loss. Infant Mental Health Journal 16(2): 102–111

Drotar D, Irving N 1979 Disturbed maternal bereavement following infant death. Child Care, Health and Development 5: 239–247

Field T, Morrow C, Healy B, Foster T, Adlestein D, Goldstein S 1991 Mothers with zero Beck depression scores act more 'depressed' with their infants. Development and Psychopathology 3: 253–262

Forrest G C, Standish E, Baum J D 1982 Support after perinatal death: a study of support and counselling after perinatal bereavement. British Medical Journal 285: 1475–1479

Giles P 1970 Reaction of women to perinatal death. Australian and New Zealand Journal of Obstetrics and Gynaecology 10: 207–210

Gilson G J 1976 Care of the family who has lost a newborn. Postgraduate Medicine 60: 67–70

Goldberg S, Perrotta M, Minde K K, Carter C 1986 Maternal behaviour and attachment in low-birth-weight twins and singletons. Child Development 57: 34–46

Green M, Solnit A J 1964 Reactions to the threatened loss of a child. Pediatrics 34: 58–66

Harmon R J, Glicken A D, Siegel R E 1984 Neonatal loss in the intensive care nursery: effects of maternal grieving and a program for intervention. Journal of the American Academy of Child Psychiatry 23: 68–71

Helmrath T A, Steinitz E 1978 Death of an infant: parental grieving and the failure of social support. Journal of Family Process 6: 785–790

Hopper E 1991 Shattered dreams. Nursing Standard 6(4): 20–21

Jensen S J, Zahourek R 1972 Depression in mothers who have lost a newborn. Rocky Mountain Medical Journal 71: 61–63

Jolly H 1976 Family reactions to child bereavement. Proceedings of the Royal Society of Medicine 69: 835–837

Kennell J H, Slyter H, Klaus M 1970 The mourning response of parents to the death of a newborn infant. New England Journal of Medicine 283(7): 344–348

Khong T Y, Hill F, Chambers H M, Staples A, Harry C 1993 Acceptance of mementoes of fetal and perinatal loss in a South Australian population. Australian and New Zealand Journal of Obstetrics and Gynaecology 33(4): 392–394

Kirk E P 1984 Psychological effects and management of perinatal loss. American Journal of Obstetrics and Gynaecology 149: 46–51

Kirkley Best E, VanDevere C 1986 The hidden family grief: an overview of grief in the family following perinatal death. International Journal of Family Psychiatry 7(4): 419–437

Kubler-Ross E 1970 On death and dying. Macmillan, New York

Lake M, Knuppel R, Murphy J, Johnson T 1983 The role of a grief support team following stillbirth. American Journal of Obstetrics and Gynaecology 146: 877–881

LaRoche C, Lalinec-Michaud M, Engelsmann F, Fuller N, Copp M, McQuade-Soldatos L, Azima R 1984 Grief reactions to perinatal death: a follow up study. Canadian Journal of Psychiatry 29: 14–19

Lasker J N, Toedter L J 1991 Acute versus chronic grief: the case of pregnancy loss. American Journal of Orthopsychiatry 61(4): 510–522

Leon I 1990 When a baby dies: psychotherapy for pregnancy and newborn death. Yale University Press, New Haven, Connecticut

Leon I 1992 Choreographing loss on the obstetric unit. American Journal of Orthopsychiatry 62: 7–8

Lewis E 1976 The management of stillbirth: coping with an unreality. Lancet 2: 619–620

Lewis E 1979 Mourning by the family after stillbirth or neonatal death. Archives of Disease in Childhood 54: 303–306

Lewis E, Page A 1978 Failure to mourn a stillbirth: an overlooked catastrophe. British Journal of Medical Psychology 51: 237–241

Lindemann E 1944 The symptomatology and management of acute grief. American Journal of Psychiatry 101: 141–149

Lockwood S, Lewis I C 1980 Management of grieving after stillbirth. Medical Journal of Australia 2: 308–311

Mammen O K 1995 Women's reaction to perinatal loss in India: an exploratory, descriptive study. Infant Mental Health Journal 16(2): 94–101

Mandell F, McAnulty E H, Carlson A 1983 Unexpected death of an infant sibling. Pediatrics 72(5): 652–657

Mekosh-Rosenbaum V, Lasker J N 1995 Effects of pregnancy outcome on marital satisfaction: a longitudinal study of birth and loss. Infant Mental Health Journal 16(2): 127–143

Nicol M T, Tompkins J R, Campbell N A, Syme G J 1986 Maternal grieving response after perinatal death. Medical Journal of Australia 144: 287–289

Oglethorpe R J L 1989 Parenting after perinatal bereavement: a review of the literature. Journal of Reproductive and Infant Psychology 7: 227–244

Office of Population Censuses and Surveys 1995 May OPCS monitor. HMSO, London, p 5

Osterweis M, Solomon F, Green M (eds) 1987 Bereavement: reactions, consequences and care. National Academic Press, Washington DC

Parkes C M 1965 Bereavement and mental illness, Part III. A classification of bereavement reactions. British Journal of Medical Psychology 38: 13–26

Peppers L G, Knapp R J 1980 Maternal reactions to involuntary fetal-infant death. Psychiatry 43(2): 155–159

Phipps S 1982 Mourning response and intervention in stillbirth: an alternative genetic counselling approach. Social Biology 28(1–2): 1–13

Phipps S 1985 The subsequent pregnancy after stillbirth: anticipatory parenthood in the face of uncertainty. International Journal of Psychiatric Medicine 15: 243–264

Rowe J, Clyman R, Green C 1978 Follow-up of families who experience a perinatal death. Pediatrics 62(2): 66–170

Rubin J D, Ferencz C 1985 Subsequent pregnancy in mothers of infants with congenital heart disease. Pediatrics 76: 371–374

Stillbirth and Neonatal Death Society (SANDS) 1991 Miscarriage, stillbirth and neonatal death: guidelines for professionals. SANDS, London

Theut S K, Pederson F A, Zaslow M J, Rabinovich B A 1988 Pregnancy subsequent to perinatal loss: parental anxiety and depression. Journal of the Academy of Child and Adolescent Psychiatry 27: 289–292

Toedter L J, Lasker J N, Alhadeff J M 1988 The perinatal grief scale: development and initial validation. American Journal of Orthopsychiatry 58: 435–449

Tooley K 1975 The choice of surviving sibling as 'scapegoat' in some cases of maternal bereavement: a case report. Journal of Child Psychology and Psychiatry 16: 331–339

Tudehope D I, Iredell J, Rodgers D, Gunn A 1986 Neonatal death: grieving families. Medical Journal of Australia 144: 290–292

Vance J C, Najman J M, Boyle F M 1994 Alcohol and drug usage in parents soon after stillbirth, neonatal death or SIDS. Journal of Paediatrics and Child Health 30: 269–272

Vogel H P, Knox E G 1975 Reproductive patterns after stillbirth and early infant death. Journal of Biosocial Science 7: 103–111

Wilson A L, Fenton L J, Stevens D C 1982 The death of a newborn twin: an analysis of parental bereavement. Pediatrics 70(4): 587–591

Wolff J R, Nielson P E, Schiller P 1970 The emotional reaction to a stillbirth. American Journal of Obstetrics and Gynecology 108: 73–77

Zeanah C 1989 Adaptation following perinatal loss: a critical review. Journal of the American Academy of Child and Adolescent Psychiatry 28(3): 467–480

Zeanah C, Danis B, Hirshberg L, Dietz L 1995 Initial adaptation in mothers and fathers following perinatal loss. Infant Mental Health Journal 16(2): 80–93

FURTHER READING AND VIEWING

Bourne S, Lewis E 1992 Psychological aspects of stillbirth and neonatal death: an annotated bibliography. Tavistock Clinic, Weavers Press Publishing, London

Leon I 1990 When a baby dies: psychotherapy for pregnancy and newborn death. Yale University Press, New Haven, Connecticut

Hopper E, Cleverly D Not too small to mourn: a video of management of perinatal loss. Available from D. Cleverly, Academic Services, St. George's Hospital Medical School, Cranmer Terrace, London SW17 ORE

Further reading on termination of pregnancy due to foetal abnormality

Black R 1989 A 1 month and 6 month follow up of prenatal diagnosis patients who lost pregnancies. Prenatal Diagnosis 9: 795–804

Leon I G 1995 Pregnancy termination due to fetal anomaly: clinical considerations. Infant Mental Health Journal 16(2): 112–126

Niswander K, Patterson R 1967 Psychological reactions to therapeutic abortion. Obstetrics and Gynaecology 29: 702–706

White-van Mourik M, Connor J, Ferguson-Smith M 1992 The psychosocial sequelae of a second trimester termination for fetal abnormality. Prenatal Diagnosis 12: 189–204

Zeanah C, Dailey J, Rosenblatt M, Saller D 1993 Do women grieve after terminating pregnancies because of fetal abnormalities? A controlled investigation. Obstetrics and Gynaecology 82: 270–275

9

Special care babies and their carers: experiences, needs and relationships

Anne McFadyen

INTRODUCTION

The birth of any child acts as a stressor on the family system, but if the baby arrives prematurely, or is sick or damaged in some way, this stress is felt acutely. Admission of the baby to a special care baby unit has appropriately been referred to as 'the crisis of neonatal intensive care' (Affleck et al 1990).

In this chapter, I want to consider the experiences, needs and relationships of those involved in this crisis. My clinical experience as a mental health professional who has consulted to several neonatal units, and my research experience in this area inform this account. My illustrations of particular themes come directly from mothers' own narratives of their experience.

Each infant's experience is unique, as is each family's. Nonetheless, I believe it is possible, by drawing attention to particular experiences, to highlight some common needs which may have implications for practice. Similarly, a midwife's or other professional's experience of caring for each of her charges will feel both unique *and* familiar. Recognizing the complexity of each child's situation may be a critical key to the facilitation of both growth and the development of relationships.

In the neonatal intensive care unit, the baby is at the centre of a complex system of relationships, involving both family members and professionals. Institutional, cultural and family beliefs about prematurity, illness and disability, and infant care inform the actions of both parents and staff, but may do so in different ways. The 'fit' between parents' and professionals' understanding of what is going on and their beliefs is of paramount importance, particularly when there are significant cultural differences. Both the development of the infant and of the infant's relationships, most importantly the infant–mother relationship, may be compromised if differences or conflicts are not addressed. This relationship is vulnerable, not only because of the baby's fragility but also because of its position, at the interface between the hospital and the family system. However, it is not only the baby's context which is important but also the context of neonatal intensive care in general.

THE CONTEXT

The care of premature and sick infants has been the subject of the writings of physicians and philosophers for many centuries (Brimblecombe 1983). Technological advances have meant that babies previously regarded as non-viable are being offered life support and care. Inevitably, the ethical dilemmas of decisions about whether to support the lives of critically ill infants, often of necessity inflicting painful and stressful procedures upon them, have become increasingly complex and difficult.

More recently, there have also been controversial advances in infertility treatment and prenatal testing. While on the one hand, the possibility of choosing not to have a baby with chromosomal abnormalities or other congenital abnormalities may have led to the birth of fewer such babies, on the other, the provision of fertility treatments has led to the sometimes early birth of 'precious' singleton children, and has also contributed to an increased number of multiple births, often premature. The families of such infants will often have endured years of treatment and uncertainty, and may well have suffered previous disappointments as well as real losses.

The population of neonatal intensive care units has changed in other ways too. The impact of changes in our society manifests itself in the shape of other infants who need special care. Babies born to drug-addicted mothers, for example, will present a particular challenge as they are weaned from potentially neurologically damaging and psychotropic drugs. Their social context may be particularly hard for staff to bear, and the importance of networking with child protection and care professionals from outside the hospital will be paramount. Our multicultural society presents some families with specific problems. Many women find themselves having to abandon their traditional ways of doing things in the face of a lack of recognition of their belief systems and also a lack of family support, felt particularly acutely by refugees. Feelings of abandonment often make it very difficult for them to maintain their resilience in the face of adversity, and this may impact on their capacity to relate to both their infants and the staff who care for them.

The type of care offered in contemporary units is radically different from that given earlier this century, and is perhaps a reflection of society's changing attitude to children generally, and also our increased understanding of psychological development. In the early neonatal units, the risk of infection was seen as an important determinant of visiting practices, and parents were generally denied direct access to their infants. The work of John Bowlby and his colleagues, the Robertsons, made a significant contribution to the understanding of early relationships (Bowlby 1951), and also had a direct impact on hospital policies, which in the 1960s started to allow open access to parents of children in hospital. Others, such as Klaus & Kennell (1975), drew attention to the importance of bonding early in the puerperium. While their ideas about this having to take place at a critical time have been challenged, the important role of early relationships for later mental health has been universally accepted.

These ideas are reflected in the philosophy of care in most units today, where the service is designed first and foremost to meet the needs of the infants, and where partnership with parents refers to a recognition that parents are the primary carers and should be supported by staff in that role. The nature of this support varies in accordance with the particular situation presented by each infant and family. The birth of an infant with a congenital malformation or obvious early disability presents a complex challenge for carers (Klaus & Kennell 1983). Likewise, when a baby is born prematurely, it is not only the infant but also the parents who require the care of professionals.

THE EXPERIENCES OF INFANTS AND THEIR CARERS
The infant

The population of any special care baby unit will include infants of different gestation with different problems. Some have relatively minor problems and require observation for 1 or 2 days only. Others may have congenital abnormalities requiring surgical intervention and life support. The majority of the longer-stay population, however, will be infants of less than 32 weeks' gestation, with some being born as early as 23 weeks and requiring to stay in the unit for several months if they survive. A smaller number of less premature but growth-retarded infants will also require 'special care'.

Although our understanding of the experiences and needs of premature babies is becoming increasingly sophisticated, we are still faced with the dilemma of knowing that infants are supposed to be born at around 40 weeks' gestation and therefore having no natural source of knowledge about those born too soon. What should we expect of them? How much do they perceive of what is going on around them? We cannot really know the answers to these questions, especially as they relate to very low birth weight (VLBW) babies, that is those weighing less than 1500 grams. There is no *right* way to care for them. However, it is important to try to think about what these babies experience in order to best support their emotional and psychological, as well as their physical development.

The study of the fetus has contributed much to our understanding. The existence of prenatal mental functioning has been supported by the research of MacFarlane (1977), for example, who has demonstrated the response to different sorts of stimulation such as light, sound and vibration. In utero, the fetus demonstrates these 'evoked' responses, in addition to more primitive reflex movements, from very early on, and later these take on a more purposive character including self-stimulation and possibly also self-soothing. The baby's development, and in particular its neurological maturation, is thought to depend on both the development of appropriate structures and their use or stimulation (Graves 1989). In the ordinary course of events, crucial changes in brain growth and maturation occur in the last few weeks of gestation. In premature babies these will occur postnatally provided that adequate respiratory, circulatory and nutritional support is present. Ideally this should be accompanied by an appropriate 'functional' expectation too, for if the baby's brain is not stimulated by a range of sensory experiences to which it can respond, this maturational process may be less than optimal.

Piontelli's observational studies of babies (1992), carried out initially in utero via ultrasound, appear to demonstrate both the existence of some sort of individuality from around the end of the first trimester and continuities in personality or temperament between pre- and postnatal life. They support the idea that infants do have the capacity to perceive and respond to their environment well before 40 weeks' gestation. This clearly has implications for our understanding of the experiences of babies born before this.

As adults, we rely on nonverbal as well as verbal communication to both convey and infer meaning. This nonverbal communication can take the form of gesture or at a more basic level observed physiological changes, for example in skin colour or respiration rate. The acknowledgement of this level of communication lends itself well to our attempts to understand the world of any baby, and in particular that of the premature baby. Gorski (1983) is among those who support the idea that even very premature babies experience the world around them and communicate that experience to their carers.

'High-risk prematurely born infants exhibit behavioral responses that represent signals for neurophysiologic stability, disorganization or distress. These cues may precede less subtle, more costly physiologic crises that caregivers commonly recognize as calls for caregiver reaction.' (Gorski 1983, p. 258). These behavioural cues include withdrawal, sometimes to the extent of falling asleep, grimacing, and crying. At a cruder level, continuously monitored vital signs may also be thought of as a communication. Increased heart rate, altered skin tone and decreased oxygen tension are all indications that the baby is stressed (Field 1990).

Premature babies are neurologically less mature than their term counterparts, and may not yet have developed rooting or sucking reflexes. Until the latter appear these infants will have difficulties feeding without compromising their precarious cardiopulmonary functioning. Later, feeding may continue to be difficult for some babies who cannot tolerate too much contact or stimulation. Most appear jittery and exhibit many startles, shudders and involuntary movements early on (Newman 1981). Their spontaneous movements are often difficult to interpret, particularly as they are constrained by splints, tubes and wires. However, some of their movements do seem purposeful. Newman (1981), for example, has described 'range-finding' activity, 'intentional action aimed at maximizing contact with hard surfaces' and thought to help the infant to define its boundaries. Similarly, non-nutritive sucking 'probably plays a major role in safeguarding continuity of salient stimuli from intrauterine to extrauterine experiences' (Freud 1989, p. 494). These actions seem to help the infant to hold itself together emotionally and can be seen as self-regulatory or protective.

Premature babies do seem to need to be held emotionally in some way. They find it less easy to shut out unwanted stimuli than older more mature infants and seem to be 'at the mercy of environmental stimuli of all kind' (Brazelton & Cramer 1991, p. 67). Their inability to habituate to bright light and noise is related to their less mature sleep patterns, which have less well-defined cycles and fewer periods of deep sleep, and also contributes to the fact that they are so readily awakened. The end result is that they have far less 'deep sleep' than ordinary babies, thus missing out on its restorative function. When premature babies are handled and stimulated, many of them appear to try to withdraw, but often do not manage this. They seem to have only a limited ability to control their state (Patteson & Barnard 1990), and when they have exhausted this, catastrophic physiological reactions may follow.

All of this suggests that these babies must be doubly disadvantaged by life in a contemporary intensive care unit. Not only are they much less able than more mature babies to regulate their internal environments, but they are also disadvantaged by being in a very demanding external environment. This milieu will be familiar to many readers – there are usually several nurseries, often referred to as 'hot' rooms and 'cool' rooms or 'growing' rooms; the 'cool' rooms are hot and the 'hot' rooms are very hot. These rooms are often bright, lit with strong, raw lighting; and they seem stuffy and airless, even though they are ventilated. There is usually lots of noise: steady beep-beep noises, erratic buzzing alarm noises that pierce through the other noise, the noise of talking amongst staff, the noise of chinking and clanking connected to procedures. In the background there may be music, usually radio pop. A number of authors have commented on how lost and remote babies often seem in this environment (Richards 1979, Szur 1981), while others have commented on the noise. Newman (1981) found a noise level ranging from 60 to 65 decibels inside the cots of preterm babies, and noted that, especially during the first week, they were continually aroused and startled by apparently random sounds. She speculated that this might cause unnecessary and clinically significant energy expenditure.

These infants are also subjected to a number of invasive and painful procedures as well as to routine caregiving activities such as cleaning and nappy changes. Jones (1982), for example, found that high-risk premature babies received direct contact from staff for 6.1 hours per day. This was usually accompanied by personal attention, but strikingly, 'preferred' infants received more nurturing and less impersonal care than other infants. My own observations suggest that, at times, there may be poor coordination of activities, so that babies have to endure quite intensive periods when different professionals interact with them.

The parents

In one sense, the parents' relationship with their child begins long before conception. With the discovery of pregnancy comes a flood of feelings and expectations about the birth, the baby, and the future life of the family. The baby's arrival may be anticipated with joy, or with anxiety and dread, but in most cases the news will be met with a mixture of feelings. The parents' own childhood and early relationships, life experience and satisfaction in their present situation will influence their reactions to the pregnancy and to the actual birth of the child. Brazelton & Cramer (1991) have described this as the 'prehistory of attachment'.

While the birth of any child has the potential to stir up unresolved feelings from the parent's own early life, the birth of a premature or damaged baby often does this in a much more dramatic way. The baby's fragility and vulnerability are potent catalysts which may trigger feelings of deprivation – the baby's dependency reminding the adults of their own wish to be looked after. While this is true in part for many parents, for some the reality of their social situation will mean that this is felt even more acutely. A disproportionate number of young women from disadvantaged backgrounds have premature or small-for-dates babies. Their wish to have a baby may have been related to their own unmet emotional needs and real experience of deprivation, and their hopes of having a satisfying and loving relationship with that baby may, in these circumstances, fail to be fulfilled.

As family relationships are thrown into sharp relief (as they are with the birth of any child), the stress of the crisis and the amount of time parents are forced to spend enduring uncertainty often precipitate a psychological revisiting of the past. In some cases, this can be a comfort and a source of support, but often this revisiting is distressing, especially when the parents are seeking confirmation from their own life that they have done something to deserve what has happened. It is not uncommon in the special care situation for parents, mothers in particular, to seek to understand their current experience and give it meaning. Indeed, this is probably one of the ways they have of surviving the crisis. Affleck et al (1990) have clearly demonstrated that the attribution of meaning to this stressful event is associated with better mental health and coping for most mothers. However, this meaning of necessity is based on their experience and belief systems, and in cases where they believe that they have failed, their explanation may be framed in terms of their dissatisfaction with their own lives. Both the stress of the current crisis and the parents' perceptions of the importance of their past experiences inform their way of coping. The relationship between these different influences is often complex and difficult for outsiders to make sense of.

Parents' past or current relationships with their own parents, or other people in authority, may be re-enacted with staff. Nurses and midwives, in particular, may be seen as critical or judgmental no matter how helpful they are trying to be. This seems to be linked in many cases to the mother's relationship with her own mother, and is fuelled by doubts about her own capacity to look after her baby well enough. For staff the experience of being avoided, or criticized may be perplexing. If they can begin to understand how vulnerable a parent might feel in this situation, they can often put up with hostility or rejection of their efforts to help. Recognizing that they are being responded to as if they were someone else may be helpful (see Case study 9.1).

At another level, higher-order beliefs may affect the way in which the crisis is managed. An example of this is when an overriding religious belief informs the parent's interpretation of events but is difficult for others to understand (Case study 9.2).

It is also important to acknowledge the impact of the most recent trauma, that of the birth. Elsewhere in this book (Ch. 7) Suzanne Lyons has discussed the possibility that some women may be suffering from post-traumatic stress disorder after the birth of their child. Women who have given birth prematurely may well fall into this category. Some of them will have been quite unprepared for the timing of the birth, while others will have been in a

---

Case study 9.1 Ms M

Ms M had had a difficult early life, and described her mother as critical and self-absorbed. She seemed to constantly reaffirm Ms M's own doubts about her capacity to manage. Her daughter's birth at 27 weeks was a sudden and traumatic event. Ms M found it difficult to relate to the fragile creature in the incubator, and was afraid that she would somehow damage her. When nurses tried to help her to care for the baby she felt that they were asking too much. She felt that she did not know what to do and would never get it right. Very quickly she came to perceive the staff as judgmental and critical of her. She tried to avoid them, often visiting at staff handover times, or sneaking out of the unit when they weren't looking. Interestingly, the staff sensed her hostility and also felt criticized by her. They started commenting on how little she did for the baby and how uncooperative she was. Locked into a cycle of mistrust, the situation became almost intolerable, with the baby in the middle receiving less and less attention from either party. For Ms M, her unworthiness and failure was confirmed by the staff's behaviour and she was left feeling abandoned and uncared for, as well as criticized. When some of the nurses were able to think about how Ms M's past experience and her relationship with her own mother influenced her behaviour on the unit, they were able to put aside their judgmental stance and renew their efforts to support her.

Case study 9.2 Mrs S

Mrs S was a refugee from a war-torn African country. Only some of her family had escaped to this country. Her baby was born at 24 weeks after 5 weeks of bleeding. Her sense of herself as helpless seemed to have been confirmed by recent events. She visited infrequently, and made little attempt to talk to or touch her baby. This behaviour distressed the nurses who were caring for the infant and many of them found it difficult to relate to her. The baby was not given a name for some time, and again this was difficult for them to understand. In due course it was discovered that Mrs S had a strong religious belief – she believed that God decided what would happen, no matter what the doctors, nurses or she herself did to try to help the baby, God would decide whether he lived or died. She said 'If the baby's destined to be alive, he will be whether I come to see him or not. Really, God takes care of little babies. He'll decide – no one has the power to heal but God.' Her strong religious beliefs stemmed from childhood, but had probably been reinforced by her real persecution in her country of origin, where the only way of making sense of that awful experience may have been to see it as God's will. She had not only been helpless then but was helpless now. However, she did have a way of making sense of things which probably protected her in some way. Her behaviour seemed strange to most of the staff but once they were aware of her beliefs they were able to respect them. This included the practice of not naming the infant until the eighth day which was the usual practice in her culture.

---

state of expectancy for weeks, or possibly since the beginning of the pregnancy if there is a past history of miscarriage or neonatal death. These women may have had a number of bleeds and been hospitalized and given drugs to try to help them to keep the pregnancy going a little longer until their infant is viable. In this situation, many will have little expectation that a live baby will be born at the end of this period. The final series of events surrounding a complicated birth often takes place at an alarming rate, with the consequence that communication may not always be as clear as it should be. Parents are often left feeling in the dark about the prognosis for both baby and mother. Many women fear that they will die, and while their partners may be more available for medical staff to talk with, they too may believe that the mother is in a life-threatening situation. The impact of all of this on how these parents then behave on the Special Care Baby Unit will sometimes be obvious. Some parents are able to share their feelings and experience, but many will be too shocked to do this or may never have been able to confide in others or seek emotional support. These women in particular may find it difficult to relate to either their baby or the staff. They may be preoccupied with memories of the birth, feelings of loss and a sense of failure. In this state, they may be sharply confronted with quite overwhelming feelings each time they visit their baby. These feelings are both about the baby and in identification with, or on behalf of, the baby. Their perception of the infant as helpless and bewildered may resonate with their own feelings of helplessness, anxiety and confusion making it difficult for them to begin to get to know their baby.

For the family, the experience of having to cope with this life-threatening event comes at a point in the family life cycle when it is least expected. In the more ordinary course of events it is a time when parents have left their own families of origin to form new relationships and create their own families. It is a creative phase, and the illness, disability or death of a child contrasts sharply with the anticipated celebration of new life. Friends and relatives often do not know what to do when a baby is born damaged or disabled, and this adds to the parents' sense of isolation. There are often few flowers or cards, and those which do arrive may not quite address the parent's confusion about what to feel. In this situation, an obvious disability or deformity may add to the parents' difficulties in getting to know their baby.

What are the implications of our growing understanding of the experiences of babies and their parents?

A range of interventions addressing the various needs of infants and parents have been developed to promote the growth, and cognitive and emotional development of premature infants and to support their developing relationships with their parents. These have been reviewed by a number of authors (e.g. McFadyen 1994, Wolke 1991). *Premature Infants and Their Families: Developmental Interventions* specifically addresses intervention in the special care baby unit (Wyly 1995). Interventions can take place at a number of levels, but will always be in the context of the technological advances in medical care which have led to more accurate assessment and prediction of outcome, and increasingly sophisticated treatment of potentially damaging conditions.

'Developmental support' is a term which has come to refer specifically to interventions which promote the development of particular aspects of the baby's sensory and motor functioning. An awareness of the needs of the developing nervous system initially led to an indiscriminate use of sensory stimulation, but this has now been replaced with a sensitivity to the uniqueness of each infant's experience. Wyly's (1995) guidelines are helpful. The first step is to tune in to where the baby is; staff need to learn to recognize the signs of stress in infants, who may only communicate via their physiological state. The second step is to consider the advantages and disadvantages of active intervention; in some cases it may be appropriate to leave the infants to develop their own capacity to self-regulate initially. If interventions either to promote specific functions or to help self-regulation are thought to be necessary, they must be designed with care to meet the infant's precise needs. One of the most important interventions early in the life of the preterm infant may be to help the parents to understand their baby's signals. Many will feel guilty because they are afraid to touch or hold their infant, yet their gut feeling that they may cause some damage may be accurate. Many infants indicate that they do not wish to be touched. They may withdraw into sleep or turn away, or more alarmingly may become physiologically compromised, in response to medical intervention or attempts to engage or stimulate them.

Nonetheless, many developmental interventions used in the correct way can be helpful. These range from simply turning down the lights while infants are sleeping, to the more elaborate use of particular visual patterns to promote their neurological development. Research in this area has also addressed the impact of caregiving and invasive, often painful, procedures and has clearly demonstrated that a reduction in handling and attention to the number and timing of procedures can lead to reduced episodes of hypoxaemia and increased growth in VLBW infants. Other supplementary interventions such as the use of dummies or pacifiers to encourage non-nutritive sucking also help infants to regulate their state at times of stress (Field 1990).

Assessment itself can be useful in helping parents to know how to relate to their infants and to feel pride in their achievements. The Neonatal Behavioral Assessment Scale (Brazelton 1984) is used to facilitate parents' understanding of their particular baby, as well as to identify neonates whose behaviour might make them difficult to handle (Brazelton & Cramer 1991). Preconceived ideas about premature babies' functioning, 'the prematurity stereotype' (Stern & Karraker 1992), can be gently challenged in this situation.

Other attempts to support the developing parent–infant relationship have been shown to be of benefit in the long term. A wide range of interventions, from the purely educative to the broadly supportive, may be helpful. Reviewing these, Patteson & Barnard (1990) interestingly concluded that 'the content of the intervention seemed less important than the interaction involved and the development of a relationship between parents and the intervener' (1990, p. 52). Affleck et al (1990), in their large study of a consultation model of support, also found that this relationship was important. Further, their findings highlighted the need for intervention to be tailored to mothers' specific needs, as the provision of high levels of support seemed to threaten rather than improve the adaptation of those who were less distressed.

The feeding of very premature babies is a complex issue. Early on their reflexes are poorly developed, they are unable to suck or swallow and have to be fed by nasogastric or orogastric tube. The mother is deprived of the intimacy of the feeding relationship, and despite great encouragement in most centres it is often only a minority who manage to establish breast-feeding. A specific intervention which has been shown to improve the quality of the early relationship and promote breast-feeding is 'Kangaroo care' (Anderson 1989). Babies are held in skin-to-skin contact with their mother, and sometimes their father, for differing periods of time each day depending on their needs. This contact has been linked to increased oxygenation and thermoregulation in the baby, as well as improved lactation and satisfaction in the mother (Wyly 1995).

Many special care baby units have mental health professionals and social workers as part of their staff group. Child psychotherapists, psychiatrists and psychologists can provide more intensive therapeutic support in cases where there are particular concerns about parental coping or the developing relationship. Often they will also take a more general overview helping staff to identify concerns. A psychosocial ward round provides an opportunity for all staff to discuss various aspects of the care of the babies and their families. This includes consideration of feeding which may be addressed by a feeding adviser, who can give more time to mothers having difficulty. Often a liaison health visitor will join these meetings providing a critical link to the support system outside the hospital.

The presence of mental health professionals on the unit can be both worrying and reassuring for parents. Some may fear that the offer of support signifies a belief that they are mentally ill, and it is important that the preventive aspects of the work are explained. These professionals can provide help in a number of ways. By showing a genuine interest in the baby, they can often help a parent to identify the child's strengths and temperamental characteristics, establishing the infant's identity as a unique human being. The act of observing infants is in itself an intervention as it often gives the parent permission to study the baby and wonder about what he or she is actually experiencing. Getting in touch in this way is a very important step in the development of the relationship.

Similarly, by listening to the story of the pregnancy, the birth and the baby's history to date, they offer parents an opportunity to talk about and make sense of their experience, and to acknowledge their fears and anxieties. Of course, nurses and midwives also have a key role in this area. Their increasing awareness of the importance of 'debriefing' has led to the incorporation of this kind of work into their everyday practice. However, staff on the neonatal unit may not always be able to give the time, and in some cases the more specialist approach which is needed, to this task in the same way as trained mental health workers. Parents' groups can also provide an opportunity for the sharing of experience, and this may lead to practical suggestions about particular difficulties as well as the giving and taking of emotional support. Including fathers in these initiatives is particularly important as they often have little chance to share their feelings with other parents, and in particular other men.

Staff experiences and needs

The task of caring for very premature or damaged infants is emotionally taxing. Not only do staff have to focus on keeping these infants alive, if possible minimizing future disability by providing an optimal physiological environment, they also have to care for their families in an emotionally sensitive way which will facilitate the development of their intimate relationships. They are required to be at ease with increasingly sophisticated and highly technological methods of care *and* to be warm and empathic in their style of relating. These two functions are often difficult to perform simultaneously, and many staff experience a subjective sense of conflict about their role. The support they receive from their fellow professionals and from parents will affect their sense of self-worth, and may counteract some of the symptoms of stress experienced in such a demanding work environment.

As neonatal units provide care for younger and smaller preterm babies, staff have to face increasingly complex ethical dilemmas about whether to support the lives of these babies. Senior staff are often actively involved in the decision-making about the care of particular infants, and this may help them to manage their feelings about carrying out invasive and painful procedures on their helpless charges. More junior staff, however, may be afforded little opportunity to air their distress, or may hold on to their difficult feelings for fear of being seen as not coping. This perception may be reinforced by the awareness that ethical debates often focus on the child's suffering and potential future disability, or the parents' distress, rather than the emotional needs of staff in the front line. Lee et al (1991) asked parents, paediatricians and nurses whether they thought that active treatment should be offered to potentially severely disabled VLBW infants. Nurses were most opposed to active intervention, a finding which the authors related to the nurses' lack of later contact with the children. It is equally important to remember, I think, that nurses will have been most in touch with the infants' suffering early on.

Attention has been drawn to the conflicts and anxieties borne by staff working in neonatal intensive care (Bender 1981). This has been related not only to the demands placed on them by the infants, but also the fact that they often have to cope with the emotional responses of parents to their situation. Although aware of parents' feelings of being traumatized, professional caregivers may still find it hard to bear their hostility and criticism. The feeling of not being valued may manifest itself in low morale, absenteeism and 'burnout' (Oehler et al 1991). Preventive interventions include the promotion of an atmosphere where tensions and conflicts can be discussed, as well as practical measures to ensure, for example, that staff are not working long hours without relief, or are not left unsupported when parents are expressing their anger or hostility. Staff support groups work well in some centres, but in others more educative interventions geared to help staff to understand the psychological processes involved in this life-or-death situation are more helpful.

COMPLEMENTARITY AND FIT

In this section I want to draw attention to the impact that the relationships between the various participants can have on other relationships. This is best exemplified by thinking about the way that the caregiver–baby, the mother–baby and the caregiver–mother relationship affect each other. This triangle can perhaps be seen as representing the larger and more complex relationship between family and hospital.

How staff and parents get on is influenced by their perceptions of each other, and also by the projection of other real or fantasized characteristics which belong elsewhere. This is easily seen in situations where a mother, for example, is able to acknowledge that she feels the nurse handles her infant too roughly or is always telling her off for doing the wrong thing. In this situation an atmosphere of mistrust can build up and the mother may feel not only unsupported but may also have her feelings of failure reinforced and withdraw from the baby and the staff. The perceived caregiver–baby and caregiver–mother relationships affect the mother–baby relationship. Alternatively, a professional who finds a particular mother rude and hostile may find herself becoming critical and begin to avoid her and her baby except when absolutely necessary. Or, as in the example given earlier, if a mother is not seen to be making any effort to reach or care for her infant, staff may be confused and angry and find it difficult to know how to relate to her.

There have been a number of studies which have sought to find out about parents' experience of special care (e.g. Rosenblatt & Redshaw 1984, Stewart 1989). As well as drawing attention to the fact that mothers in particular may well be preoccupied with an expectation of loss, doubts about who owns the baby, fears for their own lives and feelings of having failed, these studies have highlighted more practical problems. Concerns about communication are repeatedly reported, with parents often feeling left in the dark, misunderstood, or confused about the apparently conflicting advice they have received. Some of these criticisms may well be justified, but others are perhaps best understood in the context of this emotionally overwhelming event, which probably makes it difficult for parents to hear what is being said. The reality of the situation is also that it is usually a time of great uncertainty with the baby's prognosis often changing from hour to hour. Added to this is the enormous potential for confusion when parents' personal contexts, past experiences and belief systems are unknown. Tensions can arise in this crucial staff–parent relationship very quickly, and if unchecked can develop into mistrust and suspicion. The impact of this on the care and developing relationships of the neonate is potentially enormous. Conversely, a good fit between staff and parents is often apparent in the ease of communication and the relaxed but competent care given by both parties to the baby. In particular, a good caregiver–mother relationship will facilitate the development of the mother's confidence and sense of relatedness to her baby.

Key points for caregivers

- Special care babies are at the centre of a complex set of relationships. Their growth and their developing relationships may be facilitated if a number of ideas are kept in mind.
- The admission of a baby to neonatal intensive care represents a crisis for family members who then find themselves having to cope with an experience which might be quite unfamiliar.

Key points for caregivers *(Cont'd)*

- There is a need for careful attention to the fit between carers, and between carer and infant. Each infant and his or her family present a unique set of issues which have to be acknowledged, and should inform their care when practically possible.
- Developmental interventions should be tailored to meet the specific needs of each infant, and should be informed by the baby's behavioural cues.
- Staff should try to remember that mothers in particular may be suffering from post-traumatic stress disorder and may find it difficult to hear and remember what is being said to them.
- As authority figures, staff members may remind parents of previous relationships and they may behave accordingly. It is important to try to find out about past relationships and beliefs which may be affecting how parents are responding to the current situation.
- Staff at all levels need to acknowledge the personal stress inherent in the task of caring for these infants and families.

REFERENCES

Affleck G, Tennen H, Rowe J 1990 Infants in crisis: how parents cope with newborn intensive care and its aftermath. Springer Verlag, New York

Anderson G C 1989 Skin to skin: kangaroo care in Western Europe. American Journal of Nursing 89: 662–666

Bender H 1981 Experiences in running a staff group. Journal of Child Psychotherapy 7: 152–159

Bowlby J 1951 Maternal care and mental health. World Health Organization, Geneva

Brazelton T B 1984 Neonatal Behavioral Assessment Scale, 2nd edition. Blackwell, London

Brazelton T B, Cramer G 1991 The earliest relationship: parents, infants, and the drama of early attachment. Karnac Books, London

Brimblecombe F S W 1983 Evolution of special care baby units. In: Davis J A, Richards M P M, Roberton N R C (eds) Parent–baby attachment in premature infants. Croom Helm, London

Field T M 1990 Alleviating stress in newborn infants in the intensive care unit. Clinics in Perinatology 17: 1–9

Freud W E 1989 Notes on some psychological aspects of neonatal intensive care. In: Greenspan S I, Pollock G H (eds) The course of life, volume 1: infancy. International University Press, Madison

Gorski P A 1983 Premature infant behavioral and physiological response to caregiving interventions in the intensive care nursery. In: Call J D, Galenson E, Tyson R L (eds) Frontiers of infant psychiatry. Basic Books, New York, vol 1

Graves P L 1989 The functional fetus. In: Greenspan S I, Pollock G H (eds) The course of life, volume 1: infancy. International University Press, Madison

Jones C L 1982 Environmental analysis of neonatal intensive care. Journal of Nervous and Mental Disease 170: 130–142

Klaus M, Kennell J 1975 Maternal–infant bonding. Mosby, St Louis

Klaus M, Kennell J 1983 Care for the family of an infant with a congenital malformation. In: Davis J A, Richards M P M, Roberton N C R (eds) Parent–baby attachment in premature infants. Croom Helm, London

Lee S K, Penner P L, Cox M 1991 Comparison of the attitudes of health care professionals and parents towards active treatment of very low birth weight babies. Pediatrics 116: 620–626

MacFarlane A 1977 The psychology of childbirth. Fontana/Open Books, London

McFadyen A 1994 Special care babies and their developing relationships. Routledge, London

Newman L F 1981 Social and sensory environment of low birth weight infants in a special care nursery: an anthropological investigation. Journal of Nervous and Mental Disease 169: 448–455

Oehler J M, Davidson M G, Starr L E, Lee D A 1991 Burnout, job stress, anxiety, and perceived social support in neonatal nurses. Heart and Lung 20: 500–505

Patteson D M, Barnard K E 1990 Parenting of low birth weight infants: a review of issues and interventions. Infant Mental Health Journal 11: 37–56

Piontelli A 1992 From fetus to child: an observational and psychoanalytic study. Routledge, London

Richards M P M 1979 Effects on development of medical intervention and the separation of newborns from their parents. In: Shaffer D, Dunn J (eds) The first year of life: psychological and medical implications of early experience. John Wiley, Chichester

Rosenblatt D B, Redshaw M E 1984 Factors influencing the psychological adjustment of mothers to the birth of a preterm infant. In: Call J D, Galenson E, Tyson R L (eds) Frontiers of infant psychiatry. Basic Books, New York, vol 1

Stern M, Karraker K H 1992 Modifying the prematurity stereotype in mothers of premature and ill full-term infants. Journal of Clinical Child Psychology 21: 76–82

Stewart A 1989 Having a baby on a neonatal unit: what do parents feel? How can health visitors help? Health Visitor 62: 374–377

Szur R 1981 Infants in hospital. Journal of Child Psychotherapy 7: 137–140

Wolke D 1991 Annotation: supporting the development of low birthweight infants. Journal of Child Psychology and Psychiatry 32: 723–741

Wyly M V 1995 Premature infants and their families: developmental interventions. Singular Publishing Group, London

FURTHER READING

Affleck G, Tennen H, Rowe J 1990 Infants in crisis: how parents cope with newborn intensive care and its aftermath. Springer Verlag, New York

Brazelton T B, Cramer G 1991 The earliest relationship: parents, infants, and the drama of early attachment. Karnac Books, London

Goldberg S, DiVitto B 1983 Born too soon: preterm birth and early development. Freeman, San Francisco

Hudson G B 1985 You and your special care baby. Sheldon Press, London

McFadyen A 1994 Special care babies and their developing relationships. Routledge, London

Wolke D 1991 Annotation: supporting the development of low birthweight infants. Journal of Child Psychology and Psychiatry 32: 723–741

Wyly M V 1995 Premature infants and their families: developmental interventions. Singular Publishing Group, London

10

Working with breastfeeding mothers: the psychosocial context

Mary Smale

INTRODUCTION

Breastfeeding has potential for delighting or disappointing both helper and helped. This chapter looks at some of the psychological aspects of caring, from both perspectives. Only 63% of women put the baby to the breast on even one occasion in Great Britain in 1990 (White et al 1992). The rates vary between an initiation rate of 74% in London and the South East and 50% in Scotland (White et al 1992). 6 weeks after birth 38% of babies who began breastfeeding were being fully bottle-fed in Great Britain. Breastfeeding rates in many industrialized countries are low and statistics are often not collected or published. Around 50% of French babies are breastfed initially, with 15% still feeding at 3 months. In selected regions of Italy 62% of mothers breastfeed with 46% still doing so at 3 months (Baby Milk Action 1993). Only in Scandinavia is the situation very different, for example up to 98% of Norwegian women begin breastfeeding and 75% are still breastfeeding at 6 months, as compared with the 21% still breastfeeding in Great Britain (Austveg & Sundby 1995, White et al 1992). Breastfeeding rates here are not responding to advocacy and many women find the experience one of failure. There is also fear that in non-industrialized nations bottle-feeding will continue to grow in popularity. The priority of this chapter is to assist health professionals to help women who wish to breastfeed in a way which allows a sense of success and autonomy.

Current attempts to translate biomedical knowledge into policy tend to focus on clinical management of breastfeeding during the first few days after birth, a time when expert help is seen as essential. However, there is still a gap between medical 'rhetoric' about the superiority of breastfeeding and finding ways to achieve its 'reality' (MacIntyre 1982). Women who begin breastfeeding have a daily choice to make about exclusive breastfeeding. Bottles and formula are seen as reasonably safe and socially acceptable in most western societies where breastfeeding tends to be viewed as ideal, but impractical in the long term, for the majority of women. Well-informed health professionals know physiological facts which might help breastfeeding women, but know they struggle against cultural confusion about issues including the feasibility, value and styles of breastfeeding, which makes the information difficult to put into practice.

Knowledge about the psychosocial context of breastfeeding has only recently been considered by those interested in changing practice (e.g. Health Visitors Association and Royal College of Midwives 1995). While there is much published material dealing with these aspects of breastfeeding, it is not widely available as a discrete body of knowledge and has not been so systematically disseminated as biomedical or demographic findings which have reached health workers via study days and publications such as *Successful Breastfeeding* (Royal College of Midwives 1991).

Different lenses for viewing breastfeeding

A 'wide-angle' view of breastfeeding has been provided by demographic quantitative work. This has considered correlations between breastfeeding behaviour and other factors such as education in a 'long distance' view of how socially differentiated groups of women behave. Explanations for low rates of breastfeeding include misleading learning associated with exposure to a bottle-feeding culture, commercial promotion by formula manufacturers, the public invisibility of breastfeeding women and low confidence through decades of failure due in part to iatrogenic interventions – all factors with psychological components. 'Close-up' scrutiny of breastfeeding has concentrated on physical aspects such as initial positioning of the baby at the breast which has been recognized as vitally important.

This chapter takes a 'middle-focus' view. It is vital to consider social and psychosocial aspects of an area as emotive as breastfeeding. It is recognized that women are open to 'a variety of conscious and unconscious psychological influences' (Raphael-Leff 1991, p. 338). Statements collected from women overtly reflect such elements, when, for example, embarrassment or distaste are cited as reasons for not breastfeeding. Ideas about breastfeeding also need to be seen in the context of birth and personal and social agendas in mothering. These agendas include issues such as fatigue, managing other expected tasks, questions as to whose needs take priority and the 'disciplining' of babies. Beliefs about such issues, often implicit and under-researched, transmitted by psychological influence, affect not only whether women breastfeed, but also the 'style' of breastfeeding from the beginning of a baby's life. Breastfeeding 'style' encompasses many things, including the frequency and duration of feeds, and some styles can make breastfeeding very difficult (Quandt 1995).

There are missing areas in this part of the picture, however. Psychosocial influences have largely been discussed in relation to women's choices and decision-making, especially in the initial breast–bottle decision. This approach fails to recognize that women's feelings about breastfeeding can be the result of the influence of health professionals and implies that health professionals themselves are immune to psychological influences, and simply pass on current practices. There has been a particular lack of interest in psychological factors in women and health professionals which might help or prevent the sustaining of women's breastfeeding 'in the social setting of their homes' (Wylie 1992). It has been suggested that 'the difference between those who are capable [of breastfeeding] and those who succeed may pinpoint weaknesses among those who support them rather than the women themselves' (Royal College of Midwives 1991). Almost half of all babies in British hospitals in 1990 were given complementary feeds, although this is known to shorten the duration of breastfeeding (White et al 1992). It is hard to see practices which appear so resistant to research-based information as being caused simply by ignorance. They may rather offer evidence of insecurity in the beliefs of women and/or those around them, including their caregivers, about the feasibility or even the desirability of breastfeeding; thus the 'weaknesses' may be of psychosocial origin.

It is understandable that proposed solutions to the problems of breastfeeding have focused on challenging unhelpful practices with biomedical facts, rather than addressing more complex areas such as attitudes. The 'middle ground' lens can usefully focus on awareness of how the transfer of social desires about breastfeeding and breastfeeding style are mediated to women by others interpersonally and perhaps find ways to alter ingrained messages.

A challenge for health professionals

Research is not always easily assimilated into practice especially, I suggest, where there is much associated psychosocial meaning. For instance a newborn's weight is often recorded very soon after birth and carries significance for parents, health professionals and others as a part of a rite of passage. De Chateau and colleagues reported how hard it was initially to alter delivery routines when the detrimental effect on breastfeeding of separation caused by weighing was identified. Yet, once nurses involved in this research had seen the difference, they did not wish to return to the old order (de Chateau et al 1977).

I suggest that health professionals now have a challenge to extend their thinking beyond practices to the importance to mothers and others of the beliefs upon which behaviour is based. However, recognizing the need to consider psychosocial influence on professional practice and examining the meaning of personal experiences may not be easy.

A WIDE RANGE OF MATERIAL WITH A PSYCHOLOGICAL VIEWPOINT

Although I have highlighted the lack and narrowness of psychological material relating specifically to the interaction between caregiver and woman, there is a wide range of material that includes some reference to the psychological context of breastfeeding for mothers. It is difficult to isolate psychological aspects of breastfeeding by selecting research from particular journals, just as links between physical and psychological dimensions are intertwined in the everyday experience of breastfeeding – matters of 'mind over milk' – so these are often linked in the literature. For example there are many questions about the giving of complementary feeds. Is this simply a matter of the baby becoming accustomed physiologically to suck rather than suckle and a matter of appetite and supply inhibition? Or does it involve the psychological aspects of a baby's learning about instant rewards rather than waiting for let-down, and the transmission of low confidence from one person to another about the adequacy of breast milk to satisfy babies? Subjective differences in meaning do appear to be important in this area. For example, in a study of women assigned randomly to receive a once-a-day supplementary bottle or to expect no supplementary bottle, breastfeeding was perceived as more problematic where bottles had not been planned (Kearney et al 1990).

Research described below in a brief review of some of the psychological aspects of breastfeeding confirms how difficult it is to disentangle the personal, physical and social meaning of breastfeeding and the process of caring for breastfeeding women.

Babies' abilities

Research has found out much about what a baby can do at birth and immediately afterwards which has implications for delivery room practices. Babies exhibit a series of preparatory acts in the first sensitive period after a normal birth – including salivating, mouthing, rooting and moving to achieve successful fixing at the breast, which suggest an optimal time for the first feed (Righard & Alade 1990). Such research findings may make women and their caregivers anxious if a first breastfeed is not achieved soon after delivery, but it is worth bearing in mind that many mothers are separated from their babies from necessity at birth and still breastfeed. Babies who miss out on this opportunity then sleep, rather than feed, may also sometimes be stimulated by being in skin-to-skin contact with the mother and both may be enabled to go through the process of discovering one another. Babies have been shown to prefer an unwashed to a washed breast, suggesting the use of a sense of smell to find the mother's breast (Porter R, unpublished work, 1995). The effect of narcotic analgesia on babies' abilities to root and suckle has also been demonstrated (Righard & Alade 1990). Women whose caesarean sections were accompanied by a general anaesthetic have a lower rate of breastfeeding than those who had an epidural (White et al 1992). This may not mean that epidural anaesthetic is without effect itself. Rajan (1994) suggests that caregivers need to be aware that women whose babies have received drugs may well need extra help. They may also benefit from reassurance that their babies will neither dehydrate nor starve while sleeping off the effects of the sedation or pain relievers. Enabling the baby and mother to re-enact the skin-to-skin contact which would have been ideally possible after birth in an unhurried atmosphere may be helpful when he or she wakes.

Research by physiologists and psychologists has shown that babies are able to regulate their calorific intake appropriately and can best organize feeds without time intervention (Royal College of Midwives 1991). Research also indicates that there are typical changes in feeding patterns as babies grow, and suggests that the feeding patterns of boys and girls may also differ (Wright 1988). Such information may help mothers. Women often compare their babies with others and worry that differences, especially during so-called 'growth spurts' where supply is ensured or increased through periods of very intense feeding, may mean something is wrong, and it is always worth reminding them of their babies' individuality.

Mothers' responses

Breastfeeding is often seen as an instinctive and natural facet of motherhood, but paradoxically one which can easily fail. For example, the squeezing out of milk from cell-clusters within the breast, usually known as let-down, happens sometimes simply in response to the cry of (any) baby, but early psychological research involving plunging women's feet into icy water showed that this impaired the let-down reflex (Newton & Newton 1948). From this finding it has been extrapolated that all kinds of stress can lead to the end of breastfeeding. The need for a mother to learn breastfeeding as a skill is now rarely questioned. It is worth pointing out that there is little research on how women intending to breastfeed behave towards their infants immediately after birth. This is a part of a wider lack of research into how women succeed in breastfeeding, especially into how they manage their own and their family's emotions and wider social constraints in order to breastfeed.

In an interesting study of the immediate postnatal period, the presence of fathers in the delivery room seemed to make baby–mother contact more animated, while the presence of health professionals distracted the mother from the baby as she sought reassurance, but no implications for breastfeeding were drawn – indeed the subject was not mentioned (Dunn 1981). Research on this aspect of the environment and its effects on the initiation of breastfeeding would be useful.

Choices

Initiating breastfeeding

Quantitative research about women's choices in infant feeding has identified a number of factors associated with breastfeeding, but often raises many questions. For example, a woman whose mother or friends have breastfed is more likely to do so herself (White et al 1992). Mechanisms to account for this association need more exploration. Individual goals and feelings about breastfeeding, for example intended length of breastfeeding and motivation levels, appear to be more important than (although not necessarily unshaped by) socioeconomic factors (Coreil & Murphy 1988). This suggests that if we wish to know how much support women are likely to need it may be useful to talk with women antenatally and identify what their own goals and levels of confidence are, rather than simply ticking one box or another about the intention to breastfeed.

Various ways of thinking about decision-making have been proposed in relation to women's infant feeding. Personal construct theory, in which broad beliefs about anticipated events are understood to influence behaviour, has been described as a useful model for infant feeding choices (Price & Price 1995). Health belief models are suggested as being important by other researchers, who take into account an individual's perception of the seriousness of any ill-effects, the benefits of any action and the barriers likely to be associated with an action being carried out (Sweeney & Gulino 1987). Cognitive orientation theory proposes that it is possible, with knowledge of an individual's goals, rules and norms, beliefs about herself and general beliefs about others and the environment, to predict likely behaviours. This theory was used by researchers to show that it was possible to determine important themes for breastfeeding women, without mentioning breastfeeding directly, and, potentially, to suggest ways of modifying behaviour (Kreitler & Kreitler 1990). These models confirm the important influence of the overarching beliefs held by an individual and suggest that it is important to be able to envisage their modification. These beliefs may include ideas about related themes such as physical contact, bodies, food and sex. Discussing women's feelings about breastfeeding may be helpful in sustaining breastfeeding through difficult times. For example, a mother who has always liked the idea of prolonged breastfeeding because it means closeness, but who finds her breastfeeding temporarily under threat, might be helped not only by practical suggestions, but also by having her original aim taken into consideration by her caregiver and by being asked to imagine how she thinks she might feel later if she succeeds in breastfeeding or if she stops in the middle of the crisis.

The decision about whether to breastfeed depends on many factors, not just women's perceptions of the benefits of breastfeeding for their babies. In one general practice 94% of pregnant women agreed that breast milk was better than formula but only 76% intended breastfeeding (Hawthorne 1994). Psychosocial obstacles can also be important. For example, in a study of mainly middle-class women in America, 98% of women whose partners strongly approved of breastfeeding began breastfeeding, compared to only 27% of those whose partners were indifferent (Littman et al 1994). While many writers suggest that the decision to breastfeed or not is made in early pregnancy, research suggests strong ideas are already held in childhood about issues such as whether breastfeeding is 'rude' or best for babies (Gregg 1989). Such research can make us question whether there is any point in trying to persuade women to consider breastfeeding. Rather than simply reiterating what is best for her baby, it may be useful to offer the mother an opportunity to articulate the influences she sees as important on her decision-making, to find out whether or not she is making an 'automatic' choice. It may also be helpful to talk about realistic interpersonal strategies for managing breastfeeding as a psychosocial process, including identifying who she will turn to for support. A woman may appreciate further information about the benefits of breastfeeding to use herself later as a way of helping explain her decision to others.

Continuing breastfeeding

The two main reasons women give for discontinuing breastfeeding are the perception that they have insufficient milk, and sore nipples (White et al 1992). Discussion about the psychological context of the perception of milk insufficiency could fill a whole chapter. In one study no objective weight gain difference was found between babies of mothers who stopped breastfeeding and those who did not (Wylie & Verber 1994). It is probable, once technical difficulties such as incorrect positioning have been eliminated, that the problem is to some extent one of perception – the woman's or another's – or it may represent the offering of an acceptable explanation rather than articulating a complex set of other reasons for discontinuing. While women may not wish to discuss their reasons in detail with health professionals or breastfeeding support workers, particularly if they see them as likely to condemn their choice, it is important that they do have someone to talk to. A great deal of trust may be needed to help women to articulate the complexities of their motivations and so come to terms with their decision to stop. Cultural and personal beliefs about an appropriate time to end breastfeeding vary greatly and may well influence caregivers' opinions, as well as those of women, about whether it is time to stop, especially when a baby becomes a toddler. The woman's intentions, and her interpretation of her baby's wishes, should remain central whether she is ending or struggling to continue breastfeeding, whatever the age of the baby.

The elusive breastfeeding 'type'

Some health education material seems to suggest that women must change their personality to be able to breastfeed, becoming passive, relaxed, even cowlike! One summary of research on the ideal breastfeeding mother included the need to be calm, mature, instinctive, independent, accepting of the giving of oneself, involved in the mothering role, respectful of her own needs and flexible (Kearney 1988). Some research suggests that pregnant women who choose breastfeeding tend to be antenatally less neurotic and to report more happy episodes than those who do not (Adler & Bancroft 1988). Other research has identified assertiveness as an important factor in breastfeeding (Wright 1988). Barnes and colleagues (1993) found that women with no clear-cut sense of identity were more likely to bottle-feed. Such associations may reflect, in part, varying views of what 'proper' mothers should be like in a particular culture at a particular time. It might be useful to help a woman identify what aspects of her previous experience or personality she feels may help her to enjoy breastfeeding, such as perseverance, as well as aspects which might make it difficult.

Child-centred reasons for breastfeeding such as infant health benefits and women-centred ones such as convenience are sometimes differentiated, the first being more likely to lead to breastfeeding. The decision to breastfeed is often explained by mothers as being the best for their babies (e.g. Bacon & Wylie 1976). When women describe making women-centred decisions they may be seen as selfish, but this takes no account of social pressure and psychological needs and resources. It is easy to see the characteristics of breastfeeders as static, whereas, for example, experience suggests that the most unexpected breastfeeder may find, after a period of adjustment, that it is possible to respond more 'instinctively' with support which acknowledges her difficulties. Wright (1988) points out that breastfed babies control both pace and duration of feeds in a way which in bottle-feeding is more under the mother's direction. Raphael-Leff (1984) describes a continuum between two types of women – 'regulators' who need a high degree of control over their babies' lives and 'facilitators' who are able easily to follow their babies' needs. Such a model is useful for empathizing with a woman who finds demand feeding difficult.

Attempts to define women into polarized types who do or do not breastfeed may not be helpful. The first faltering may lead to a 'diagnosis' of inadequacy in the woman rather than raising suspicions about technical or supportive help needed. Typing a woman as someone who never would have been able or could not really have wanted to breastfeed may make it easier for a caregiver to come to terms with early termination of breastfeeding, which would otherwise have been seen as a shared responsibility, but does not take account of the complexity of her decision-making.

MEANINGS OF BREASTFEEDING FOR WOMEN AND OTHERS
Women's feelings

Confidence in their breastfeeding in many women is fragile, often started 'if I can' and maintained by 'good luck'. Many women speak of feeling 'drained' or tired by breastfeeding. Is this a part of recovery after childbirth, low blood sugar in a woman who has not allowed herself to snack while giving several feeds, a normal sleepiness in response to a release of prolactin, or fear, of social or personal origin, that the baby who wishes to feed more than 4-hourly will wear out the woman and make her unable to fulfil her other tasks? This calls for careful listening to understand the meaning, experience and expectation behind the words.

Some women may find breastfeeding impossible for deep-rooted reasons. One woman's distaste may alert the caregiver to the possibility of previous abuse, while another's embarrassment may suggest a need for help with assertiveness or practical strategies against social norms. Wanting one's body back is also sometimes given as a contributory factor in the decision to bottle-feed. One study suggested that many women saw breastfeeding in some sense as a 'sacrifice' even when they felt this was worthwhile (Hewat & Ellis 1984, p. 443). Given that in some cultures breastfeeding is almost universal, even where bottle-feeding is comparatively safe, it seems that not only physical, but psychological pathology in women is rarely enough to stop its course, although social or personal experiences may make the process emotionally challenging for some women. Listening for individual meanings with a non-judgmental approach which reflects the woman's own position and allows her to explore her fears and fantasies about breastfeeding is essential.

Breastfeeding, with its demands upon the exclusive resources of one person for nurture, can become the focus of a response to enormous changes in lifestyle. The range of sometimes ambivalent emotions experienced by a woman as she breastfeeds is well explored by Raphael-Leff (1991), varying from boredom to feelings of being trapped, doubt, delight and fear. Feelings and attributions may shift from hour to hour – breastfeeding being blamed for tiredness or depression, for example, or being clung to as the only part of mothering which is going well. Some women may feel negative towards breastfeeding all the time, others occasionally, and it is important that such feelings are accepted as valid for that woman by health professionals and other supporters before any other help is offered, whether physical or psychological to enable breastfeeding to continue or end. Whatever the direct or vicarious experience of the helper, it needs to be set aside. It may be difficult for caregivers to do this if they have not had their own experience heard in a non-judgmental way elsewhere.

Research about whether breastfeeding is helpful or unhelpful to women's mental health is equivocal; some (retrospective) research found women who fed for more than 3 months reported more depressive symptoms than those who did not and the effect on sexuality was more marked still. Yet other studies have shown that breastfeeding women who persist are less 'neurotic' than those who give up (Adler & Bancoft 1988). It is hard to know in which way any cause and effect may flow when postnatal depression follows the premature ending of breastfeeding.

Positive effects of breastfeeding include the possibility that it can be a reparative experience for women with little confidence in their bodies after being unable to give birth without intervention (Laufer 1990). Rajan (1994) suggests that the mother's first impressions of her baby's responsiveness may have long-term effects on their relationship and emphasizes the need to try to ensure a good first meeting. Locklin & Naber (1993) describe a process of empowerment in a group of low-income women who experienced increased self-esteem, mutual support, reliance on their own judgment and other positive feelings through successful breastfeeding. It has also been suggested that breastfeeding can prevent an expected exacerbation in panic attacks postpartum (Klein 1994).

There is little language to describe the range of pleasure possible from breastfeeding, from delight in the baby's contentment and health to hormonally stimulated sexual sensations. Deutsch comments on one extreme end of a continuum: 'the nursing mother can bear almost anything more easily than the confusion of conscious, sexual emotions with the tender, loving action of nursing'– another, rarely mentioned, area which may be of concern to mothers (Deutsch 1945, p. 290).

Women's own view of breastfeeding as successful or comfortable is what is important – it is easy to see a beautiful baby and expect a mother to be pleased to feed him or her, or to see one who is hungry every hour and imagine that the mother must want to stop breastfeeding, but these assumptions may not reflect reality.

Pregnancy, labour, birth, breastfeeding and the postnatal period are sometimes seen as separate in research and in the organization of the maternity services, but women's lives may feel more continuous, despite the drama of birth. For women who choose to breastfeed the way this goes is a crucial part of their mothering. Several hours will be taken up in each day – and night – by a task for which a first-time breastfeeding woman cannot practice, in a process which is almost unimaginable either for a mother, father and many caregivers, for whom simply making milk can be hard to envisage. Her many new tasks include attempting to control time and keep everyone who is concerned with her and the baby happy, including health professionals. Lomas (1967) gives a useful account of the changes needed for a woman's acceptance of her new status, including changes in her relationship with her partner, her in capacity because of the baby's needs, accepting more help and tolerating success as work is future. It can be seen that breastfeeding is central in all these tasks. Breastfed baby 'snacking' is apparently irrational in a social context which prescribes definite 'meals', although it is much more like adult eating and drinking than many care to admit and, like them, reflects as many psychological needs as nutritional.

At 8 weeks the woman's experience of her baby is still dominated by the need to stabilize the baby's psychobiological waking states (Niven 1992). Time was found to be of central importance in accounts of breastfeeding concerns, used by both family members and health professionals descriptively, proscriptively and prescriptively (Smale 1996). This suggests that mothers need realistic expectations of the changing needs of their baby and a great deal of support to defend their decision to begin or continue breastfeeding. Much advice still involves time despite the apparent disappearance of traditional advice to feed every 4 hours for 10 minutes on each side. Some actions may be seen as a way of ensuring good weight gain or a settled baby but also work to rationalize time, for example offering bottles controls weight increase in relation to time, or extends the time between feeds. Such actions offer a way of circumventing some of the necessarily unquantifiable aspects of this transitional period but have deleterious effects on breastfeeding in the longer term and their implications need to be explained to women. Achieving some sense of 'routine' is socially expected and may be a way of attempting to regain control, especially where a woman has had a previous career in which she was in charge of her own time and tasks. Women need time to come to terms with the enormous changes which a baby brings and a caregiver can help here by listening and empathizing with the mother's sense of disorder, as well as explaining the baby's apparent irrationality as a coherent response to his or her needs.

Meanings for partnerships

Raphael-Leff (1991) has explored issues around breastfeeding and sexuality and the dilemmas which women face, caused by contradictory demands. Other literature explores the difficulties men may face in accepting their partners' breastfeeding. These include embarrassment when breastfeeding becomes visible in mixed company and jealousy both in terms of the ownership of breasts and the ability of the woman alone to satisfy the baby's needs. Various researchers have identified problems with the return to sexual relationships in breastfeeding women. Breastfeeding is understood to be one aspect of women's psychosexual experience. In one study women who reported insufficient milk were also found to be experiencing more negative feelings towards sexual desire than those who were not (Hillervik-Lindquist 1992). Sensitive discussion about such areas may be helpful.

Women can, however, sometimes make inaccurate assumptions about their partners' wishes, whether for intercourse or care and attention, and can be usefully encouraged to find time to talk and explore these issues with their partners. Freed et al (1993) found that women's guesses about their partners' ideas about breastfeeding antenatally were little more accurate than random guessing. There is even less time for discussion postnatally.

The wider family and friendships

Grandmothers and others, especially those who found regimented breastfeeding unsuccessful, may have a low level of confidence in the process of breastfeeding and may bombard new mothers with their own unresolved concerns. The new mother may find it helpful to rehearse how she will deal with comments and consider where she can gain support, for example from other mothers who are breastfeeding with a similar style to her own. It may be helpful to suggest that the woman encourages those who undermine her breastfeeding to talk about their own experience so that they both come to understand what happened and why, and begin to see how different their circumstances are – in other words to make explicit the principles on which each is working.

WHO CAN HELP MOTHERS?

The ideal qualities of a breastfeeding supporter have not been researched as extensively as the ideal attributes of a breastfeeding woman. The quality and quantity of help which may be valuable means that various levels of intervention are appropriate at different times, from information-giving to counselling skills. The supportive health worker may need to address the varying and possibly conflicting psychosocial needs of more than one member of the family, as well as the influence of those beyond the family.

Partners

Raphael argues that breastfeeding women initially need a 'doula', someone to mother them and make space in which their breastfeeding can happen without interruption or stress, and suggests that the woman's partner may usefully take this role (Raphael 1975). In Britain men often attend delivery and antenatal classes. Mobile nuclear families are common and there may already be some expectation for the father to take the role of supporter for his partner and her breastfeeding.

The identified difficulties of men may sometimes, however, make it hard for them to act supportively towards their partners' breastfeeding. They may simply find the process distasteful or place physical limits on where it should take place so as to restrict the number of people who see it. The imperative some men feel to undertake shared care for the baby and their desire to nurture may clash with a belief in the superiority of breast milk and lead to the introduction of bottles, whether of formula or expressed breast milk. Just dismissing these urges with a suggestion about the father's role in nappy-changing is unlikely to address this issue sufficiently. Both ingenuity and sensitivity may be needed where partners feel that they have no part to play other than the giving of a bottle.

Partners may be helped to resolve any feelings about being uninvolved, by encouraging them to think out loud about their own needs for support in the postnatal period, as well as the support they might be asked for. Where partners do not attend antenatal visits or classes it may be possible to send ideas for talking together home with the pregnant woman.

The role of the health professional

Antenatal help

Health professional intervention can be seen as a replacement for the bottle-educated or distant family. It is known that having information about breastfeeding helps mothers continue (Rentschler 1991). Jenner (1988) used very basic information to help women sustain breastfeeding effectively, especially explaining that it was normal for breastfeeding babies to cry more than bottle-fed babies. It is certainly important for women to know that they are not doing something wrong or that their milk is not weak or failing if their baby wants to feed more often, or for longer than is socially desirable.

It has also been suggested that it is important that caregivers should offer information not only about how breastfeeding works, but also about what might go wrong and how to deal with problems. This raises issues about the balance between speaking of breastfeeding as natural and easy and giving information in case of crisis. We do not yet know what are the best educational strategies for enabling breastfeeding. For example, is breastfeeding best learnt by 'observation and practice' (Royal College of Midwives 1996)? Such experience is not easily obtained in many industrialized countries and is usually replaced by teaching or reading. Losch and colleagues (1995) note that teenagers who have contact with breastfeeding women are more likely to breastfeed themselves. Raphael-Leff (1991) suggests that some of the unfamiliarity of breastfeeding might be overcome by the use of videos. It is worth using sections which do not simply concentrate on a clinically correct breast–baby contact but give women's – and their partners' – perspectives on breastfeeding as an everyday normality. The role of different styles of assistance (for example with and without physical contact) in breastfeeding initiation is, extraordinarily, unresearched. Effective help in the early stages of breastfeeding can be given both by health professionals and voluntary supporters who use no physical contact but rather emphasize the empowerment of women to find their own route to comfortable positioning with minimal suggestions. Women are known to dislike having their babies forcibly attached to their breasts (Green et al 1988). Where attempts to position babies at the mother's breast are strenuous, normal behaviour may be disrupted (Renfrew & McGill 1996). Some women express surprise at the ease with which caregivers may assume access to their breasts. Permission to handle a woman's breast should always be sought.

Winicoff and colleagues (1987) wrote that those least likely to sustain breastfeeding are those most likely to rely on information from health professionals. Anticipatory guidance – that is explaining about the value and management of breastfeeding – has not always been found to encourage breastfeeding (Shand & Kosawa 1984). The contradictory nature of the findings in this area suggest that it may be less-quantifiable factors than simply the content of information given which influence the outcomes, such as the nature of the relationships between the woman and her caregivers or women's perception of the caregivers' beliefs about breastfeeding.

Helping in decision-making

From an educational point of view it may be most helpful to allow women to articulate their own reasons for their choices. Some researchers have suggested emphasizing women-centred reasons such as the practicality of breastfeeding. Women who offered child-centred reasons for breastfeeding were found in one study to have more lactation crises (Hillervik-Lindquist 1992). It may help to find out not only the level of understanding a woman has before offering information but asking where she feels she is in the process of thinking about feeding. This will give her the possibility of developing her ideas in the light of information from health professionals and other women. Though very few women currently do change their minds after early pregnancy about whether or not to breastfeed, we do not know if they might if their concerns were heard and understood. Open-ended questions and good listening skills should help here. If women are cajoled into breastfeeding against their unexplored inclination and then give up breast-feeding, their 'failure' may perpetuate negative societal beliefs about breastfeeding.

Support after the birth

We know that support from friends and family can be helpful to women. A study of low-income women found that those who succeeded in breastfeeding had support systems similar to successful breastfeeders in the more affluent groups (Grossman et al 1990). We are less sure what the 'recipe' for such help is – approval, encouragement, problem-solving ideas, offers of meals and child care all may contribute. Postnatal support from health professionals has been shown to help women wishing to breastfeed (Houston 1984). Although, again, what it was about the support which made it work so well has not been clearly identified. Information and practice are usually included in the package of help caregivers provide, but little is known about the interpersonal skills used. An exception is research by a psychologist who shared her experience of both breastfeeding and bottle-feeding with a group of low-income women as a part of unconditional support using counselling skills (Jenner 1988). The group who received such help were significantly more successful in breastfeeding than those who did not.

Health professionals may have a useful role in helping both parents to identify (and if necessary to facilitate reconciliation between) their long-term wishes in the light of their experience, and to achieve their goals by giving information and support for choices made at all points.

Caring in failure

In many industrialized countries much of the caring role is inevitably directed towards women whose breastfeeding has, in the woman's own terms, 'failed'. Almost half of the women who began breastfeeding in one general practice had stopped by 8 weeks (Hawthorne 1994). Where breastfeeding ends before the woman wishes, or this is anticipated, it is important that negative feelings are accepted and not dismissed. It may be tempting to offer inaccurate statements about breastfeeding as 'excuses', but perpetuating myths helps neither the woman nor those she will talk to. Where the woman experiences the baby as rejecting her as the baby begins to prefer other sources of food or comfort to the breast, at whatever age, sensitivity is especially necessary.

WOMEN'S IDEAS ABOUT WHAT IS HELPFUL AND UNHELPFUL

Women's own feelings about the help they have received is another under-researched area. A review of women's experience of support in breastfeeding lists being listened to, feeling cared for and having been given time as being especially important (Cronenwett & Reinhardt 1987). Breastfeeding women have been shown to be more concerned than bottle-feeding mothers about the quality of the 'psychological environment' as they feed (Wright 1988).

Inconsistency of advice has been especially singled out as disturbing breastfeeding mothers in several studies (Green et al 1988). It may be that this is not simply a matter of confusion about what is the practice to adopt, but the difficulty of complying with more than one person's contradictory advice at a time when peace and a low profile are sought.

Some women report feeling that they have been too readily rescued from difficulties such as babies crying at night in hospital when they were tired. Helping women to breastfeed – and explaining why an odd bottle may adversely affect future breastfeeding – often takes more time than giving a bottle, or cup. It can be difficult to justify time spent on relatively passive activities, such as listening, in comparison with other more intensive acts, like bottle-feeding, which are often more readily seen as 'real' work.

It was clear from my counselling records that women can describe vividly, in great detail, the words said to them by caregivers and the tone of the words (Smale 1996). For example, a woman whose baby is not gaining weight quickly enough and who is told 'we can take him and make him put weight on', may not remember further discussion as she is so distressed by the power relations implied by the caregiver. The normal vocabulary of breastfeeding has been shaped by a culture which did not approve of its 'demands', building in, by the use of this word, a description which implies unreasonable behaviour by the baby and a passive response by the mother. It may be possible to work with women to find new, more positive metaphors which suggest generosity and responsiveness and remove medical language.

Dilemmas in support – women or breastfeeding?

There are questions about how far caregivers should go in offering arguments for the initiation or continuation of what is increasingly seen as a health behaviour. There is a tightrope between encouragement which sustains and cheerleading which makes a woman unable to contemplate failure without shame and so jeopardizes future trust. There is a narrow and useful balance for caregivers between conveying that they believe that breastfeeding is both a valuable activity and a genuine possibility for most women and not pressurizing women to sustain it to please someone else.

Health professionals are sometimes reluctant to use health knowledge, such as health benefits to baby and mother, to encourage breastfeeding owing to concerns about making women feel guilty if they fail (Beeken 1990). Such reluctance needs exploration in the light of the comparative ease with which, for example, knowledge of the hazards of cigarettes is passed on to parents.

HEALTH PROFESSIONALS' ATTITUDES AND THEIR HELP

Raphael-Leff (1991) suggests that breastfeeding is a highly emotive situation for the observer. Caregivers can experience a wide range of responses including feelings of frustration, exclusion from the intimacy of breastfeeding, or a need to rescue the woman from a situation similar to their own earlier failure. They may also experience both delight at gratitude, and disappointment at anger from mothers in relation to the breastfeeding help received. However, research tells us little about health professionals' emotions or needs in this area. The first step is to recognize potential complexities: 'Maybe it is a sign of insight and knowledge to concede that this work is difficult' (Bergman et al 1993).

Some caregivers may simply feel unconfident; for example trainee paediatricians in one US hospital were found to be (appropriately) unsure of their level of knowledge (Williams & Hammer 1995). It is clear that many health professionals feel a responsibility for breastfeeding. For example, Beeken & Waterston (1992) found that although 71% of staff wanted wider publicity for breastfeeding support groups only 45% felt it appropriate to allow 'lay' breastfeeding supporters into hospital wards.

The wide range of opposing ideas about breastfeeding shows it to be an issue around which much tension exists. Is it, for example, normal and natural, reliable and clean or abnormal, unreliable and impure? It is not surprising that some of these tensions are reflected as ambivalences in health professionals' attitudes. For example Beeken & Waterston (1992) found that while almost all health professionals agreed that breast milk was healthier for babies, 37% disagreed that the type of feeding affected the health of the baby. Anderson & Geden (1991) found that although health workers who had breastfed themselves had more information than those who had not, this may not always be based on a positive experience of breastfeeding. Research done two decades ago showed that some caregivers who had breastfed their own children experienced it as impractical and so discouraged mothers who they cared for (Kurtz 1980). It is to be hoped that as more health professionals find breastfeeding a successful experience, they will bring more positive attitudes about the feasibility of breastfeeding to their relationships with women and share the realities of their breastfeeding experience with colleagues. There is, however, a tendency to deny the relevance of personal knowledge. For example, McCaughan (1993) found that three-quarters of the staff in one hospital felt it was not as important as clinical experience.

Research also tells us little about breastfeeding helpers as feeding mothers. However, one study found that midwives in Northern Ireland began breastfeeding at a much higher rate than the average for their population, but stopped for the same reasons as other women (McMulkin S & Malone R, unpublished, 1993). Many health professionals will have been bottle-fed and so may have to cope with some feelings of disloyalty in describing the benefits of breastfeeding. There may be many feelings for caregivers to work through before they can unconditionally help women to make their own decisions. It may be especially hard to come to terms with failure in breastfeeding as a health professional and to recognize that iatrogenic intervention from colleagues may have played a part in this failure. Seeing overenthusiastic forcible attachment of a baby to the mother's breast can be upsetting not only to mother and baby but to professionals who have breastfed but feel that they can say nothing. Many health workers have sacrificed their own ideal breastfeeding experience in order to return to work or study and may have this loss to discuss. One British health visitor has written vividly about the lack of a safe place to take unresolved feelings from one's own breastfeeding experience (Crawford 1992). Support groups, similar to those sometimes set up to help caregivers working with bereaved parents, have been suggested as useful for health professionals working with breastfeeding mothers (Lee 1995). Alternatively a consistent person who will give time uncritically to a helper's own feelings may free her or him to offer what Raphael-Leff calls a 'quiet space in which to savour the feeding interchange rather than turning it into a regimented means of getting milk into the baby' (Raphael-Leff 1991, p. 348).

Many attempts to run education programmes for health professionals have been described, some suggesting success in terms of new information absorbed, others arguing that programmes need repeating regularly. Health professionals appear to gain much from an interdisciplinary forum involving, for example, midwives, health visitors, general practitioners and volunteer breastfeeding supporters, offering feedback for caregivers who may usually only see the quickly changing early stages of breastfeeding. Health professionals in initial and in-service training are also likely to benefit from meeting breastfeeding mothers, with and without problems, to request feedback about the help received and strategies used.

Enabling change in other health professionals

As well as working to improve their own care of breastfeeding women, caregivers may also wish to enable change in other health professionals. Various suggestions have been made including offering of accurate information and giving opportunities for leadership. As with mothers, it may help to listen to the story of a caregiver who is finding it difficult to give enabling assistance to breastfeeding mothers. Unwilling adoption of practices by caregivers may simply lead to superficial change, with unhelpful underlying messages still being conveyed to women by the use of particular words, tone, or body language.

CONCLUSION

Current research about the psychosocial context of breastfeeding has few answers for many of the important issues for those caring for breastfeeding women, having largely concentrated on how women fail. It can, nevertheless, open our eyes to wider meanings than our own limited experiences. More research on how women succeed, especially how they manage emotions and social pressures is needed.

Health professionals have a challenging set of tasks in enabling breastfeeding – not only to convey to parents the superiority of breast milk and the feasibility of breastfeeding, but also, paradoxically, to empower women to become less dependent upon their help. These tasks involve both caring (for the woman, her baby and their relationship) and not caring (that she complies with prescriptive advice if she finds another way to solve her problem).

Being cared for as a breastfeeding woman is a different experience from being shown how to use a bottle and formula without seriously risking a baby's health. There is potential for a more complex biopsychosocial interplay between the woman, her baby and those around them. Caregivers may convey a greater anxiety about checking that all is well when working with breastfeeding women than they do with those who are bottle-feeding, as breastfeeding is so inevitably invisible. Caring for the breastfeeding woman is a different experience for health professionals too. The demands made in relation to nurturing, allowing 'failure' or 'success' and other tasks may mean that the carer may well benefit from time for support for herself.

Key points for caregivers

- Emotional as well as technical support is needed to promote independence, wherever possible, since breastfeeding is something which mainly happens outside the medical arena. Counselling skills may well be more appropriate than advice-giving in the majority of situations. These skills include non-judgmental acceptance, allowing distress to be aired and listening to the woman's agenda. Such skills are not natural for most people and benefit from practice.
- There are good psychological, as well as physiological, reasons for enabling the first feed to be a time of unhurried intimacy, offering the opportunity for breastfeeding or preliminary licking to be initiated in an uninterrupted period of skin-to-skin contact, without anxiety about instant fixing.
- Simple changes from a medical, to a less directive, model can be helpful. This may include explaining how the baby takes the breast and encouraging the woman to work out for herself what to do. Caregivers might usefully change statements beginning with 'you should' to ones starting with 'it may help if . . .'. Avoid suggesting that certain feeding positions are 'wrong', especially if the woman does not report any problems. Watching how a woman positions her baby at first is helpful and, with the woman's permission, observing how a whole feed goes is an investment saving time for the future.
- If problems arise the woman's perception of her situation is important, as she is aware of her own long-term as well as short-term goals and meanings, as well as those of her partner and family. For example, ask women for their own ideas about the cause of any problems and ideas for improving the situation and what other people have suggested already. Recognize the enormous variation possible in any encounter between two people whose personal history and cultural pressures may have led to very different ideas about breastfeeding. Fuller communication between caregivers and women and among caregivers is necessary, addressing the psychosocial context of infant feeding as well as biomedical issues. Such communication will help to prevent the apparent conflict of practice and principle.

Key points for caregivers *(Cont'd)*

- To promote continued breastfeeding it may be useful to help women to think about breastfeeding beyond the early postnatal period, for example considering how they might mobilize the support they need or rehearsing basic assertiveness.
- Look critically at feeding practices and policies in the light of psychosocial as well as biomedical research. Consider writing awareness of psychosocial factors into local breastfeeding policies.
- Caregivers may find it helpful to seek out supportive opportunities for coming to terms with their personal experience of breastfeeding. This will help them to avoid bringing their own unmet needs into the breastfeeding support they provide.

REFERENCES

Adler E, Bancoft J 1988 The relationship between breast feeding persistence, sexuality and mood in postpartum women. Psychological Medicine 18: 389–396
Anderson E, Geden E 1991 Nurses' knowledge of breastfeeding. Journal of Gynecological and Neonatal Nursing 20(1): 58–63
Austveg B, Sundby J 1995 The case of breastfeeding in Norway: empowerment of women. Norwegian Breastfeeding Association, Oslo
Baby Milk Action 1993 National governmental statistics and regional reports. Baby Milk Action, Cambridge
Bacon C J, Wylie J M 1976 Attitudes to infant feeding at Newcastle General Hospital in summer 1975. British Medical Journal 1: 308–309
Barnes J, Leggett J, Durham T 1993 Breastfeeders versus bottlefeeders: differences in femininity perceptions. Maternal–Child Nursing Journal 21(1): 15–19
Beeken S 1990 An evaluation of professionals' attitudes and practices concerning breast feeding. Undergraduate dissertation, University of Newcastle upon Tyne
Beeken S, Waterston T 1992 Health service support of breastfeeding: are we practicing what we preach? British Medical Journal 305: 285–287
Bergman V, Larson S, Lomberg H, Moller A, Staffan M 1993 A survey of Swedish mothers' views on breastfeeding and experiences of social and professional support. Scandinavian Journal of Caring Sciences 7(1): 47–52
Coreil J, Murphy J 1988 Maternal commitment, lactation practices, and breastfeeding duration. Journal of Gynecological and Neonatal Nursing 17(4): 273–278
Crawford J 1992 Understanding our own breastfeeding experiences. Newsletter of the Joint Breastfeeding Initiative 4(1): 1–2
Cronenwett L R, Reinhardt R 1987 Support and breastfeeding: a review. Birth 14(4): 199–203
de Chateau P, Homberg H, Jakobsson K, Winberg J 1977 A study of factors promoting and inhibiting lactation. Developmental Medicine and Child Neurology 19: 575–584
Deutsch H 1945 The psychology of women, volume 2, motherhood. Grune & Stratton, New York
Dunn D 1981 Interactions of mothers with their newborns in the first half hour of life. Journal of Advanced Nursing 6: 271–275
Freed G, Fraley J K, Schanler R J 1993 Accuracy of expectant mothers' predictions of fathers' attitudes regarding breastfeeding. Journal of Family Practice 37(2): 148–152
Green J M, Coupland V A, Kitzinger J V 1988 Great expectations: a prospective study of women's expectations and experiences of childbirth. Childcare and Development Group, University of Cambridge, Cambridge
Gregg J 1989 Attitudes of teenagers in Liverpool to breastfeeding. British Medical Journal 299: 147–148
Grossman L K, Fitzsimmons S M, Larsen-Alexander J B, Sachs L, Harter C 1990 The infant feeding decision in low and upper income women. Clinical Pediatrics 29(1): 30–37
Hawthorne K 1994 Intention and reality in infant feeding. Modern Midwife March: 24–28
Health Visitors Association and Royal College of Midwives 1995 Invest in breast together. HVA and RCM, London

Hewat R J, Ellis D J 1984 Breastfeeding as a maternal–child team effort: women's perceptions. Health care for Women International 5: 437–452

Hillervick-Lindquist C 1992 Studies on perceived breast-milk insufficiency: relation to attitude and practice. Journal of Biosocial Science 24(3) (Special Issue): 413–425

Houston M J 1984 Home support for the breastfeeding mother. In: Houston M J (ed.) Maternal and infant health care: recent advances in nursing. Churchill Livingstone, London

Jenner S 1988 The influence of additional information, advice and support on the success of breast feeding in working class primiparas. Child: Care, Health and Development 14: 319–328

Jones D A, West R R, Newcombe R G 1986 Maternal characteristics associated with the duration of breastfeeding. Midwifery 2: 141–146

Kearney M 1988 Identifying psychosocial obstacles to breastfeeding success. Journal of Gynecological and Neonatal Nursing March–April: 98–105

Kearney M, Cronenwett L R, Barrett J A 1990 Breastfeeding problems in the first week postpartum. Nursing Research 39(2): 90–95

Klein D F 1994 Pregnancy and panic disorder. Journal of Clinical Psychiatry 55(7): 293–294

Kreitler S, Kreitler H 1990 The cognitive–motivational determinants of breastfeeding. International Journal of Prenatal and Perinatal Studies 2(2): 161–169

Kurtz Z 1980 Medical and nursing staff attitudes to breast feeding: some implications for health education. Journal of the Institute of Health Education 18(4): 106–112

Laufer A B 1990 Breastfeeding, towards resolution of the unsatisfying birth experience. Journal of Nurse-Midwifery 35(1): 42–5

Lee B 1995 Breastfeeding: report of forum on maternity and the newborn, 27 October 1994. Journal of the Royal Society of Medicine 88(9): 537

Littman H, Medendorp S, Goldfarb J 1994 The decision to breastfeed: the importance of fathers' approval. Clinical Pediatrics 33(4): 214–219

Locklin M P, Naber S J 1993 Does breastfeeding empower women? Insights from a select group of educated, low-income, minority women. Birth 20: 30–35

Lomas P 1967 The significance of post-partum breakdown. In: Lomas P (ed) The predicament of the family. Hogarth Press, London

Losch M, Dungay C I, Russell D et al 1995 Impact of attitudes on maternal decisions regarding infant feeding. Journal of Pediatrics 126(4): 507–514

McCaughan D 1993 The role of the voluntary breastfeeding counsellor in the provision of support for breastfeeding on hospital wards. Master's dissertation, King's College, London

MacIntyre S 1982 Rhetoric and reality: mothers' breastfeeding intentions and experiences. Research and the Midwife Conference Proceedings: 39–62

Newton M, Newton N R 1948 The letdown reflex in human lactation. Journal of Pediatrics 33: 698–704

Niven C 1992 Psychological care for families: before, during and after birth. Butterworth Heinemann, Oxford

Price A, Price B 1995 How do women choose to breastfeed? Modern Midwife May: 10–14

Quandt S 1995 Sociocultural aspects of the lactation process. In: Stuart-Macadam P, Dettwyler K A (eds) Breastfeeding: biocultural perspectives. Aldine de Gruyter, New York

Rajan L 1994 The impact of obstetric procedures and analgesia/anaesthesia during labour and delivery on breast feeding. Midwifery 10: 87–103

Raphael D 1975 Being female: reproduction, power and change. Mouton, The Hague

Raphael-Leff J 1984 Varying needs. Nursing Mirror 158(2): v–vii

Raphael-Leff J 1991 Psychological processes of childbearing. Chapman & Hall, London

Renfrew M J, McGill H R 1996 Enabling women to breastfeed: interventions which support or inhibit breastfeeding: a structured review of the evidence. Unpublished report for the Department of Health, University of Leeds

Rentschler D D 1991 Correlates of successful breastfeeding. Image, the Journal of Nursing Scholarship 23(3): 151–154

Righard L, Alade M O 1990 Effect of delivery room routines on success of first breastfeed. Lancet 336: 1105–1107

Royal College of Midwives 1991 Successful breastfeeding, 2nd edn. Churchill Livingstone, London

Royal College of Midwives 1996 Breastfeeding: coping with the first week. (video) Mark-it Television Associates, Bristol

Shand N, Kosawa Y 1984 Breastfeeding as cultural or personal decision: sources of information and actual success in Japan and the United States. Journal of Biosocial Science 16: 65–80

Smale M 1996 Women's breastfeeding experiences. Doctoral thesis, University of Bradford

Sweeney M A, Gulino C 1987 The health belief model as an explanation for breastfeeding practices in a Hispanic population. Journal of Advanced Nursing Science 9(4): 35–50

White A, Freeth S, O'Brien M 1992 Infant feeding 1990. HMSO, London

Williams E L, Hammer L D 1995 Breastfeeding attitudes and knowledge of pediatricians-in-training. American Journal of Preventative Medicine 11(1): 26–33

Winicoff B, Myers D, Laukeran V, Stone R 1987 Overcoming obstacles to breastfeeding in a large municipal hospital: application of lessons learned. Pediatrics 80(3): 423–433

Wright P 1988 Learning experiences in feeding behaviour during infancy. Journal of Psychosomatic Research 32(6): 613–619

Wylie A 1992 Health service support of breastfeeding. British Medical Journal 305: 523

Wylie J, Verber I J 1994 Why women fail to breastfeed: a prospective study from booking to 28 days post-partum. International Journal of Human Nutrition and Dietetics 7: 115–120

FURTHER READING

Bottorff J L 1990 Persistence in breastfeeding: a phenomenological investigation. Journal of Advanced Nursing 15: 201–209

Bostock Y 1993 Pregnancy, childbirth and coping with motherhood. What women want from the maternity services. Report for the Framework for Action Working Group on Maternity Services, Edinburgh

Harrison M J, Prowse M 1985 Successful breastfeeding: the mother's dilemma. Journal of Advanced Nursing 10: 261–269

Lewis E, Bradley E 1992 Health service support of breastfeeding. British Medical Journal 305: 523

Millard A V 1990 The place of the clock in pediatric advice: rationales, cultural themes, and impediments to breastfeeding. Social Science and Medicine 31(2): 211–221

Raphael-Leff J 1991 Psychological processes of childbearing. Chapman & Hall, London

Widstrom A Breastfeeding: the baby's choice. (video) Dept. of International Health Care Research, Karolinksa Institute, Box 60400, S–104 01, Stockholm, Sweden, or Ace Graphics, PO Box 173, Sevenoaks, Kent, TN14 5ZT

11

Women's experience of postnatal support

Jane Podkolinski

INTRODUCTION

Student: All women need to be pampered after they have had a baby.
Tutor: Why? It is a normal physiological event.

This exchange took place in a seminar between myself and my tutor whilst I was studying for the Diploma in Professional Studies of Midwifery. I made the statement because of:

1. My observations and experience as a midwife working with women at home and in hospital. Many women appeared to be tired and exhausted. It seemed that they had not been made to feel special. They also appeared to gain a sense of achievement from resuming household chores as soon as possible after giving birth.
2. An awareness of traditional rituals in other cultures which enable a woman to recuperate after birth (Jordan 1993, Vincent Priya 1992).

At the time I had no research-based evidence to back up my statement. Therefore I used the opportunity my MSc dissertation gave me to explore it more fully. What follows is a résumé of the work done as part of the MSc study.

Midwifery texts refer to the midwife's role in 'supporting' women both throughout the pregnancy and the postnatal period. Support at both stages is considered to be crucial. Furthermore, the British Government's policy document 'Changing Childbirth' (DoH 1993, p. 38), the principles of which underpin the delivery of maternity services within the National Health Service, refers to the midwife's support role: 'The midwife is able to offer a woman and her family support and encouragement during a time of great change.'

Whilst there appears to be consensus between midwifery experts and policy makers that a notion of support is important to women and their families at the time of childbirth, any detail as to what is considered to constitute the concept of 'support' is glossed over. What is 'support'? Does it include a notion of pampering? What is it that women themselves want in terms of support? Is there a shortfall in the quantity and quality of support that women receive in the postnatal period? It is with these questions in mind that I set out to explore women's experience of postnatal support.

SUPPORT

Childbirth and becoming a mother may be fulfilling experiences for many women but they also involve change and are acknowledged to be stressful events in parents' lives. How parents cope with this transition has come under scrutiny by investigators, and the notion of 'support' has been identified by researchers as a key factor in easing the stressors of that transition.

The dictionary definition of 'support' is 'to give strength to', 'to encourage', 'to keep from falling or sinking or failing'. Studies which have investigated the concept of 'support' around childbirth often refer to the social nature of the support given. Its study has become increasingly popular amongst researchers because of the current belief in the crucial role of social networks and friendship to health. Price (1988, p. 119), a psychiatrist, concludes from her work with women that: 'Young motherhood is often a time of "discovering" female friendship and learning to value its emotional and practical support'.

However, the concept of 'social support' has remained elusive, not easy to define and researchers have struggled to give it a precise meaning. Oakley explored the concept in detail for her own longitudinal study into social support and motherhood. Following her analysis she gives what she refers to as 'a negative definition' (Oakley 1992, p. 144) of the concept, defining it as not being clinical care or health education. However, she does state that it includes listening and being sensitive to women's individual needs. Majewski (1987, p. 400) used the following definition of 'social support' for her own research into social support and the transition to the maternal role: 'Factors that buffer an individual from physiological or psychological consequences that are often present as the individual makes the transition from not being a mother to the maternal role'.

Ball (1987), a midwife, investigated the factors which affect women's well-being postpartum, because she wanted to learn more about their emotional needs as they adjusted to motherhood and how midwives could best help them. She surveyed 279 women and examined the quality of support given by others during the postnatal period, and considered how that could affect postnatal well-being. Her findings identified a 'flexible supportive environment' (Ball 1987, p. 133) to be crucial to the woman adjusting successfully to her new role and found that lack of rest, sleep and social support were significantly related to low emotional well-being. The results of other research also demonstrate that 'social support' in pregnancy and postpartum has an important influence on health outcomes (Majewski 1987, Oakley 1992). Furthermore, research suggests that the benefits of social support intervention can continue to affect the family in a positive way for years in terms of the child's development and health and the mother's physical and emotional well-being (Oakley et al 1996).

POSTNATAL CARE

Research into postnatal care has not been afforded the same level of interest as research into antenatal care and care in labour. The House of Commons Health Committee's report (House of Commons 1992) which preceded that of the Expert Maternity Group (DoH 1993) concluded from the evidence presented to it that there was a lack of research into postnatal care on which to base good practice. Reviews of the available research can be found in Enkin et al (1989) and Alexander et al (1990). They cover various aspects of the physical and emotional care of both the mother and the baby, and mention support in the context of postnatal education and postnatal depression.

New policies are often introduced before being effectively evaluated. For example, early discharge from hospital was introduced in the 1980s, and has been defended in terms of 'women's choice', but in fact was introduced in many units in order to save money. Today many women stay in hospital for no longer than 2 or 3 days after the baby is born and some women leave hospital within 6 hours of the birth. 'Lying-in' periods of 8 days or more are long gone (Towler & Bramall 1986). When early discharge from hospital was introduced the value of 'lying-in' periods, in terms of rest, the support women received from other women and the opportunity for women to be nurtured, were ignored.

Arms (1994) quotes Faye, a mother, grandmother and midwife who mourns the demise of the 'lying-in' period. Faye does, however, acknowledge that there were disadvantages of keeping women in hospital for long periods, for example minimal contact with partners and any other children, and the increased risk of infection. Nevertheless, traditional long postnatal stays did give the women the opportunity for rest and to find support from the *community* of women in the ward and gave permission to mothers to be looked after. Faye summarizes this concept of nurturing neatly by relating it to the notion that 'if you "baby" the mother, the mother will "baby" the baby' (Arms 1994, p. 249).

In today's maternity services there is competition within the service for scarce resources. Examples of the conflicts between priorities are reported in the midwifery press and elsewhere. A victim of this competition has been postnatal care areas (Audit Commission 1997) and many services have seen a reduction in the number of midwives available to support women during this time of change. In hospital the wards are often very busy, understaffed and the women actually get very little support and rest during their hospital stays.

Ball (1987, 1994) as a result of her research into postnatal care, which has been referred to already, recommended changes in the way postnatal care is delivered both in hospitals and the community. A number of the issues she raised in her work were presented as evidence to the House of Commons Health Committee (1992) and influenced the Committee's recommendations for more schemes which offered 'continuity of care' and 'continuity of carer' to women throughout childbirth.

In her analysis Ball (1987) graphically represents the relationship between the various sources of support required by a mother to successfully adjust to motherhood by using a diagram which she refers to as the 'support system deck-chair' (see Fig. 11.1). Family and friends combine to support the new mother. Her personality and life experience affect how she copes. The maternity services, usually the midwife, provide support to the mother, her partner and any other children depending on the requirements of each family. The deck-chair rests on a bed of cultural attitudes, values and beliefs and resources.

Why postnatal care is organized in the variety of ways that it is depends on the prevailing values of the society, which in turn influence decisions about how resources are spent. Some of the cultural rituals for postnatal women in traditional societies recognize that having a baby is a spiritual and social event, and many traditional rituals are practised in order to allow the women to rest following the exertions of childbirth, and to protect from evil spirits (Vincent Priya 1992). In the UK there are no such prescribed periods of rest during which women can make the adjustment to motherhood. Furthermore women are generally required to make their own arrangements for practical help at home during the postnatal period. This will depend on the family and the family's economic circumstances. As recently as the 1950s, for those in poor or difficult circumstances, practical help from 'home helps' – women employed by local councils to provide practical help in the home to families and others in need – was available to mothers (Wynn 1995). Currently in Holland maternity aides are available to look after women and their families in their own homes for 8 days following the birth of the baby. This service enables the women to rest (Beck 1991, Tasharrofi 1993).

Michaelson's (1988, p. 10) anthropological study of childbirth in America identified notions of choice, control and individualism to be the values that generally underpin the way care in childbirth is organized and delivered. This she suggests has led to a widespread lack of social support and the paucity of 'cultural imagery that celebrates birth as a significant life experience'.

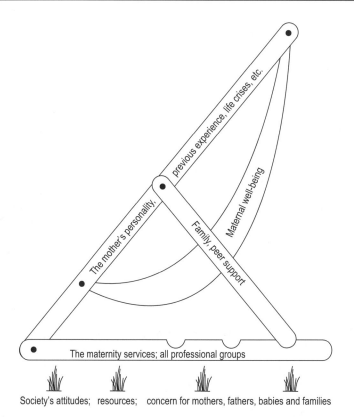

Fig. 11.1 Support system 'deck-chair' (adapted from Ball 1987, p. 121, by permission of Jean Ball).

Indeed it is those same principles which underpin the service here in the UK, as outlined in the document 'Changing Childbirth' (DoH 1993). It is therefore important to consider whether these may have influenced the nature and quality of support which the women receive in the postnatal period.

POSTNATAL 'SADNESS'

The birth of a baby is generally perceived to bring great joy to parents and their families. Pregnancy and parenthood have often been planned and carefully prepared for. However, some women experience feelings of sadness during the postnatal period, which may not be understood by their families, partners and friends, or even by the women themselves. This may make a woman feel abnormal because the birth of a baby is supposed to be a happy event according to a widely held cultural belief as represented by the following quotation from Katharina Dalton 'Babies should bring happiness but if they do not something is wrong' (Dalton 1989, p. 154).

In a society where childbirth is medicalized, women's postnatal 'sadness' is also often medicalized and referred to as 'postnatal depression' (PND). PND is one of three main types of postnatal emotional problems/difficulties. They are 'postnatal blues', PND, and puerperal psychosis. 'Postnatal blues', which is transient, occurs on about the fourth or fifth postnatal day, resolves quickly and affects about 50–80% of women. The main symptoms are tearfulness and emotional lability. PND is a 'nonpsychotic postnatal depression' which occurs in the first few weeks after delivery, is prolonged and affects between 10% and 15% of women depending on the study referred to. The symptoms/experiences of the condition include low mood, poor self-esteem, anxiety, difficulty sleeping and lack of energy. Puerperal psychosis is a psychotic disorder which affects about 0.2% of women. Delusions and hallucinations are a feature of this condition along with mood disturbances which can be high or low. The sufferer may hear voices, she may believe she has special powers, and her general functioning is impaired (Cox 1986).

Much of the experts' attention has focused on PND, because of its debilitating effects on the woman, her family and even on the development of her child which may extend well beyond her own recovery (Murray 1992) and because, unlike puerperal psychosis, it is relatively common. Possible causes of PND are reviewed in the literature (Cox 1986, Gregoire 1995, Romito 1989); they include biological/hormonal, psychological and social factors. However, there is agreement amongst the experts that there is no one cause which is responsible, but rather that the causes are multifactorial, and that there is no one treatment that is effective in all cases. Each case must be assessed individually.

In the 1950s, before researchers became seriously interested in PND, Gordon & Gordon (1959) investigated the impact of women's social history on their adaptation to motherhood. They concluded from their findings that social and environmental factors were significant to a women's postpartum well-being. Subsequent studies have identified poor social support as a contributory factor in the development of PND (Oakley & Chamberlain 1981, Paykel et al 1980, Romito 1989). Gregoire (1995, p. 100) concludes in his review of the literature that the lack of supportive social relationships with partners, families and friends is the common factor that links all three categories of postnatal emotional problems and speculates 'on the considerable importance of this factor, not so much for any specific postpartum psychiatric disorder, but for postpartum mental health generally'.

However, these studies assume that PND, or postnatal sadness is an abnormal response to childbirth. Nicolson (1990), a psychologist, adopted a different approach to the study of PND. Her aim was to contribute to the understanding of women's *normal* postnatal experience. She concluded from her results that PND can be explained within a model of loss and bereavement, so women respond to the change in role, the changes in relationships and the loss of previous identity following childbirth with a grief reaction. This perspective normalizes the sadness which many women feel in the postnatal period, and the expression of grief is seen as an essential process in the return to an equilibrium.

McIntosh's (1993) study focused on the condition itself. She defined depression as: 'the experience of depressed mood for a period of at least 2 weeks at some stage during the first nine months postpartum' (McIntosh 1993, p. 178). Using this definition she found that 63% of her study group had reported feeling depressed during the first 9 months following childbirth and did not seek help for their depressed mood. The women believed that the causes of their depression were social and economic.

These findings suggest that depression can be viewed as a normal response to childbirth, and that the feelings of sadness many women experience in the postnatal period are part of the reality of that experience. One woman who has done much to reveal the reality of women's lives through her research and writings is Ann Oakley. She believes that 'The medicalization of unhappiness as depression is one of the great disasters of the twentieth century' (Oakley 1993, p. 8).

However postnatal sadness is defined or conceptualized, persistent sadness is a painful and difficult experience for the woman and her family, and it is important to explore what role postnatal support can play in reducing the sequelae of this condition.

RITUALS

During the 20th century the escalating medicalization of childbirth and various government reports brought about the transfer of birth from home to hospital. By 1992 hospital was where 98.7% of women had their babies (Campbell & Macfarlane 1994). However, the hospitalization of women in childbirth and the takeover of birth by 'experts' has included ritualized care based on tenets of the biomedical model which ignored the social and cultural context of birth. Such care dehumanized the woman, ignored her individual needs and experience and left her bereft of choice and control. Hence pressure groups such as the National Childbirth Trust (NCT) and the Association for Improvements in Maternity Services (AIMS) challenged the medical profession's control over the birthing process and lobbied for more 'choice' and 'control' for women (Kitzinger 1990). Midwives campaigned for it too. The principles of 'choice' and 'control' are now included in the government's policy document for maternity services (DoH 1993). These developments mean that care ought to be individualized to each woman's needs and circumstances and not standardized regardless of her experience.

Choice and decision-making are important and complex issues, as discussed in Chapter 5. Making decisions and choices can sometimes be both physically and emotionally exhausting and it may be refreshing to have space in which no decisions are required to be made. The use of a ritual is in one sense a way of making space from decision-making. Liedloff (1986, p. 36) defines a ritual as: 'another form of relief from the burden of choice-making . . . The rest refreshes not only the intellect but the entire nervous system. It adds a measure of serenity to the balance against the unserenity brought about by thought'. It is in this sense that some of the postnatal rituals in other traditional cultures offer women space to recuperate from the exhaustion of childbirth (Vincent Priya 1992).

Rituals are part of a rite of passage, and a rite of passage marks the transition from one social role to another. Seel (1986) describes three phases to a rite of passage, namely 'the rite of separation', 'the liminal period' and 'the rite of incorporation'. In the first phase, the rite of separation, the person undergoing the social change is removed from his or her old environment, for example admission to hospital for a woman in childbirth. In the liminal period, those undergoing the change have no status, they are in between roles. Many procedures in hospital rob the labouring woman of her status. Seel (1986) gives the use of monitors and drips and the manner in which women's questions may not be satisfactorily answered as examples of such rituals during this liminal period. The rite of incorporation occurs when the subject adopts his or her new status, in this case as mother. Seel argues that in western cultures the first two parts of the rite of passage are fulfilled by procedures and practices during childbirth. But we fail to complete the rite of passage with any rite of incorporation, which, he maintains, causes unhappiness and which both he and Ugarriza (1992) believe may even lead to PND. The reintegration of the new mother into society is crucial for her to be valued by that society: 'there must be a welcoming climax to the rite of passage. Otherwise the participant is left high and dry, with feelings of alienation and distress' (Seel 1986, p. 184). It is possible, therefore that care which protects women from the anxiety and weariness caused by making choices and being in control, and which allows them to rest may actually be supportive in their postnatal 'journey'.

THE POSTNATAL SUPPORT PROJECT

Having reviewed the literature I defined the aims for my project as follows:

1. to explore women's experience of support in the early postnatal period
2. to highlight their experience of this episode in their lives, and record the cultural reality of their experience
3. to demonstrate what made the postnatal period a good/bad time for women.

One of the first tasks was to find a methodology which best suited the project. A search of the literature suggested feminist methodology as an appropriate approach. The appeal of this methodology was that it is non-hierarchical, interactive, acknowledges feelings and that 'all social knowledge is generated as a part and product of human social experience' (Stanley & Wise 1993, p. 192). The nature of reality would be understood from the female perspective and feminist methodology works towards change (Stanley & Wise 1993, Webb 1993). This methodology seemed to match the aims I had identified for the project:

- I wanted to reflect the reality of women's lives
- I wanted a way of knowing that was alternative to the objective scientific research paradigm
- I did not want to prove anything
- I wanted to include women's experience as a way of knowing
- I wanted to make things better for women.

Furthermore having read the following statement made by Kirkham (1986, p. 35): 'The word "midwife" seems to me to mean in concrete terms exactly what "feminist" means ideologically: with woman', it seemed to be appropriate that a midwife would be using a feminist methodology as a set of assumptions, beliefs and values to underpin a piece of midwifery research.

Three methods of data collection were used for the research, namely a profile questionnaire, self-report diaries and interviews. The questionnaire was completed for each woman participating in the project. It included basic details such as her age; occupation; partner's occupation; number of children and their ages; who was going to help in the immediate postnatal period; and how she intended to feed the baby. The questionnaire was not completed in any formal way, but rather the information was gathered during the course of my contacts with the women.

The self-report diaries and interviews were the main sources of data collection. The women completed the diaries during the first 4 weeks of the postnatal period. They were asked to make an entry in the diary each day for the first week after the birth, and then two or three entries a week for the following 3 weeks. Guidelines for the completion of the diary were included in the front and the women were asked to refer to the questions when they were completing the diary. These questions invited the women to comment on:

- who had supported them, both lay and professional support
- how they had been supported
- what they felt about the support they received

- whether they had felt special
- whether there was anything they would have liked in terms of support which they did not receive.

Whilst these guidelines provided a modicum of structure to the diary the women were encouraged to write whatever they wanted in as little or as much detail as they wished. The diaries were to be returned to the women at the end of the study.

The interviews, which were called 'conversations' to reflect the non-hierarchical interactive nature of the interview appropriate for a feminist approach, took place in the women's homes at the end of the 4-week postnatal period. The conversations were unstructured, although there was a clear focus, namely postnatal support. I had not read the diaries before I came to the conversations with the women, so the content of the interviews added rigour to the data collected from the diaries. Furthermore, for me the researcher they were an opportunity to thank the women for their part in the study; to debrief them of the experience; to identify any related problems which may have required further support from myself or other agencies and to close the relationship.

11 women were recruited to the study. One woman was excluded after the birth because of her distress. I felt it would be too much of a burden for her to consider completing a diary for my study, while she felt so emotionally challenged. Of those 10 women remaining, six of them were having their first baby and four already had children. Further details about the participants are given in Table 11.1.

The validity of the data collected was assessed in terms of its trustworthiness, and triangulation of method was used to establish this (Lincoln & Guba 1985). Cowman (1993, p. 788) defines triangulation as 'a combination of multimethods in a study of the same object or event to depict more accurately the phenomenon being investigated'. This I did using self-report diaries and 'conversations' as methods of data collection. Other ethical considerations, such as consent, confidentiality and the principles of beneficence were dealt with using the feminist perspective to underpin the decisions made.

For the purposes of this chapter the analysis of the data has been organized under four headings. I have used the women's words as much as possible to illustrate a point, but inevitably the requirement to be brief has resulted in the exclusion of some detail from the women's stories. Whilst some of the examples used can only be attributed to individual women and their own individual experience, they may also reflect concerns and experiences shared by other women.

Table 11.1   Profile of the participants in the study

Participant (partner)	Age	Parity	Mode of delivery	Nights in hospital	Help at home during day	For how long
Jane (Peter)	25	2	Normal	2	Partner Mother	Indefinitely 6 days
Sarah (John)	29	2	Normal	1	Partner	Indefinitely
Laura (Brad)	21	1	Normal	0	Mother Partner	10 days 1 week
Julie (Bret)	30	1	Ventouse	2	Partner Parents	2 days 1 week
Wendy (Mark)	25	1	Forceps	4	Partner	1 week
Jennifer (Philip)	24	1	Ventouse	2	Partner Mother	5 days 9 days
Zanna (Harry)	35	4	Normal	3	Partner	14 days
Alison (Steve)	27	1	Normal	3	Partner	1 week
Michelle (Doug)	25	1	Forceps	2	Partner Parents	2 days 1 week
Katy (Sam)	28	2	Normal	1	Mother Partner	3 days 1 week

FINDINGS

Who offers support?

From Table 11.1 it can be seen that at home the women's main source of support for 24 hours a day came from a combination of their partners and their mothers. The length of time that this source of intensive support was available to them varied from 6 to 17 days. For eight of the women in the study the husband was their primary source of support in the immediate postnatal period. The other two women had arranged for their mothers to come and help from the time they arrived home from hospital. Katy's mother was only able to come for 3 days but Laura's mother came to *look after* her and her new baby for 10 days. Reading Laura's diary 'look after' are the operative words here. Zanna had only her husband to help and her eldest daughter who is 14, because she said that from past experience her mother was 'too dogmatic' and more of a 'hindrance' than a help.

All the women identified the midwife as an important source of support both in the hospital and at home. Without exception in those first few days at home, the women mentioned both in their diaries and in the conversations the value they placed on the daily visit from the midwife – most of the women in the study received daily visits from the midwife for the first 10 postnatal days. Some needed and relied on their daily visits more than others and some were reassured by the availability of a midwifery 24-hour 'on-call' service – that is telephone advice and call-out service. Both Zanna and Julie used the 'on-call' service for breast-feeding problems. However, Wendy, who had great difficulty with breast-feeding, did not use the service. She said in her conversation with me, 'Because they [the midwives] came every day to start with, I thought I can cope until tomorrow morning.' The women also commented both in their diaries and in our conversations on the support they received from the maternity care assistants in hospital. These maternity care assistants provide a supporting role to the midwife in hospital. For example Alison wrote in her diary: 'the maternity assistants were always about to help or refer us to a midwife'.

Some of the women received visits from their general practitioners and listed them as a source of support. Other health professionals who were perceived as being supportive in the community were the health visitors. Julie also included the student who visited her with the health visitor as being supportive because she was 'obviously a married mum' (Julie's diary). However, the young student midwife who came with her midwife was not seen as supportive because of her 'young age'.

Other sources of support came from other female relatives, friends and neighbours. However, they were not regular offers of help and most of the women found it difficult to accept their help. Zanna perceived accepting help from other women as 'exploitation'. Julie was simply not used to asking people for help, and others believed they ought to be able to cope on their own.

Other women who were sharing the same experiences at the same time were perceived as supportive. Alison wrote:

I feel supported by those new mothers/fathers within the ward environment. You can guarantee that if you have a certain problem or are feeling a certain emotion then there are two or three more individuals in the same boat.

Julie found the women from her parentcraft group especially supportive and particularly in the postnatal period. In fact it was their support that she 'most valued'. Networking with other women who had babies and/or small children was an important component of the women's support framework. This contact relieved their isolation both in physical and emotional terms.

What type of support – practical or emotional?

In the early days all the women needed practical support with household chores. The help offered included making meals, housework, washing, ironing, shopping, caring for any other children and looking after the baby so that a couple could have space to just be together, or to go Christmas shopping, for example. Partners continued to offer practical help when back at work albeit at a lower level.

The support offered by midwives included:

- information and practical advice on the care of the baby, demonstrating a baby bath and how to change nappies
- advice about how to cope with a crying baby
- encouragement and advice during breast-feeds
- advice about pain relief and self-care.

The midwives also gave praise and reassurance, bolstered flagging confidence, and answered questions and concerns about the baby. The last four features of support in particular, were valued by the women. For example Sarah desperately needed reassurance that 'she was doing well' this time because she was 'depressed' after her first baby. But for Katy it was not reassurance that she needed this time. She commented in our conversation:

I need somebody to do the cooking, the cleaning, walk the dogs and (laughs) . . . but it's just a question of organization.

In fact a number of the women referred to 'organization' and 'routine' as the key to coping with a baby.

Emotional support from partners did not always meet the women's expectations/needs. For example Julie experienced a lack of understanding from her partner, who at 4 weeks after the birth expected her to have recovered and to be ready to leave the baby with someone and to go out to the cinema with him (Julie was breast-feeding and at 4 weeks her baby had not yet regained his birth weight, which was a source of great anxiety to her). Alison's experience was different. She was fortunate to enjoy both the practical and emotional support of her partner and the words she wrote in her diary reflect how important the emotional support was at this time:

I feel emotionally supported by him . . . someone to share my feelings with which is so important at the moment when everything is so new.

Emotional support from other women was welcomed particularly when the partner did not appear to understand. It included sharing experiences, feelings and discovering that they were not alone when they felt tired, tearful and emotionally drained. It confirmed for them that they were not abnormal.

Being made to feel special was perceived as 'support'. For example receiving flowers, cards and presents because as Wendy wrote in her diary, 'it made me feel that everyone was thinking of me.' Visitors were generally welcome and for Alison if they were also parents they were 'supportive, knowing that they had been through the same experience'.

Other small acts were perceived as support in that they made the women feel special. For example Wendy mentions in her diary the 'strip wash' she was given by 'a lady' after the birth. She writes: 'She was very gentle and chatted to me which was nice. I felt much better afterwards . . .'. Also in hospital Laura wrote in her diary:

I was very pleased to find my bath towel, flannels, etc. on radiator to dry. That I thought was an extremely homely and thoughtful gesture. Also stuff out of my bag in cupboard.

Just becoming a mother was enough to make some of them feel special. Jennifer wrote in her diary: 'Today I felt special just because I am a mum'. If the baby was gaining weight and appeared to be settled this also was perceived as support and made the women feel special. Alison wrote:

being able to feed the baby myself . . . I feel a great sense of achievement that I'm able to provide the very best nourishment for him.

What makes the support good/bad?

In the main it was the way in which support was offered and delivered which affected how the women experienced the support. For example in the early days at home Wendy felt her husband was trying to 'impress her' with everything he was doing for them, when she was unable to do anything other than feed the baby, because of breast-feeding difficulties. She wrote:

I felt I needed to do just one thing even if it was to just put the washing out . . . it made me feel that I could do other things as well as just look after him (the baby).

On the other hand her sister, who is also a mother, did the ironing for her. She commented in her diary: 'She didn't make a big deal out of it . . . She was so relaxed'.

There was sometimes a thin line between support being experienced as 'interference' which was unhelpful and support which was helpful. Occasionally help from their mothers was perceived as interference but mothers-in-law were particularly vulnerable to this accusation. Women described them giving inappropriate advice, or advice that had not been asked for. They were also sometimes perceived as being too dominant or threatened their daughter-in-law's ability to cope.

The support offered by the professionals, particularly the midwives in hospital, was also not immune from criticism. The amount of support offered was right for some and not others. For example Laura asked for help to sort her baby out when he had a very dirty nappy. She was left for half an hour whilst the midwives' handover was completed. She would have appreciated more prompt assistance:

I thought this was disappointing and would have very much liked someone to help sort him out sooner.

Furthermore, when she wanted to go home earlier than the hospital midwives thought suitable for a first-time mother, she found their care, offered in the guise of support, to be intrusive and inappropriate. This suggests that it is unhelpful to categorize women as 'first-time mothers' and to make assumptions about the type of support they need, rather than listening to them as individuals. Alison's experience of what sounded like a similar level of support was different. She wrote in her diary:

the amount of support was about right – the staff have always been around but not too intrusive, letting us do things in our time and space.

The women censured the midwives' attitudes and described how they affected the experience of support. Michelle felt the midwives in the hospital made her feel 'stupid' and 'silly'. When she asked someone to help her change a nappy on her first night after the birth, she wrote in her diary: 'She (the midwife) looked at me as if I should have got on with it myself'. This experience discouraged her from asking for help again. Wendy commented in her diary about a midwife who showed her how to change a nappy: 'She was a bit bossy and sarcastic'. Zanna found midwives' emphasis on breast-feeding to be unhelpful as she felt it induced 'guilt' in the mother. However, she found the friendly atmosphere in hospital supportive.

The long length of the visits offered by community midwives was appreciated. Women described it as 'brilliant', 'excellent'; 'she didn't seem to rush her visits and made me feel I had all the time I needed'. Wendy enjoyed the health visitor's visits. She wrote:

She's really friendly and helpful. She makes little jokes and comments which makes it more relaxing and less worrying.

Care offered by doctors received a mixed reception when considering support, which was again often due to some women being made to feel inadequate or stupid.

Feeling special and acknowledgement by others of what they had gone through was important to the women. Having visitors contributed to this by marking the birth of the baby. However, sometimes visitors were a mixed blessing, overstaying their welcome and handing the baby round from person to person 'like a little toy' (Wendy's diary), contributing to feelings of tiredness and distress. Wendy would have welcomed more 'strict' visiting hours in hospital to control their excesses. On the other hand Zanna had no visitors and this made her feel depressed.

Katy's partner did not give her the recognition she needed 'of the difficulty' that she had been through in the birth (Katy's diary). For her this second baby was a more exhausting labour and birth than her first child. Her partner thought it was easier. This made her feel 'robbed' when she did not get enough 'sympathy'.

If Laura and Wendy's stories of their homecoming with their babies are compared it appears that having someone at home who has previous experience of babies and whom the mother trusts can make a difference. Wendy, who had only her husband to help, recorded their feelings in her diary 'we were both really scared'; on the other hand Laura, whose mother was at home on her return from hospital, wrote 'I knew I'd be safe'.

Do women want/need support postnatally?

All the women regardless of whether it was their first or a subsequent baby anticipated some change in their lives after the birth of the baby and expected to need some support during the postnatal period. They had all made their own arrangements for support as described earlier. All the women in the study commented on the impact the arrival of a new baby had on their lives. Their comments included not just the obvious physical changes but also the emotional and psychological effects which influenced their feeling of well-being. The first-time mothers in particular were surprised by the extent of the change. They referred to the new skills they needed to learn to meet the physical needs of a baby and how their relationships with the partner, other family members and friends were all affected. They also referred to the loss of self-esteem, blows to confidence, changes in appearance, the isolation of being at home with a baby and loss of control over their time. These feelings led to unhappiness, which was exacerbated by tiredness, but improved when they had enough sleep and the baby thrived. In our conversation Julie said:

I didn't anticipate feeling so overwhelmed by the baby . . . when you first come home and you cry all the time and I never thought I would feel like that. People said that is what happens, but you have to feel it, experience it to believe it really . . .

At 5 weeks after the birth Julie was still struggling to cope. She had refused most offers of help from friends because she thought she should be coping and her husband thought she should be over it, but in her diary she wrote:

I think more information should be thrust at men, as Bret doesn't seem to understand what I'm feeling. It's all I can do to wash up the breakfast dishes each day. I would value more support and understanding from him as this adds more emotional stress to an already difficult time.

Wendy referred to the change as 'a completely different lifestyle'. Zanna, who had just had her fourth baby, said:

It is the continual dependency of a baby that is the hardest thing, along with very little sleep . . .

Katy, who had given birth to her second baby, summed up the women's feelings when she said:

I think a lot of women say it's not going to affect me. I won't change. I'll still be the same person. But you're not. It is hard. It is a huge . . . it's an enormous change . . . your second baby's another change again, another big change.

Without exception the women needed support during the postnatal period, but the length of time the women needed support and the type of support that was needed varied between women. No single 'support package' could meet each woman's needs. They were all very individual. For example Julie still needed a high level of both practical and emotional support particularly from her partner 4 weeks after the birth, but it was not forthcoming. Katy and

Zanna would have welcomed more practical help with household chores and child care. Sarah needed frequent reassurance that she was coping.

Community midwife and health visitor visits did not help to relieve the isolation and physical and emotional exhaustion experienced by some. Also, when the midwife discharges a woman from her care at 28 days following the birth it is often assumed by others that the woman should have recovered from the birth. For those that established a routine early, they began to feel that they were beginning to cope with the demands a new baby brings. But for some, help in terms of practical and emotional support beyond 4 weeks would have been welcomed. The popular notion that women were meant to cope alone led to offers of help from family and friends tailing off and prevented the women from either accepting help or asking for it.

DISCUSSION

'Having a baby changes everything, both within and around a woman. Nothing is the same again and that overwhelming unfamiliarity is frightening to even the most capable and supported of people' (Price 1988, p. 126). The women's experience of 'support' in this study gives a glimpse of the differences between women in their experiences. Those differences can be attributed to the differences in their experience of birth, different relationships with relatives and friends, different personal beliefs and values, and different personalities. These differences may account for my finding that some women appear to cope better than others despite similar levels of 'support'.

However, despite the differences, the women had a shared experience. They all commented on the change having a baby had brought to their lives. They discussed the change both in terms of the gains and the losses they experienced from their change in role. They had all expected some change and therefore anticipated needing some support. Apart from the support the women had from the professionals, they had all organized support at home for the immediate postnatal period. In all cases the partner was involved in providing that support. However, the support given by partners did not always meet the women's physical and emotional needs and the women sought support, particularly emotional support, from other women. It did not matter whether they were relatives, friends or professionals. If they had a shared experience it gave the women reassurance and support in the sense that they were not alone or abnormal in their feelings. Such supportive relationships with other women were not what some of the women in the study had expected, but they are what they valued. This is akin to the notion of 'companionship' which Oakley (1992) refers to in her search for a definition for 'social support'. Furthermore these relationships helped the women understand their own experience in the absence of any formal rite of passage.

Change is about 'loss', and not just loss associated with death and bereavement (Marris 1974). The women talked about 'loss' and several had periods of unhappiness in the 4-week postnatal period under study. Bowlby (1980) argued that for loss to occur attachment needs to have taken place and 'grief' is the emotional response to loss (Jacob 1993). Attachment need not be with an individual but can also occur with images, fantasies and lifestyle. Therefore it is not unusual for a new mother to assess her new situation in terms of loss and her response to be the sadness which is normally associated with grief.

Ball's (1987) diagram the 'Support system deck-chair' reproduced in Figure 11.1 is a useful tool to facilitate a deeper understanding of how these findings could affect the women's experience of support. If the cultural beliefs and values on which Ball's deck-chair rests were changed, and the women's postnatal experience viewed both in terms of gains and losses, as Nicolson (1990) suggests, then it should follow that the nature of support offered to them would be affected. Instead of society believing that having a baby is solely a happy time for new parents and that unhappiness means that the woman is depressed, the unhappiness should be recognized as a normal response to the change in role and more should be done to acknowledge that change than the mere giving of cards and presents. The support may include appropriate rituals to complete the rite of passage which Seel (1986) believes are so important to postnatal emotional well-being.

The medicalization of childbirth, the transfer of birth from home to hospital, and the framework of society built around the nuclear family mean that the 'experts' have replaced the 'mothers' of the past. Family and friends often do not know how to respond to the needs of new parents and the 'rituals' they adopt are the hallmark of a capitalist and materialistic society. The midwife has the potential to be a key player in bringing about change to these cultural attitudes, expectations, values and beliefs. She could set an example to the rest of a woman's support network, indeed society generally, by enabling women, indeed giving them permission, to ask for help. Midwives could facilitate women's own support networks, make women feel special, ensure that they know they need not cope alone, pamper and nurture them and allow them mental space from the pressures of day-to-day living by supporting them in an appropriate way whilst they are in our care. As midwives we have the privilege to *listen* to women's stories, to *know* the reality of their lives and to be in a position to make things better for them.

CONCLUSION

Now let me return to my original statement 'Women need pampering after they have had a baby'. If I replace 'pampering' with 'mothering' and understand 'mothering' as 'support' in terms of 'nurturing', companionship, women sharing experiences, knowledge and skills, which is what the women in the study needed, then my original statement gains credibility.

However, my study also highlights that issues of 'mothering' or 'support' are very complex, and how it is experienced will depend not only on the needs of the helped, but also on the perceived motivations of the helper. There is a need to strike a balance between supporting the new mother and enabling her to achieve things herself, just as any parents do with their children as they grow to independence.

Obviously the study has its limitations, in particular the transferability of its findings to other women's situations. However, the findings could be used and applied where deemed appropriate on the judgment of the user (Lincoln & Guba 1985). Perhaps some of the ideas generated from the data can be tested by readers on others' experience and be of value in offering an interpretation of that experience.

Key points for caregivers

- The postnatal period should be viewed in terms of loss as well as gain, and this time should be acknowledged more formally as a rite of passage, the successful completion of which is considered to be crucial to women's emotional well-being.
- It is important to consider the role of the midwifery advanced practitioner and other caregivers not solely in terms of technical skills but also in terms of nurturing/caring skills. These latter skills were those of midwives in the past, but owing to the combined influence of the development of technology and midwifery training moving to higher education these caring skills may well have been devalued.
- The role of maternity care assistants within the service should be considered in terms of the support that they can offer women because of a 'shared experience' and a 'mothering' role which women may find of value. Their role in the community is currently under study (Kargar 1997).
- The content of midwifery courses should be reviewed to ensure that they include a cultural perspective on midwifery as well as sociological, psychological and medical perspectives, because it too has a role in determining society's beliefs and values which affect how we care.
- The maternity service is constantly under review to find opportunities for making savings. Therefore midwives must be clear about what the aims and objectives of postnatal care are so that they know and can argue for which parts of the service they wish to defend against any sweeping cuts.
- In many areas selective visiting by midwives as opposed to daily visiting has become the norm in the first 10 postnatal days, and there may be no midwifery visits offered beyond 10 days. These changes in policy may well have been led by the economic demands of the service rather than the needs of the women. Midwives must be able to defend to those who shape the service the frequency and length of their postnatal visits in terms of the needs and the long-term well-being of the women in their care.

REFERENCES

Alexander J, Levy V, Roch S (eds) 1990 Postnatal care: a research-based approach. Macmillan Education, London

Arms S 1994 Immaculate deception II: a fresh look at childbirth. Celestial Arts, Berkley, California

Audit Commission 1997 First class delivery: improving maternity services in England and Wales. Audit Commission Publications, Abingdon

Ball J A 1987 Reactions to motherhood: the role of postnatal care. Cambridge University Press, Cambridge

Ball J A 1994 Reactions to motherhood: the role of postnatal care, 2nd edn. Books for Midwives Press, Hale, Cheshire

Beck M 1991 Independent midwifery in Amsterdam. Midwives Chronicle 104(1238): 72–75

Bowlby J 1980 Attachment and loss Vol 3 Loss: sadness and depression. Penguin, Hogarth Press, London

Campbell R, Macfarlane A 1994 Where to be born? 2nd edn. National Perinatal Epidemiology Unit, Oxford

Cowman S 1993 Triangulation: a means of reconciliation in nursing research. Journal of Advanced Nursing 18: 788–792

Cox J L 1986 Postnatal depression: a guide for health professionals. Churchill Livingstone, London

Dalton K 1989 Depression after childbirth, 2nd edn. Oxford University Press, Oxford

Department of Health 1993 Changing childbirth: report of the Expert Maternity Group. (Cumberlege Report) HMSO, London

Enkin M, Keirse M J N C, Chalmers I 1989 A guide to effective care in pregnancy and childbirth. Oxford University Press, Oxford

Gordon R E, Gordon K K 1959 Social factors in the prediction and treatment of emotional disorders of pregnancy. American Journal of Obstetrics and Gynaecology 77(5): 1074–1083

Gregoire A 1995 Hormones and postnatal depression. British Journal of Midwifery 3(2): 99–103

House of Commons 1992 Health committee second report: maternity services. (Winterton Report) HMSO, London, vol 1

Jacob S R 1993 An analysis of the concept of grief. Journal of Advanced Nursing 18: 1787–1794

Jordan B 1993 Birth in four cultures, 4th edn. Waveland Press, Illinois

Kargar I 1997 Winter National Meeting. Midwifery Matters 72: 26–30

Kirkham M 1986 A feminist perspective in midwifery. In: Webb C (ed) Feminist practice in women's health care. Wiley, Chichester

Kitzinger J 1990 Strategies of the early childbirth movement: a case-study of the National Childbirth Trust. In: Garcia J, Kilpatrick R, Richards M (eds) The politics of maternity care. Clarendon Press, Oxford, ch 5

Liedloff J 1986 The continuum concept, 2nd edn. Penguin Books, Harmondsworth

Lincoln Y S, Guba E G 1985 Naturalistic inquiry. Sage, London

McIntosh J 1993 Postpartum depression: women's help-seeking behaviour and perceptions of cause. Journal of Advanced Nursing 18: 178–184

Majewski J 1987 Social support and the transition to the maternal role. Health Care for Women International 8: 397–407

Marris P 1974 Loss and change. Routledge, London

Michaelson K L 1988 Childbirth in America: anthropological perspectives. Bergin & Garvey, Massachusetts

Murray L 1992 The impact of postnatal depression on infant development. Journal of Child Psychology and Psychiatry 33: 543–562

Nicolson P 1990 Understanding postnatal depression: a mother centred approach. Journal of Advanced Nursing 15: 689–695

Oakley A 1992 Social support and motherhood: a natural history of a research project. Blackwell, Oxford

Oakley A 1993 Beyond the yellow wallpaper. In: Oakley A Essays on women, medicine and health. Edinburgh University Press, Edinburgh

Oakley A, Chamberlain G 1981 Medical and social factors in postpartum depression. Journal of Obstetrics and Gynaecology 1: 182–187

Oakley A, Hickey D, Rajan L, Rigby A 1996 Social support in pregnancy: does it have long-term effects? Journal of Reproductive and Infant Psychology 14: 7–22

Paykel E S, Emms E M, Fletcher J et al 1980 Life events and social support in puerperal depression. British Journal of Psychology 136: 339–346

Price J 1988 Motherhood: what it does to your mind. Pandora, London

Romito P 1989 Unhappiness after childbirth. In: Chalmers I, Enkin M, Keirse M (eds) Effective care in pregnancy and childbirth. Oxford Medical Publications, Oxford, vol 2, ch 86

Seel R 1986 Birth rite. Health Visitor 59(6): 182–184
Stanley L, Wise S 1993 Breaking out again: feminist ontology and epistemology, 2nd edn. Routledge, London
Tasharrofi A 1993 Midwifery care in the Netherlands. Midwives Chronicle 106(1267): 286–288
Towler J, Bramall J 1986 Midwives in history and society. Croom Helm, London
Ugarriza D N 1992 Postpartum affective disorders: incidence and treatment. Journal of Psychosocial Nursing and Mental Health Services 30(5): 29–32
Vincent Priya J 1992 Birth traditions and modern pregnancy care. Element Books, Shaftesbury
Webb C 1993 Feminist research: definitions, methodology, methods and evaluation. Journal of Advanced Nursing 18: 416–423
Wynn M 1995 Has there ever been a better time to have a baby? Modern Midwife 5(2): 37–38

FURTHER READING

Ball J A 1994 Reactions to motherhood: the role of postnatal care, 2nd edn. Books for Midwives Press, Hale, Cheshire
Majewski J 1987 Social support and the transition to the maternal role. Health Care for Women International 8: 397–407
Nicolson P 1990 Understanding postnatal depression: a mother centred approach. Journal of Advanced Nursing 15: 689–695
Oakley A 1992 Social support and motherhood: a natural history of a research project. Blackwell, Oxford
Vincent Priya J 1992 Birth traditions and modern pregnancy care. Element Books, Shaftesbury

12

Men becoming fathers: 'Sometimes I wonder how I'll cope'

Jo Sullivan-Lyons

INTRODUCTION

In this chapter I will be outlining and discussing some of the literature about fathers and fatherhood. I will also be describing some findings of a study I am undertaking into the mental health of fathers in the transition to fatherhood. Maternity care is generally seen as the care of the mother and her baby, and so it may seem surprising to have a whole chapter devoted to fathers in a book of this kind. Indeed, until recent times there was very little interest in the needs of fathers. Whilst there has been some research into the importance of fathers in relation to their partners during pregnancy, labour and in the postnatal period, much of the research about fathers is focused on absent fathers. The difficulties that may be created for women and children when a father is not available, or willing, to take an active part in their children's lives, are undoubtedly important. The number of single-parent families in Great Britain has tripled since 1972 and 20% of all children now live in single-parent families, mainly headed by women. However, the majority of children live in *two*-parent families, and live with both their parents. Consequently, it is vital that researchers begin to focus their efforts on examining fathers who are present, as well as absent, and it is with this in mind that the chapter has been written.

The experiences of men as they become fathers is a very broad topic, and it is not possible to cover all aspects of this topic in one chapter. Consequently this chapter focuses on specific aspects, namely men's psychological health in pregnancy, during childbirth and after the birth, and their physical health during pregnancy, including the couvade syndrome. I highlight the issue of how we can measure or assess men's psychological health and how men and women differ in the way they express psychological distress. The chapter ends with a discussion of the caregiver's role in working with men in the perinatal period. Other chapters in this book cover some of the other important aspects of the partner's role, needs and experiences before and after childbirth.

THE MEN BECOMING FATHERS STUDY

I will be discussing some of the research that I have carried out looking at the needs of first-time expectant fathers, in relation to their physical and psychological health. This study collected data during pregnancy from couples expecting their first child and the sample population came from a general hospital in South London. 30 couples were approached consecutively at the routine antenatal scan in the 18th week of pregnancy, and none refused to participate. Participants completed postal questionnaires consisting of an affect balance scale, a depression inventory, a health questionnaire, a measure of the relationship between themselves and their partner, and an assessment of their satisfaction with their lifestyle, with particular reference to housing, financial position, distribution of household chores and employment.

The data from these questionnaire responses were analysed using SPSS (a statistical computer package) and where a statistically significant result occurred I shall refer to it as a 'difference'. In addition to the questionnaires, 10 of the couples were also interviewed. The man and his pregnant partner were interviewed separately, in their own home, about how they felt that things were going to change or stay the same once their baby was born. Various aspects of their lives were discussed including housing situation, financial position, their relationship with their family, and also with their partner, and their feelings about their health. The couples were also asked about their experiences of maternity and paternity care. Interviews took place between the 21st and 24th weeks of pregnancy and the quotation in the title of this chapter comes from one of the men I interviewed. However, this chapter will mainly focus on the information collected from the postal questionnaires.

MEASURING PSYCHOLOGICAL HEALTH

This section outlines some general points about the use of questionnaire measures with men and women, with specific reference to the measures used in the Men Becoming Fathers Study. The use of questionnaires to assess mood and mental health has increased considerably over the past 10 years, with caregivers using questionnaires to assess whether clients are at risk of a particular disorder. Self-report questionnaires allow the individuals to report their symptoms directly and allow professional time to be used effectively by identifying those clients who are most at risk of a particular condition. It must be remembered, however, that the majority of questionnaires are not designed to diagnose illness. Most depression questionnaires, for example, are designed to highlight those clients who appear to be most at risk of depression, but that does not mean that other clients are not suffering from depression, or that all those clients highlighted by the questionnaires are depressed. Questionnaires must always be used in conjunction with a face-to-face assessment by the caregiver.

Depression questionnaires

Caregivers are naturally interested in being able to assess whether people are depressed. A common method of doing so is to ask clients to complete self-report questionnaires that can be scored by the caregiver. By comparing a person's score with the standard scores in a normal population it is possible to assess the likelihood that the person is depressed. There are numerous depression questionnaires available, some measuring only depression (e.g. Beck Depression Inventory); some measuring both anxiety and depression at the same time (e.g. Hospital Anxiety and Depression Inventory); and some that assess psychological symptoms on a variety of dimensions (e.g. SCL-90, General Health Questionnaire). In the Men Becoming Fathers Study, I used both the Hospital Anxiety and Depression Scale (HADS), and the 28-item version of the General Health Questionnaire(GHQ-28). Half the subjects completed the HADS, the other half the GHQ-28, with both members of a couple completing the same questionnaire. Both questionnaires have been validated for use amongst several different populations including for use with pregnant women (Kitamura et al 1994).

Hospital Anxiety and Depression Scale

This 14-item questionnaire measures anxiety and depression by using two seven-item scales and was developed by Zigmond & Snaith (1983). The advantages of the HADS are that it is short and that people find it easy to complete and understand. Despite its name, the HADS has been validated for use with people in the general population.

General Health Questionnaire (28-item)

The GHQ-28 assesses psychological health using four subscales: social dysfunction, severe depression, anxiety and somatism (Goldberg & Hillier 1979). There are several forms of the GHQ, and the GHQ-28 was chosen for this study because it assesses anxiety and depression separately. This allowed response differences between the HADS and the GHQ-28 to be compared and any differences between men and women, in responses to the two questionnaires, to be examined.

Edinburgh Postnatal Depression Scale

The Edinburgh Postnatal Depression Scale (EPDS) is a 10-item self-rating depression scale, widely used by professionals investigating the mental health of women in the transition to parenthood. The EPDS was developed by Cox et al (1987) and has been found to be effective in identifying women with severe depression, but less effective at identifying women with minor depression (Murray & Cox 1990). It is quick and easy to administer and it can be presented in a variety of languages and formats.

Although the EPDS was originally validated for use with women in the postnatal period, it is now used with other populations including pregnant women and fathers (both antenatally and postnatally). Unfortunately the EPDS has not been thoroughly validated for use with these populations and this may lead to spurious and misleading results. Thorpe (1993) examined the use of the EPDS with mothers and fathers outside the postpartum year by looking at the incidence of depression in parents of toddlers. Although there appeared to be satisfactory validity for the EPDS with mothers, the number of measured cases of depression in fathers was too small for any definitive evaluation to be made of the validity of the EPDS with this group. Although it is possible that fathers of children in this age group do not suffer from depression, it seems more likely that the type of questions asked by the EPDS simply did not have sufficient sensitivity for measuring depression in fathers.

The EPDS should be used with caution when exploring psychological problems in parents. Firstly, it should be remembered that it was developed and validated for use in postnatal populations of women, and it has not been adequately validated for use with antenatal women, and neither has it been properly validated for use with fathers. It is for these reasons that the EPDS was not suitable for my study. Care must be taken to ensure that the EPDS is suitable for the task for which it is being used, and caregivers must be wary of using the EPDS as a diagnostic tool in populations outside those for which it was intended.

Affect Scale

Bradburn (1969) developed the Affect Balance Scale to measure the levels of positive and negative affect (feelings or mood). The 18-item questionnaire asks people about how they have been feeling in the past few weeks, how they are interacting with other people and how cheerful they have been feeling. The Bradburn Affect Balance Questionnaire consists of two scales: one scale asking about negative affect, for example 'Have you felt annoyed with someone?' 'Have you felt lonely or remote from other people?'; and the other scale asks about positive affect, for example 'Have you felt that you were really enjoying yourself?' 'Have you felt confident about the future?'. Usually the scores on the positive and negative affect scales are combined to give a measure of psychological well-being, although the scores on the two scales can be used separately. Bradburn suggested that positive and negative affect could be used as indicators of psychological well-being. The two scales were found to be statistically independent, and the implication of this is that positive and negative feelings influence well-being in different ways. This statistical independence has been found consistently (Warr et al 1983). I used the Bradburn Affect Balance Scale to explore whether men and women differ in the extent to which they express positive and negative feelings, and in how willing they are to express emotion.

Psychosomatic symptoms

Illnesses and pain that, whilst real in terms of the symptoms experienced by the individual, originate not from physical disorder but as a result of mental distress, are described as psychosomatic. It must be remembered that, firstly, even if the origins of an illness are psychological, the symptoms experienced by the patient can be extremely unpleasant. Secondly, symptoms that appear to have no physical origin can provide an insight into the mental health of a person, even in the absence of clinical features of depression or other psychological problems. The link between psychological problems and psychosomatic symptoms is so strong that many depression and anxiety questionnaires ask people to report these types of physical symptoms (Watson & Pennebaker 1989).

In the Men Becoming Fathers Study, the participants were asked to indicate if they had been diagnosed as suffering from any persistent health problems such as high blood pressure, heart trouble, stroke, chronic bronchitis or asthma, arthritis or rheumatism, liver trouble, epilepsy, diabetes, tuberculosis, stomach ulcer, gall bladder trouble or hernia. The participants were also asked to report any symptoms in the past few weeks such as frequent pains in the legs, pains in the heart or heaviness in the chest, frequent headaches, constant coughing or frequent heavy chest colds, trouble breathing or shortness of breath, swollen ankles, repeated pains in the stomach, paralysis of any kind, stiffness or aching in any joint or muscle, pains in the back, or getting tired in a very short period of time. It should be noted that some of the psychosomatic symptoms in the second list are the kind of discomfort that many women suffer from whilst pregnant. This explains, in part, why the pregnant women in this study suffer from significantly more of these symptoms than their male counterparts ($p = 0.05$). Although research suggests that women tend to report more psychosomatic symptoms than men anyway

(Popay et al 1993), some or all of the sex difference found in pregnancy could be due to the physical changes of pregnancy.

SEX DIFFERENCES

Differences between men and women in terms of their expressiveness, and their psychological and physical health are known to be important in the aetiology and diagnosis of illness. It is generally accepted that men are less expressive of both psychological and physical symptoms (Mirowsky & Ross 1995, Vingerhoets & Van Heck 1990) and this undoubtedly affects the diagnosis of mental and physical illness. Traditionally, women have used health services more than men, but men are more likely to die prematurely and have a shorter life expectancy than women. Pregnancy is a time when a woman can expect her health to receive particular attention, and yet this is not the case for men, even though both parents may be experiencing similar strains on their psychological health. In this section I will be highlighting some general points about sex differences. It is worth noting that studies rarely report sex differences found during analysis of data, and this raises questions about whether researchers take the issues created by sex differences seriously enough.

Depression and expression of affect

In the Men Becoming Fathers Study, I examined sex differences in the rates of depression, and in the expression of affect, in the sample of first-time expectant mothers and fathers.

It is well documented that women appear to experience depression more often than their male counterparts. Pajer (1995) concluded that women were twice as likely as men to suffer from depression. This sex difference in the rate of depression persists across many countries and historical evidence suggests that women have always appeared to experience depression to a greater extent than men (Weissman et al 1993). It is also widely accepted that men tend to be less expressive than women, and that men express less affect than women. It has also been suggested that women report significantly more negative affect than men (Fujita et al 1991).

I examined sex differences in the prevalence of depression in this group of first-time expectant parents, as well as sex differences in the expression of positive and negative affect.

The hypotheses for this part of the study were that:

1. Women will report more positive affect, negative affect and total affect than men.
2. There will be a significant difference between the numbers of men and women who are depressed, and that it will be women who are more likely to be depressed.

Table 12.1 Means for expression of negative affect

Sex	Number	Mean
Male	20	2.8
Female	22	5.09

The minimum score on this scale is 0, and the maximum possible score is 9.

Completed questionnaires were received from 22 women and 20 men. Independent samples t tests were used to explore sex differences in the expression of affect. There were no differences between men and women in the reporting of total affect expressed ($p = 0.06$) but there was a trend in the data to suggest that men express less affect than women. There were also no sex differences for the expression of positive affect ($p = 0.34$). However, there was a difference in the reporting of negative affect ($p < 0.001$), with women expressing more negative affect (see Table 12.1).

Finally, a chi-squared test was conducted to see if women were more likely to be depressed than men (if depression was more associated with being a woman than being a man). The scores from the GHQ-28 and the HADS depression scale were categorized as not depressed, depressed, and severely depressed. The outcome of the chi-squared test was that there were no sex differences for the self-reporting of depression.

No difference in the total affect expressed or in the rates of depression were found in this group of first-time parents. These results suggest that it is not always the case that women express more affect than men, or that women are more likely to be depressed than men. For this sample of first-time parents at least, the only significant difference was for the amount of negative affect expressed, with women expressing significantly more than their male counterparts.

It is possible that since the men and women in this sample are both going through similar psychological stresses that some of the sex differences that are usually reported in the expression of affect and incidence of depression do not occur. This supports the idea that the origins of depression are often social in nature (Brown & Harris 1978) and that the causes of depression are not necessarily different for men and women.

Sex differences and depression questionnaires

The content of different depression questionnaires is usually very similar, with typical questions asking people about how worthwhile they feel they are, how they are relating to other people and how they are feeling physically. The fact that depression questionnaires are so similar in their content may give the impression that there is one unified theory of the characteristics of depression, but this is not the case.

I have two main criticisms of these questionnaires. Firstly, my research shows that there is a significant association between a person's score on a depression questionnaire and the total amount of affect expressed ($p = 0.01$). Men generally express less affect and consequently they will always appear to be less depressed than women. The second criticism is that another factor that is significantly associated with a person's score on a depression questionnaire is the amount of negative affect they express ($p = 0.01$). Since men express considerably less negative affect than women, they will never appear to be as depressed as women when depression questionnaires are used to assess psychological health.

From the wording of the questions in depression questionnaires, it could be argued that what the questionnaires measure is actually the amount of negative affect that individuals express. It would be over-simplistic to suggest that depression is really just expressing a lot of negative feelings, and it is much more likely that depression is characterized by a person experiencing more negative feelings, as well as fewer positive feelings. It is quite possible that, since men do not express feelings or approach the completion of depression questionnaires in the same way as women (Page & Bennesch 1993), men may express decreasing amounts of emotion the more depressed they become. Consequently lack of expressed feelings could be as good an indicator of depression in a man as expressing lots of negative feelings are in a woman.

Couvade

Fathers-to-be who suffer from physical symptoms related to their partner's pregnancy are said to be exhibiting characteristics of the couvade syndrome or 'sympathetic pregnancy'. I examined the prevalence and characteristics of physical symptoms in my sample of first-time expectant fathers and the results suggest that 'couvade' could be seen as an expression of anxiety.

The couvade syndrome has been described from the psychodynamic, anthropological, biological and social crisis viewpoints (Elwood & Mason 1994) and some of the common somatic symptoms that have been highlighted in this context are indigestion, increased or decreased appetite, weight gain, diarrhoea or constipation, headache and toothache (Klein 1991).

Estimates of the prevalence of the syndrome among fathers vary from around 10% to as high as 61% (Khanobdee et al 1993). First-time fathers are known to suffer from more physical symptoms than experienced fathers or married men who are not fathers (Teichman & Lahov 1987), but men's physical symptoms do not always exactly mimic those of their pregnant partners.

There is evidence of a relationship between levels of psychosomatic symptoms and anxiety (Hiller et al 1995) and one of the hypotheses in the Men Becoming Fathers Study was that the psychosomatic symptoms men suffered from during their partner's pregnancy would be positively associated with the level of anxiety experienced by these men.

The 20 men in this study completed the health questionnaire described earlier to measure both physical disorders and the level of psychosomatic symptoms. Half the participants also completed the Hospital Anxiety and Depression Scale (n = 10), and the other half completed the General Health Questionnaire 28-item (n = 10). All of these questionnaires were completed between the 18th and 22nd week of their partner's pregnancy.

65% of these first-time fathers were suffering from physical symptoms. Statistical analyses showed that there was a significant correlation between the number of reported psychosomatic symptoms and the GHQ anxiety and insomnia subscale ($p < 0.05$). There was also a tentative relationship between the number of physical symptoms reported by men and scores on the GHQ depression scale ($p < 0.09$). There were no associations between reported physical symptoms and either of the HADS anxiety or depression subscales.

The results outlined here indicate that psychosomatic symptoms exhibited in the couvade syndrome could possibly be an expression of anxiety and depression in expectant fathers. In this context, the GHQ-28 seems to be a more sensitive measure for men than the HADS. Since worry and physical symptoms are known to be related, further work should explore the role of worry in the association between psychosomatic symptoms and anxiety in first-time fathers, perhaps using a worry scale such as the Worry Domains Questionnaire (Tallis et al 1992).

Men's psychological health after the birth

There is an abundance of literature examining the phenomenon of postnatal depression in women. These studies generally find rates of around 15% of women becoming depressed at some point after the birth of their child and around 6% of women suffering from a major depressive episode. However, many of these studies find depression in women whose children are as old as 20 months. It is vital that as researchers we consider carefully what constitutes the term *postnatal* and it seems to be appropriate to define postnatal as the period of 1 year after childbirth (Atkinson & Rickel 1983).

Several risk factors have been identified that increase the risk of women suffering from postnatal depression. A poor marital relationship, negative life events, lack of social support, previous psychiatric history and poor housing are all risk factors that have been consistently found to be associated with the development of postnatal depression.

It is only in recent times that researchers have begun to examine whether men might suffer from postnatal depression too. Ballard and colleagues (1994) examined the prevalence of postnatal depression in 200 postnatal couples and found 9% of fathers were depressed at 6 weeks postpartum, and 5.4% were depressed at 6 months postpartum. The literature relating to fathers' health after childbirth shows men do suffer unpleasant physical and psychological symptoms postnatally, as well as during their partner's pregnancy. Ferketich & Mercer (1989) found that men's perception of their health status was significantly poorer at 8 months after the birth of their baby, than during their partner's pregnancy, or during early postpartum. Similarly Quill et al (1984) found that, although men visited the doctor more after the birth than during the pregnancy, the types of physical symptoms experienced by these men did not change over time.

RELATIONSHIP

The couple relationship between a man and a women is an important indicator of their psychological and physical health and a robust association between depression and marital distress has been demonstrated (Beach et al 1994). It is generally accepted that where one member of the couple is depressed, the other is more likely to be depressed and report lower satisfaction with the relationship. For example, Ballard et al (1994) found that if a woman is depressed in the postnatal year, her partner is significantly more likely to be depressed. Difficulties in the couple's relationship are associated with postnatal depression, both on their own and in combination with other factors. However, one criticism of the research into the association between depressive illness and relationship difficulties is that studies have not established the direction of the association. That is, it could be that feeling depressed causes relationship difficulties or alternatively, that relationship difficulties increase people's feelings of depression.

Zaslow et al (1985) found that 62% of first-time fathers reported experiencing depressed mood at some point after the birth of their baby. Hossain et al (1994) found that 3- to 6-month-old infants of depressed mothers interacted more with their non-depressed fathers than with their mothers. This study suggested that non-depressed fathers may buffer the effects of infants having depressed mothers and highlights the need for caregivers to find ways of supporting fathers with depressed partners.

It is vital that caregivers encourage both parents of the child to discuss any difficulties they may be having, both as a couple and individually, in the transition to parenthood.

Birth attendance

In the past two decades men attending the birth of their child has become increasingly accepted. Although there are no official government statistics, in a study 98% of the men taking part said that they intended to be present during their partner's labour (Royal College of Midwives, unpublished, 1994).

The suggestion in the early 1960s that fathers should be encouraged to attend the birth of their child, was initially rejected because the medical profession believed that the presence of the father in the labour room would increase infection rates, men would be likely to faint, and the fathers might disagree and contradict the advice of the doctor (Brown 1982).

Interest in the father's experience of labour and birth is relatively recent (Nichols 1993). Hall (1993), suggests that the benefits for the labouring woman of her partner attending the birth have yet to be conclusively demonstrated. What is clear is that women who have a birth partner, in addition to the midwife and obstetrician, report less pain, are less likely to require an epidural, need less medication and have shorter labours (Niven 1985). Much of the research in this area focuses on the benefits for the woman, but not the impact that attending the birth has on the father of the baby.

Draper (Draper J, University of Hull, personal communication, 1996) found that birth attendance is the culmination of months of preparation for fatherhood. Men express their wish to be close to their labouring partners and to see the birth of a new life. From an anthropological viewpoint, being at the birth of his baby can confirm the man as the father of the baby (Seal R, author, personal communication, 1995). Fathers often report that attending the birth facilitated a close relationship with the child and that it makes it easier for them to be involved in the day-to-day care of their baby (Palkovitz 1987).

It should be noted that fathers attending births is not universally supported. There is some concern that men may inhibit the labouring women, and if there are problems in the couple's relationship, emotional and physical support may be difficult to give and take (Draper J, University of Hull, personal communication, 1996). The woman may feel she has to support a reluctant partner, or one who finds it difficult to cope with the sight of his partner in pain (Hall 1993). It has also been suggested that attending the birth of his baby may cause problems for the father himself and does not necessarily help the father to establish positive father–infant relationships. Whilst it seems clear that women benefit from the presence of a birth companion, whether it is necessary for this to be the father of the baby is uncertain. It may be that women are more effective as birth companions than men. Further, whether attending the birth is a beneficial experience for the father of a baby is very unclear.

CAREGIVER'S ROLE IN WORKING WITH FATHERS

As we move towards the next century, the economic and social structures of Great Britain and other industrial countries are changing dramatically. The number of part-time jobs, and double-income families, is ever increasing. More companies now offer paternity leave, as well as endeavouring to provide more flexibility in work practices to allow fathers to fulfil their role as parents. These changes mean that men have more opportunity to be involved in the day-to-day care of their babies.

In this section I will be offering suggestions to caregivers about how they can reinforce the role of fathers, and encourage men to see themselves not just as providers, but also as parents. The theme that comes from all the literature about men becoming fathers is that men need not just to be educated about the practicalities of pregnancy and parenting, but also to be given opportunities to ask questions and talk about how they are feeling in an environment in which their contributions are valued.

The main times when maternity caregivers have contact with fathers are during ultrasound scans in pregnancy, at antenatal classes, at the birth and during postnatal visits.

Scans

Antenatal scanning has now become routine in Great Britain and many other countries, with the majority of pregnant women scanned between the 16th and 20th week of pregnancy. 16 of the 20 men in the Men Becoming Fathers Study attended their partner's scan, and they could be observed afterwards admiring the picture produced of the baby, often stroking and touching the photograph, and it was almost always the man who took responsibility for the care of the photo by putting it in a place of safety. It appeared from the fathers' reactions that attending the ultrasound scan offers an experience that induces a real sense of involvement in the pregnancy. However, the men in my study were rarely informed directly that they were welcome to attend the scan appointment, and they often asked whether they were 'allowed' to attend the scan. It would be helpful if hospitals could mention in the appointment letter, and midwives at the booking appointment, that partners are welcomed at the scan. By doing this, from the very first contact with the hospital, fathers would be made to feel involved.

Antenatal classes

Antenatal classes offer the opportunity for parents to meet and make social contact with other parents at the same stage of pregnancy. However, all the men interviewed in the Men Becoming Fathers Study reported that they had had unpleasant experiences at the antenatal classes. Some reported feeling that the midwives did not want them there, others that they felt that by showing videos of birth at the first class the midwives were trying to embarrass the fathers. Both the men and women indicated that the men did not ask many questions at these classes, mainly because of not wishing to appear ignorant about pregnancy and labour, but also because they felt embarrassed to do so. These findings are very similar to those of Barbour (1990) who found that little opportunity was given to fathers to have informal discussions with other fathers, and that men felt awkward talking about personal matters in front of the predominately female audience.

Hospitals often run antenatal classes during working hours, which limits the possibility of men attending since fathers are not generally given time off work to attend antenatal appointments. However, it may be that antenatal classes organized for the benefit of pregnant women are not the most appropriate setting for men to ask questions and talk about any worries they have about the pregnancy, labour or becoming a father. Caregivers could consider having parallel sessions for fathers where they may feel less intimidated by the presence of women. Caregivers must be wary of their efforts to include fathers becoming tokenistic. Fathers need to be made to feel welcomed at classes, whatever the organization of these might be, and they must be helped to feel that they are involved in the pregnancy not only for the benefit of their partner and baby, but also for themselves.

Childbirth

Men who attend the birth of their baby are becoming the norm and men who do not attend the birth are often viewed with suspicion by the medical and midwifery professions (Draper J, University of Hull, personal communication, 1996). They are expected to provide emotional and physical support to their labouring partner, often with little or no 'training'. Fathers are sometimes viewed by midwives and doctors as helping them in their task, and women sometimes view their partners as mediators between themselves and their caregivers. However, the father attending the birth of his child also has needs of his own. He can be unsure about when and how to assert himself on behalf of his partner, and can perceive himself as a hindrance to the health professionals attending his partner. Furthermore, men can find it distressing to see their labouring partner in pain and can feel totally inadequate in their ability to help.

Providing information about the biology of childbirth is only the beginning of the support that men may need in order to benefit from attending the birth of their child. Whether or not the woman has a birth partner, and who this birth partner is, must be an informed choice made by the expectant couple. Whatever their decision, caregivers should remember that parents whose emotional needs have been fulfilled are far more likely to find the transition to parenthood a positive experience. Men's fears about attending the birth of their child are often dismissed by caregivers and women alike by comparing his anxieties with the pain and exhaustion suffered by the labouring woman. This only serves to encourage men not to talk about their concerns, and increases the possibility of the birth becoming a distressing experience for them. Caring for the father, both before and during the birth, will not necessarily increase the workload of caregivers, because providing the man with appropriate support enables him to help and support his partner to the maximum benefit of both them and their baby. Caregivers need to ask men before and during the birth if they understand everything that is happening, if they would like to help their partner with pain relief by using massage and alternative methods of pain relief, if there is anything with which they would like to be particularly involved, such as the cutting of the umbilical cord, and whether they have any questions. Offering practical suggestions will encourage a man to feel capable in the support of his partner, and may help him to discuss his own feelings.

Men and postnatal depression

Caregivers are generally aware of the need to identify postnatal depression in new mothers. Recent evidence has suggested that children whose mothers are depressed can have long-term difficulties (Sharp et al 1995), and since partners are often simultaneously suffering from psychological problems, it is vital that fathers are considered to be an important influence on the overall environment into which an infant is born.

There are factors that seem to predispose women to postnatal illness and there is no reason to suppose that these influences do not impact on the father. As men are not always present during postnatal visits and, if they are present, they often tend to hover in the background, caregivers can encounter problems in establishing how men are coping with the transition to fatherhood. However, women's reports of their partner's psychological and physical health have been found to be reliable (Briscoe 1980) and Lemmer (1987) emphasizes the need to sensitize caregivers to the needs of fathers. This can particularly focus on the couple's adjustment to pregnancy, their expectations of birth and the physical and emotional needs of fathers during early parenting. Caregivers can enquire how the woman's partner is, whether he seems to be enthusiastic about the baby, if he has been suffering from any health problems, and how the couple's relationship seems to be going.

Caregivers should be particularly aware of the fact that a man who appears completely uncommunicative may be as depressed as a man who is expressing depressive feelings. Encouraging men to talk about their feelings can be difficult, especially since societal pressure dictates that men should not express emotion and that they should be 'strong'. Men can find it more acceptable to be suffering from a physical illness than a psychological problem and caregivers should bear this in mind when dealing with fathers. Minor physical complaints in fathers should be acknowledged carefully by caregivers.

Caregivers could consider the possibility of setting up groups specifically for men in the transition to parenthood. These may be invaluable for men whose partner's are depressed, and for men who are depressed themselves.

> **Key points for caregivers**
>
> - Although men do not appear to suffer from psychological problems to the same extent as women, this may be an artefact of the questionnaires typically used to measure anxiety and depression. Whilst depression inventories can give useful information about problems that people may be having, caregivers should always use information collected in this way in conjunction with a face-to-face assessment. Further, caregivers should ensure that questionnaires are only used with people for which the questionnaire has been validated.
> - Men tend to be less emotionally expressive of emotion than women, but may express emotional problems by increased levels of physical symptoms. Caregivers should try to find out how the baby's father is feeling, either by encouraging him to talk directly, or by asking his partner to report how he is coping. Caregivers should also consider that people who are having psychological problems do not always express them, and that a lack of feeling can be as indicative of psychological problems as a person expressing depressive symptoms.
> - Parenthood is not a universally positive experience and many mothers and fathers suffer from unpleasant physical and psychological symptoms both during pregnancy and after the baby is born. Caregivers should deal sympathetically with men during the transition to fatherhood by encouraging them to ask questions and feel involved in the process of becoming a parent, not only as a support to their partner, but also for their own benefit.
> - The couple's relationship has an important influence on men and women's physical and psychological health. Caregivers should encourage parents to discuss their relationship, both individually and as a couple. Becoming a parent is an enormous change in the lives of men and women. Caregivers should ensure that they do not appear to dismiss the effect these changes have on men, by comparing them to the changes in women's lives when they become mothers.
> - Caregivers should involve men throughout the transition to fatherhood. During pregnancy, men could be encouraged to attend the routine antenatal scan. Antenatal classes need to be organized so that men can attend if they wish to do so, and the content of these classes should be designed so that information and support is accessible to men, as well as to women. Men should be encouraged to consider carefully their role during labour, and this process can be supported by caregivers both before and during labour. Caregivers can continue to offer support for men postnatally by building on the relationship that has already been established between caregiver and father during pregnancy.

REFERENCES

Atkinson A K, Rickel A U 1983 Depression in women: the postpartum experience. Special issue: social and psychological problems of women: prevention and crisis intervention. Issues in Mental Health Nursing 5: 197–218

Ballard C G, Davis R, Cullen P C, Mohan R N, Dean C 1994 Prevalence of postnatal psychiatric morbidity in mothers and fathers. British Journal of Psychiatry 164: 782–788

Barbour R 1990 Fathers: the emergence of a new consumer group. In: Garcia J, Kilpatrick R, Richards M (eds) The politics of maternity care services for childbearing women in twentieth century Britain. Oxford University Press, Oxford, ch 11

Beach S R H, Smith D A, Fincham F D 1994 Marital interventions for depression: empirical foundation and future prospects. Applied and Preventative Psychology 3: 233–250

Bradburn N M 1969 The structure of psychological well-being. Aldine, Chicago

Briscoe M E 1980 Sex differences in psychological well-being. PhD Thesis, University of London

Brown A 1982 Fathers in the labour ward: medical and lay accounts. In: McKee L, O'Brien M (eds) The father figure. Tavistock Publications, New York

Brown G W, Harris T 1978 Social origins of depression. The Free Press, New York

Cox J L, Holden J M, Sagovsky R 1987 Detection of postnatal depression: development of the 10 item Edinburgh Postnatal Depression Scale. British Journal of Psychiatry 150: 782–786

Elwood R W, Mason C 1994 The couvade and the onset of paternal care: a biological perspective. Ethology and Sociobiology 15: 145–156

Ferketich S L, Mercer R T 1989 Men's health status during pregnancy and early fatherhood. Research in Nursing and Health 12: 137–148

Fujita F, Diener E, Sandvik E 1991 Gender differences in negative affect and well-being: the case for emotional intensity. Journal of Personality and Social Psychology 61: 427–434

Goldberg D P, Hillier V F 1979 A scaled version of the General Health Questionnaire. Psychological Medicine 9: 139–145

Hall J 1993 Attendance not compulsory. Nursing Times 89: 69–71

Hiller W, Rief W, Fichter M M 1995 Further evidence for a broader concept of somatization disorder using the Somatic Symptom Index. Psychosomatics 36: 285–294

Hossain Z, Field T, Gonzalez J, Malphurs J et al 1994 Infants of depressed mothers interact better with their non depressed fathers. Infant Mental Health Journal 15: 348–357

Khanobdee C, Sukratanachaiyakul V, Gay J T 1993 Couvade syndrome in expectant Thai fathers. International Journal of Nursing Studies 30: 125–131

Kitamura T, Shima S, Sugaware M, Toda M A 1994 Temporal variation of validity of self rating questionnaires: repeated use of the General Health Questionnaire and Zung's self rating depression scale among women during antenatal and postnatal periods. Acta Psychiatrica Scandinavica 90: 446–450

Klein H 1991 Couvade syndrome: male counterpart to pregnancy. International Journal of Psychiatry in Medicine 21: 57–69

Lemmer C 1987 Becoming a father: a review of nursing research on expectant fatherhood. Maternal Child Nursing Journal 16: 261–275

Mirowsky J, Ross C E 1995 Sex differences in distress: real or artefact? American Sociological Review 60: 449–468

Murray D, Cox D L 1990 Screening for depression during pregnancy with the Edinburgh Depression Scale (EPDS). Special issue: psychiatric disorders associated with childbearing. Journal of Reproductive and Infant Psychology 8: 99–107

Nichols M R 1993 Paternal perspectives of the childbirth experience. Maternal–Child Nursing Journal 21: 99–108

Niven C 1985 How helpful is the presence of the husband at childbirth? Journal of Reproductive and Infant Psychology 3: 45–53

Page S, Bennesch S 1993 Gender and reporting differences in measures of depression. Canadian Journal of Behavioural Science 25: 579–589

Pajer K 1995 New strategies in the treatment of depression in women. 147th annual meeting of the American Psychiatric Association: special challenges and strategies in the treatment of anxiety and mood disorders. Journal of Clinical Psychiatry 56: 30–37

Palkovitz R 1987 Fathers' motives for birth attendance. Maternal–Child Nursing Journal 16: 123–9

Popay J, Bartley M, Owen C 1993 Gender inequalities in health: social position, affective disorders and minor physical morbidity. Special issue: women, men and health. Social Science and Medicine 36: 21–32

Quill T E, Lipkin M, Lamb G S 1984 Health seeking by men in their spouse's pregnancy. Psychosomatic Medicine 46: 277–283

Sharp D, Hale D F, Pawlby S, Schmuker G et al 1995 The impact of postnatal depression on boys' intellectual development. Journal of Child Psychology and Psychiatry and Allied Disciplines 36: 1315–1336

Tallis F, Eysenk M W, Mathews A 1992 A questionnaire for the measurement of nonpathological worry. Personality and Individual Differences 13: 161–168

Teichman, Lahov 1987 Expectant fathers: emotional reactions, physical symptoms, and coping styles. British Journal of Medical Psychology 60: 225–232

Thorpe K 1993 A study of the use of the Edinburgh Postnatal Depression Scale with parent groups outside the postpartum period. Journal of Infant and Reproductive Psychology 11: 119–125

Vingerhoets A J, Van Heck G L 1990 Gender, coping and psychosomatic symptoms. Psychological Medicine 20: 125–135

Warr P B, Barter J, Brownbridge G 1983 On the independence of positive and negative affect. Journal of Personality and Social Psychology 44: 644–651

Watson D, Pennebaker J W 1989 Health complaints, stress and distress: exploring the central role of negative affectivity. Psychological Review 96: 234–254

Weissman M M, Bland R, Joyce P R, Newman S et al 1993 Sex differences in rates of depression: cross national perspectives. Special issue: toward a new psychobiology of depression in women. Journal of Affective Disorders 29: 77–84

Zaslow M J et al 1985 Depressed mood in new fathers: associations with parent–infant interaction. Genetic, Social and General Psychology Monographs 111: 133–150

Zigmond A S, Snaith R P 1983 The hospital anxiety and depression scale. Acta Psychiatrica Scandinavica 67: 361–370

FURTHER READING

Bothamley J 1990 Are fathers getting a fair deal? Nursing Times 86: 68–69

Duncan D 1995 Fathers have feelings, too. Modern Midwife 5: 30–31

Edey L 1992 Fathers and pregnancy: the changing face of fatherhood. Midwifery Matters 55: 5–6

Lewis C, O'Brien M 1987 Reassessing fatherhood: new observations on fathers and the modern family. Sage, London

Marks M, Lovestone S 1995 The role of the father in parental postnatal mental health. British Journal of Medical Psychology 68: 157–168

13

Teenage motherhood: experiences and relationships

Catherine Dennison   John Coleman

INTRODUCTION

In the UK, as in many other countries, the perceived social and economic consequences of teenage motherhood are currently the subject of much discussion and debate in political and media arenas. Teenage motherhood is widely seen as a 'problem' in contemporary society. A 'deficit' model of teenage parents has been constructed, whereby they are portrayed as sexually promiscuous, over-reliant on state benefits, irresponsible and possessing poor parenting skills. Though a substantial amount of research has focused upon the issues surrounding teenage parenthood, much of this has only served to reinforce negative stereotypes. This chapter aims to illustrate that such images of young mothers are misplaced and inaccurate; the reality is much less simplistic. The experiences, motivations and, indeed, aspirations of these women varies greatly. This chapter will focus particularly upon the relationships of young mothers and the impact that the presence or absence of support from those around them has upon their experiences of early motherhood.

It is necessary at the outset to place teenage parenthood in the wider context of adolescent sexuality. Findings from the past decades point to the fact that teenagers are becoming sexually active at an increasingly young age (Wellings et al 1994). Estimates suggest that around half of UK 16-year-olds and 80% of 19-year-olds have had their first sexual experience, whilst one in four males and one in six females have intercourse before they are 16 (Breakwell & Fife-

Schaw 1992, Wellings et al 1994). Earlier physical maturity, greater availability of contraceptives and societal pressures are all assumed to have contributed towards this increase (Hudson & Ineichen 1991).

Greater levels of involvement in sexual activity during the teenage years appear to be combined with high levels of contraceptive non-use. One study found that 50% of teenagers reported not using contraception the first time they had intercourse (Ineichen 1986). A lack of knowledge about reproduction and contraception, difficulties in obtaining contraceptives (Winn et al 1995), combined with characteristic adolescent risk taking, may be important factors in explaining such findings. Increasing attention is being paid to exploring the situational and attitudinal aspects also influencing contraceptive use and non-use (e.g. Abraham & Sheeran 1994).

All these findings lead us to the conclusion that unprotected sexual activity is now common amongst teenagers; thus the risk of pregnancy is real for a large proportion of young women in this age group (Moore & Rosenthal 1993). In England and Wales the conception rate for all young women under the age of 20 was 58.6 per 1000 in 1994 (OPCS 1997). Though significantly lower than the peak levels of the mid 1970s, teenage conception rates increased during the 1980s (OPCS 1997). As a response to this, the UK government singled out rates of teenage pregnancy as a cause for concern in its 'Health of the Nation' white paper (DoH 1992). This report set down targets to lower the number of conceptions in those under 16. From the 1989 baseline rate of 9.5 conceptions per 1000, the Government aims to reduce rates by at least 50% by the year 2000. Official statistics suggest that the numbers of teenage conceptions have over the past decade begun to show initial signs that the upward trend is being halted. Indeed the most recent years have seen initial signs of a decline becoming apparent (see Table 13.1). This may, to some degree, reflect the success of programmes instigated as a result of 'Health of the Nation'. However, signs of this downward trend began before the initiative and it is as yet far from clear that this will be a continuing trend.

Within the figures presented in Table 13.1 there are major differences in the conception rates according to the age of the young woman (see Table 13.2).

Table 13.1 Conceptions to teenagers in England and Wales (from OPCS 1997)

Year	Total (thousands)	Conception rate per 1000 women aged 15–19
1971	133.1	81.5
1981	115.2	57.1
1990	115.1	69.0
1991	103.3	65.1
1992	93.0	61.7
1993	86.7	59.6
1994	85.0	58.6

Table 13.2 Rates of conceptions to teenagers in England and Wales by age (from OPCS 1997)

Age	Rates per 1000 women					
	1984	1990	1991	1992	1993	1994
Under 14	1.0	1.3	1.3	1.2	1.2	1.3
14	5.5	6.5	6.6	5.9	5.9	6.1
15	19.1	21.5	19.8	19.0	18.1	17.8
16	41.8	46.3	43.4	41.0	39.6	40.3
17	61.2	69.4	65.3	61.0	60.7	61.0
18	77.6	89.2	84.6	80.8	77.8	78.1
19	89.2	100.5	95.6	91.3	89.1	88.3

The majority of conceptions occur in those over 16, the age of sexual consent. The proportion of 'schoolgirl mothers' is small. It is important to note that whilst the rate of conceptions in the 15- to 19-year-old age range has been decreasing since 1990, rates in those aged 14 and under have remained largely unaffected (OPCS 1997).

What proportion of these pregnancies lead to a maternity?

With the availability of legal abortion, the UK has seen termination become an increasingly common option for dealing with 'unwanted' pregnancies. Medical terminations have been the most frequent outcome for those under the age of 16 since the 1970s, with latest figures suggesting that around half of conceptions to this age group resulted in abortions, compared to around a third in those aged 16–19 (OPCS 1997). This trend is mirrored in the US, Australia and other parts of the world where abortion is also legal.

In part as a consequence of increased access to abortion, maternity rates have declined slightly over the last 20 years. From a high in 1971 of 51 births per 1000, current statistics suggest that there are approximately 28 births per 1000 women under 20 (OPCS 1996). In 1995, 41 900 babies were born to teenagers in England and Wales, representing 6.5% of all births (OPCS 1997).

Reviewing these statistics, it would appear that teenage pregnancy cannot realistically be described as an 'epidemic'. Indeed rates of pregnancy show signs of decreasing rather than increasing. We must at this stage add the caveat that the UK still has one of the highest rates of births to young women in the western world, exceeded only by the US. Rates have fallen much more sharply in many other European nations. For example, between 1976 and 1986, the teenage fertility rate had halved in several countries, amongst them Denmark, Sweden, West Germany and the Netherlands (Werner 1988). There are many lessons to be learnt from countries such as the Netherlands, where attitudes towards, and policies on, sex education, contraception and sexuality, in general, are a great deal more progressive.

SOCIAL AND ECONOMIC VARIATIONS

Though informative, the 'rates' of conception and pregnancies we have presented mask great variations due to geography, social and economic conditions and ethnic group. The incidence of teenage pregnancy differs between geographical regions, and also within them. In the UK, conception rates are highest amongst those in urban areas, whilst those in more rural areas have rates below the national level (Babb 1993). Several studies have shown a strong association between socio-economic status, incidence of teenage pregnancy, and maternity rates. Those from lower status families have both higher rates of pregnancy and higher rates of those who take the pregnancy to full term (Hudson & Ineichen 1991). Reviewing the current situation, Babb (1993) draws the conclusion that 'the highest levels of teenage births occur to the most socio-economically disadvantaged women'.

In the US all demographic statistics are routinely broken down by colour and ethnic group, and findings have shown it to be black women who are most likely to become teenage mothers. In Britain, there are no such national figures to illustrate if ethnic group differences are present. Phoenix (1991) suggests that a marked difference might not be expected here as young black and white people attend the same schools, live in the same areas, share the same friends and have many of their cultural practices in common. However, Phoenix does acknowledge that black and white people occupy different economic positions within society and that this is likely to affect how people live, and may have an impact upon rates of teenage pregnancy.

A commonly held belief is that large numbers of young women living in disadvantaged circumstances deliberately plan their pregnancies in order to make financial or material gains in the form of welfare payments and access to subsidized or council housing. This stereotype is challenged by the findings of several research studies which show little or no support for this idea (Clark 1989, Phoenix 1991). In fact, in Clark's (1989) study, which asked young mothers about their reasons for getting pregnant, such suggestions were met with disbelief 'It seemed laughable and tragic to them that anyone would "use" a baby to get a flat or house' (p. 11). Though several young women do report 'planning' their child, it appears that it is not due to such simplistic economic reasons, but to more complex social and psychological factors. The vast majority are, however, 'accidental' pregnancies (Macdonald & Skuse 1996, Phoenix 1991).

An important question to explore is, therefore, why do some young women choose to continue with a pregnancy and become parents whilst others have the pregnancy terminated or choose to have the child adopted? The available evidence points to it being younger teenagers, those from higher socio-economic backgrounds, and those with higher educational and occupational ambitions, who are most likely to have terminations. Peer, parental and partners' attitudes towards abortion have an impact, as do the religious beliefs held. The finding that teenagers are less likely than older women to have abortions in the earlier months of pregnancy alerts us to the issue of the possible psychological consequences of having a termination. Young women may develop an attachment to their baby and suffer feelings of loss and regret after the event. Few studies have looked at the long-term impact of abortion on the teenager; however, Sharpe (1987) argues that although most cope well, they may experience recurrent periods of guilt or depression. Having access to good counselling support is essential, though not always present.

Adoption is becoming increasingly unpopular as an option for dealing with an unwanted pregnancy. Pregnant teenagers commonly express disbelief at how anyone could 'give their child away', and how they would always wonder what happened to the child, what the child looked like, etc. Thus, if abortion is discounted, the remaining option is to continue with the pregnancy and to become a parent. For many this may not be a real choice: some young women realize that they are pregnant too late to have an abortion; others may avoid thinking about the pregnancy, or informing others, until the legal deadline has passed.

Though much stigma still remains, over the past decades society has increased in its tolerance of teenage, and single, motherhood. In stark contrast to the early 1970s few births to women under the age of 20 now occur inside marriage. Though the percentage varies greatly across the age range, the stereotypical image of the 'shotgun wedding' seems to be disappearing with only 17% of births to teenagers now occurring to married teenage women, compared with 74% in 1971 (Babb 1993). The numbers of births registered solely in the name of the mother has, however, increased only slightly in recent years, reflecting in part the wider societal trend towards cohabitation rather than marriage. Both cohabitation and marriage are more likely to be options for older adolescents; very few young women under the age of 18 share the same address as their child's father around the time of birth. The young woman is most likely to remain in the parental home for the duration of her pregnancy and at least the first months of her child's life (Phoenix 1991) and the younger the mother the more likely this is to be the case (Cooley & Unger 1991, East & Felice 1996, Spieker & Bensley 1994). Obviously, it must be remembered that the experiences and needs of a school-girl mother, drawing primarily on the support of her parents, will be in contrast to that of a mother of 19, married or cohabiting, with her own home; both women are, however, referred to as 'teenage mothers'.

Over the past two decades a wealth of material, both academic and popular, has addressed the topic of teenage pregnancy and motherhood. However, most of this originates from the US. Relatively little research has been carried out which looks specifically at the British context. Though there are exceptions (e.g. Clark 1989, Phoenix 1991), much of what has been done tends to support the view of teenage motherhood as a 'social problem', stressing negative impacts upon the health of both mother and child, the detrimental effect on the young woman's life chances and negative outcomes in terms of the development and well-being of the child.

In this vein, several research reports have isolated various psychological and social characteristics that they have found to be commonly related to teenage pregnancy. Studies, both in the UK and elsewhere, have shown that teenage mothers are more likely than non-parenting peers to have lower self-esteem, and to lack purpose in life (Barth et al 1983). Commonly they are seen as being alienated from their own mother, who was herself likely to have been a teenage parent (Birch 1987, Simms & Smith 1986). Previous to having their child they were more likely to be low achievers at school and have a history of school non-attendance or delinquency (Furstenberg et al 1989). Those with little chance of success in education and employment are portrayed as 'choosing' to become pregnant, or failing to take the precautions necessary to avoid it.

The factors that increase the risk of pregnancy continue to have negative effects on the adolescent mother after the birth of her child (Chase-Lansdale et al 1991). They are more likely to be dependent on state benefits and to live in poor housing (Simms & Smith 1986); it is more likely that they will drop out of school and not go to college or university. They are less likely to find stable and well-paid employment.

Though few studies have been conducted into the outcomes for the children of adolescent parents, existing findings seem to suggest that these children are at a disadvantage compared to those born to older mothers (Furstenberg et al 1987). They have been shown to suffer greater ill-health and be at greater risk of abuse and neglect (Burghes & Brown 1995). They are more likely to exhibit behavioural problems and suffer educational disadvantages that extend well beyond the early years (Furstenberg et al 1987, Hudson & Ineichen 1991).

Explanations for these findings look to the age of the young woman and make assumptions of immaturity and limited knowledge and experience (Moore & Rosenthal 1993). A number of studies have shown the parenting skills of young mothers to be of a poorer quality than those of older mothers. As the following illustrates, 'ignorance' of what makes for good mothering is seen as a major causal factor: 'The infants of young mothers – who themselves have had little in the way of stimulation and positive attention – are not victims of planned cruelty, but rather of innocent omissions on the part of their parents' (Hudson & Ineichen 1991, p. 105).

Young mothers are seen to have a less responsive style of parenting and to offer their children less verbal, and more physical, stimulation. Evidence suggests that such forms are those less likely to result in optimal social and cognitive development in the child.

Recent work has, however, shifted in focus somewhat and has begun to challenge the validity of the negative representations of teenage mothers found in the media, political circles, in research and among some health and welfare professionals. Such changes may reflect differing methodologies or samples. The resulting paradigm shift has resulted in a less pessimistic portrayal of young mothers as a group which, in the main, copes well with motherhood, often under very difficult circumstances (Phoenix 1991, Schofield 1994).

A number of authors have now begun to look at the social and material circumstances in which young mothers live as explanation for any negative consequences of adolescent mothering. Such conclusions are based upon the findings of research which has compared the children of adolescent and older mothers, whilst holding socio-economic factors constant. They have shown little difference between the experiences of teenage mothers and those who become mothers in their early 20s, living in similar economic and material circumstances (Phoenix 1991). The risk of physical complications surrounding the birth has been shown to be only slightly higher in teenage mothers compared with more mature women (DoH 1994). Factors related to a teenager's psychological well-being have been shown to be more strongly related to the context in which she lives, than to whether or not she is a parent (Barth et al 1983).

The work of sociologist Anne Phoenix has been notable in its contribution to current debates. Her work examined the experiences of 80 young women who became pregnant between the ages of 16 and 19, following them from late pregnancy until just before the child's second birthday. She found that they formed a heterogeneous group in terms of ethnicity, employment and educational backgrounds and in their reasons for having children. They were, however, all linked by a common experience of poverty. Findings from Phoenix's study showed that the majority of young mothers she spoke to felt that they loved their child and held their child's needs as priority, often sacrificing their own food and clothing in order to provide for their children.

Looking at the life chances of these women, Phoenix (1991) concludes, rather than being caused by early pregnancy and motherhood, the outlook for most of the teenage mothers in her study was rather dismal before the birth of their child. For example, most had experienced failing examinations, had dropped out of school and had found it difficult to find permanent jobs. Therefore, she argues, simply looking to chronological age for explanation of any negative outcomes is inadequate. Factors such as social class and poverty are of equal, if not greater, importance. The young women would have had little to gain by delaying the time of birth of their first child.

Few studies have examined the long-term effects of adolescent parenthood for both mother and child. What is known is that there are substantial obstacles to continuing education (Dawson 1994) and entering employment after the birth of their baby. Longitudinal studies have, however, shown significant disparity between the life courses of young mothers. One such study (Furstenberg et al 1987) followed 300 low-income black young mothers living in Baltimore, USA, over a period of 17 years from 1967. By the time these women had reached their mid-30s a great deal of variation in the educational and employment outcomes was apparent. More than two-thirds were employed, while about a quarter were receiving welfare payments. One-third had gained some form of post-secondary level education, while 5% had attended college. More recent research confirms that many women are able to overcome the barriers, do return to education and eventually find work and become self-supporting (Furstenberg et al 1989)

SOCIAL SUPPORT

The presence of social support for pregnant and parenting teenagers has been shown to ameliorate many of the negative effects of adolescent motherhood (Barth et al 1983, Furstenberg & Crawford 1978). Though support has been shown to facilitate successful transition into the parenting role at all ages, as discussed in the chapters on antenatal and postnatal support, it may be particularly crucial to those entering motherhood during their teenage years. Who gives the support, and when and how it is given, may be crucial factors influencing future outcomes for the adolescent mother and her baby.

Support may originate from a number of relationships; however, partners and the family are the most probable sources (Phoenix 1991). The potential for a contribution to be made by professionals, either by supporting the young woman directly or through their support of existing networks should not be underestimated.

The role of partners

The role played by the child's father in supporting young mothers and children has been much neglected by research. It is important not to underestimate the difficulty of involving them in the research process. For a number of reasons they may not want to make themselves known to health and social service professionals, which will of course include researchers (Moore & Rosenthal 1993). It is commonly assumed that young fathers do not want to take any responsibility for, or do not wish to play an active role in the upbringing of, their child. Recent findings, suggest this is often not the case. Large numbers of fathers do maintain substantial contact and play a significant role in the child's upbringing (Voran 1991). Where he is absent this may be because of ignorance of the pregnancy, disbelief that he is the father, uncertainties about his own ability to be a father and to support the child or a desire to escape responsibility. The young mothers themselves may have a significant influence on the extent of the fathers' involvement, through their role as 'gatekeepers', often restricting the part they are allowed to play. The attitudes of the father's parents may also influence whether or not he stays in contact and shares any of the responsibility. Research has shown that where the father is able to make a positive contribution, this is related to the young woman's adjustment to motherhood and positive outcomes for the child (Voran 1991).

For the women in Phoenix's (1991) sample, however, this positive contribution was rarely made. A number of relationships ended during pregnancy and where the father did remain involved, the majority did not provide the support that the women wanted, both in terms of practical and emotional support. Male partners, who were often unemployed or in low paid jobs, made little economic contribution to the households in which their children lived. Very rarely were they involved in any child care or domestic duties. In fact, the women were more likely to turn to their families and particularly their own mothers for emotional, material and child care support.

Though lots of questions relating to the role of the father still need to be answered what is becoming apparent is that many fathers would like to participate actively in the care and upbringing of their child, but find the demands and responsibilities too great and their abilities and preparation inadequate. Recognition of the strains upon the father, the need for 'training' for fatherhood and the need to support him in his role may decrease the number of absent fathers and may encourage and enable them to make a contribution that will be of benefit to mother and child.

The role of the family

The research carried out up to now has often given little more than passing attention to the family relationships and support networks of young mothers, as Judith Lask points out: 'The birth of a child to an adolescent is usually an important event for the whole family. The literature has given little attention to the wider family, in spite of the fact that it can provide practical and emotional support, as well as being a source of stress.' (Lask 1994, p. 233).

The family can have a crucial impact on outcomes for the young mother and her baby. As Phoenix's work illustrated, they may provide financial, material and emotional support frequently surpassing that offered by the child's father.

As was pointed out earlier, large numbers of young mothers continue to live in the family home. Studies have shown that between 55% and 85% of pregnant and parenting teenagers remain with their parents for at least the first months of the child's life (Chase-Lansdale et al 1991, Phoenix 1991). Continued co-residence does necessitate major adaptations to the functioning of the family unit (Ooms 1981). As well as having major practical and financial implications, the family has also to deal with the change in status of the young woman and to begin to redefine their relationships with her. This is a complex process as the teenage mother must continue to negotiate the developmental tasks of the adolescent period, amongst them the need for increasing autonomy from parents and increased decision-making powers. At the same time the baby usually causes an increased need for emotional and practical support from these same people. Such close proximity means that the baby's grandparents are potentially available to be involved in providing help with or sharing the tasks of 'parenting'.

Though there is some suggestion that the child's grandfather may have significant impact on outcomes for the child, potentially filling the 'father figure' role (Oyserman et al 1993), it is the link between the young mother and her mother that appears to be particularly crucial during the period surrounding the birth and on into the first years of the child's life. Even when mother and baby do not live in the family home, the grandmother is usually a crucial source of social support and links are generally maintained even under difficult circumstances. The majority of research uses the term 'grandmother' to refer to the young mother's mother, though often its use is extended to the paternal grandmother or other women assuming this role, e.g. aunts.

Obviously, there is much variation in the role played by the grandmother. This may be due to a number of factors including the age of the young woman, her perceived needs, involvement of both women in employment and education, living arrangements and the needs of other family members. Research findings suggest that she has a significant influence on decisions about whether the pregnancy is continued, child care and parenting practices, and further involvement in education or employment (Furstenberg 1981).

Importantly, grandmother and family support has been shown to be related to the amount of antenatal care that the young woman receives. The amount of care received appears to be linked to when the young woman informs her mother of her pregnancy, the timing of which may reflect the quality of the mother–daughter relationship and fears of her mother's reaction (Voran 1991). Many young women do report delaying telling their parents for substantial periods of time, which may increase the risks for both mother and child.

GRANDMOTHER–MOTHER–CHILD RELATIONSHIPS

Having the child's grandmother around might be expected to be a useful addition to the functioning of the mother–child dyad. East & Felice (1996), in their recent review of the role played by grandmothers, outline three reasons why this might be so. Firstly, because of her age and experience, the grandmother's parenting abilities are assumed to be greater than those of her teenage daughter. Secondly, and in combination with the former, grandmothers are expected to provide a positive role model for their daughters' parenting. Thirdly, they are thought to act as a source of social support, offering practical assistance and acting as a 'buffer' against some of the stresses and strains inherent in motherhood.

Evidence to support the above hypotheses is apparent in the findings of several research studies which link social support from grandmother to an adolescent mother's mental health, greater support being associated with fewer symptoms of postnatal depression and anxiety (Furstenberg & Crawford 1978). The relationship between support and self-esteem, depression and anxiety has been found to be stronger among parenting teenagers than among pregnant and non-parenting teenagers (Barth et al 1983).

Grandmother support has been shown to be related to favourable educational and employment outcomes for young mothers. In a sample of black American mothers, those who lived with their family of origin were more likely to complete high school and be employed than those who lived independently (Furstenberg & Crawford 1978).

Research has also shown a positive relationship between characteristics of the grandmother–mother relationship, the grandmother–infant relationship and the young mother's parenting (Brooks-Gunn & Chase-Lansdale 1991). For example, an open and flexible relationship style in grandmother–mother parenting and a nurturing style in the grandmother's interaction with the infant have been seen to be related to the presence of similar styles of parenting in the young mother (Wakschlag et al 1996).

Support for grandmother involvement as beneficial is not unequivocal and several studies have found results that appear to contradict this view. In the US, research has suggested that grandmother contact, including both assistance in child care and living arrangements, is related to more behaviour problems and less secure attachment in the infants of young mothers (Spieker & Bensley 1994, Unger & Cooley 1992). High levels of grandmother support have been shown to be related to a variety of difficulties for the teenage mother, including lower levels of self-esteem and maternal responsiveness (Voran 1991). Seemingly grandmother involvement can become an additional source of stress to a young mother. Her advice and help with child care may begin to be seen as intrusive.

The work of Chase-Lansdale and colleagues (Chase-Lansdale et al 1994) provides interesting insights into how this contradiction may be explained. They have looked primarily at African–American communities where young single motherhood is highly prevalent and, in the face of extreme poverty, the pooling of resources and sharing of child-rearing across kin networks is common. Examining a sample of 99 multigenerational families with a 3-year-old child, they observed the parenting practices in the home environments of mothers, who ranged from 13 to 25 years at the time of the birth, and grandmothers, on a number of problem-solving tasks. The results failed to show that the grandmothers' parenting practice was of a higher standard than that of their daughters and few correlations in parenting ability across the generations were present, those that existed being on negative dimensions.

Interestingly, Chase-Lansdale's work found that age itself was not a significant predictor of the quality of mothers' parenting; instead it was co-residence that was associated with poorer quality of both mother's and grandmother's parenting, as well as greater child behaviour problems. As several authors have noted (Chase-Lansdale et al 1994, East & Felice 1996), it is difficult to untangle the effects of grandmothers' involvement with parenting from the effects of co-residing in multigenerational families. Chase-Lansdale and colleagues take on this task, attempting to tease apart those factors concerned with grandmother involvement and those concerned with co-residence (Chase-Lansdale et al 1994).

Their findings suggest that the age of the young mother, when she first gives birth, is a major factor affecting the impact of co-residence. For *very* young mothers, living with their mother was found to be correlated with positive outcomes; for older young mothers it was living apart (Chase-Lansdale et al 1994). Having separate households may enable the grandmother to take on the more 'traditional' role, of pleasurable, part-time caring, whilst still providing social and emotional support. The young mother may benefit from this support, whilst being able to make her own decisions about parenting.

So what are the possible explanations for the difficulties caused by co-residence that older teenage mothers experience? It may be that co-residence, for older teens, is a necessary reaction to economic hardship, and it is the stress caused by poverty that acts as causal factor. Alternatively, it may be that higher levels of intrafamily conflict and tension result when all are forced to live under the same roof and it is this that impacts upon outcomes (Chase-Lansdale et al 1994, Spieker & Bensley 1994). A third possible explanation is that those young mothers who continue to co-reside may be those who are least able to cope with motherhood and who remain at home because their abilities to survive independently are inadequate.

These findings can be understood by attention to the developmental tasks of adolescence. The adolescent transition incorporates essential developments in the identity of the individual, the negotiation of increased autonomy from parents and the preparation for independence. Adolescent mothers who continue to live with their own mothers are more likely to continue in their adolescent role, for instance continuing to attend school and maintaining a teenager–mother relationship. Though long-term benefits may be gained from an increased opportunity to achieve educationally, this process may prevent them from paying immediate attention to tasks that are associated with the adult role, specifically forming intimate partnerships and parenting. Those who move out of the family home may be ready to take on that adult role and develop their parenting skills (Spieker & Bensley 1994). The continuation of support from her mother may act as validation of the young mother's new role. Growing amounts of evidence point to non-shared residence, but high support as the most positive circumstances for adolescent mothers and their children (Chase-Lansdale et al 1994, East & Felice 1996, Spieker & Bensley 1994).

Few studies have tried to understand how or why some young mothers and their children benefit from remaining in the parental home while others appear to suffer negative consequences. Little research has examined how adolescent parents negotiate domestic tasks and child care with their mothers when both live together, how both women adjust to the teenager's new role, and what characteristics of the relationship ensure positive outcomes. Most of the work that has addressed these issues originates from the US and utilizes methodologies which observe interactions between mothers and grandmothers on simple tasks or solely rely on data from psychological measures. Few have started from explanations given by the women themselves.

THE THREE GENERATIONS STUDY

The research that will now be described arose out of our desire to address these questions using an in-depth qualitative approach. The aim was to explore how young mothers and their mothers describe their experiences and the issues that are pertinent to them, to look in detail at the needs of these women, to what extent these are being met and to investigate the potential for contributions to be made by the range of professionals working to support these families.

A sample of 53 young mothers and their mothers were interviewed. Where the maternal grandmother was not available, the person who occupied this role participated. The study focused upon the experiences of those young mothers who had been 17 or under when they had their first child. This may have been just a few months ago or looking back over a period of a few years. Some of the young mothers had remained living with their parents, others had initially stayed there but had since established an independent household, while still others had lived apart even before the birth. Some were attending school or college, some were employed part time, others were full-time mothers. Most were from working-class backgrounds and the majority of women were white, though a number of Asian and Afro-Caribbean families also took part. They were all living in three areas of England: the Southwest, the North and the South Coast.

FINDINGS

What became apparent to us was that the experiences of the young mothers and grandmothers varied greatly. Their concerns were diverse, for example some were facing severe economic hardship and concerns over housing and finances were foremost, for others child care arrangements and the sharing of domestic duties were key issues. The following discussion will try to describe how these women collaborated and negotiated the task of bringing up the new addition to the family.

The relationship between the two women fell broadly into two groups, chiefly defined by the age of the young mother. Firstly, the mothers of the *older* young women seemed to offer practical support with housework, money and a little baby-sitting. However, they left nearly all aspects of child care to their daughters, feeling strongly that it is their responsibility. Though they enjoyed their involvement with their grandchild greatly, the impact that the child had on the structure of their lives was relatively limited. They often saw themselves as a 'safety net', there to support and help when needed.

In turn, the mother saw herself as an 'adult' and as being the one with main responsibility for the child's care and upbringing. These young mothers were keen to be independent, but knew they could draw on their own mother's help and support when they needed it:

If I didn't have my mum I don't think I'd be able to manage, 'cause my mum's always somewhere I can come back to her, she's always there if I need her for anything and if I wanna talk to her. (Clare, 17 years old, with 15-month-old)

As in the above example, the young mother was often either living apart from her mother or was planning to move out of the family home in the near future. She often had a partner, frequently the child's father, who was, to an extent, involved with the child.

The second relationship pattern, which appeared most frequently with the *younger* teenage mothers, was much more complex. Independence from the grandmother was less commonly asserted; there seemed greater dependence on her for advice, practical help and support. Several of the young women saw themselves as somewhere between 'teenager' and 'adult', for example the following response was given to the question 'so how do you see yourself, as a teenager or more of an adult?':

A bit of both really, because sometimes I feel like younger, but at other times I feel older, it depends really. But sometimes I look at other teenagers and think 'oh my God, get a grip, stop laughing at such stupid things'. (Laura, 15 years old, with 6-month-old)

Several grandmothers discussed the difficulties that ensued from having an adolescent daughter who was also a parent. They often talked about how they realized their daughter was 'only a teenager' and thus needed time to go out and enjoy herself, to be involved in *normal* teenage activities, and to be supported as a teenager. The need to relate to their daughter as a parent and in an adult role was also acknowledged. Getting the balance right seemed to be an issue for many of the women, as the following quotation illustrates:

The only way I find it quite strange is the fact that because she's so young, if she wants to go out, I have to tell her a time that she's got to be in and it seems funny to be telling someone that's a mother that 'you've got to be in at 11 p.m.'. It's strange that way. (Jan, mother of a 16-year-old young mother)

Grandmothers often saw themselves as playing a necessary role to ensure that the child received adequate care, often intervening, and offering help and advice. However, a large number of these women talked about how they were anxious not to 'take over' and were very aware of the problems that might arise if they did this. Instead they saw themselves as working in partnership with their daughters allowing the young mothers to make decisions and hold main responsibility. Grandmothers frequently validated and praised their daughters' parenting skills for example:

She takes it on fully and to the best of her ability and one of my jobs is to remind her how well she's doing! (Christine, mother of a 16-year-old young mother)

Though some young mothers did see their mother's help as 'interference', in the main they saw the necessity of this help, and wanted her to be involved. Many of the young mothers talked about how the pregnancy and birth of their child had brought their mother and themselves closer together. Few mother–daughter dyads described anything but moderate levels of disagreement and conflict. The teenagers acknowledged that without their mothers' help and support their task would have been much harder.

A common arrangement was for grandmother to look after the child whilst the young mother attended school and college and also on a number of evenings during the week. In order to do this several women had given up their jobs and a small number were consequently experiencing feelings of being 'trapped' and of having a lack of control over their own lives. Several grandmothers were themselves single and they commonly expressed feelings indicating that they lacked social support:

I was very disappointed, there was no counselling, there was nobody to support me. I feel very, unsupported is too strong a word, but I had no support from relatives or anything, so there was nobody coming round saying 'Are you coping?' so that I could say 'No, I am not physically or mentally coping.' Everything was basically done by me. (Pauline, mother of 15-year-old young mother)

Having spent a lot of time involved in their care, grandmothers often were very emotionally attached to their grandchild. Many of the women looked to the time when the young woman would be ready to move out of the family home, and were working to prepare their daughter for this. However, many grandmothers in this position feared how they would react when this finally came about:

I think one day she'll want to leave home – I do worry about that because obviously I'm getting more and more attached to him. When the time comes that they both leave, I don't know how I'll feel about that. You know, I look at him as being part of my family now. That will be hard. I think about that because she'll always be my child and they can never do things right for you, can they? I'd be worried 'my God, what's she doing with him now'. (Mary, mother of a 16-year-old young mother)

Of all the young mothers, the majority expressed positive feelings towards their child. Few pregnancies had been planned, but by the birth all had been 'wanted' children. The young women, though realistic about the difficult task they faced, described deriving much pleasure from their child:

Exhausting! Although it is fun seeing Jack do funny things and that, and I do enjoy having him and that, I do enjoy it even though I do have regrets and that, but I wouldn't give him up for anything. (Shona, 16 years old, with a 12-month-old)
It's tiring, but it's definitely worth it in the end. To begin with, when you first bring your baby home, it's like a struggle because they hardly sleep through the night and stuff, but as they get older it's definitely worth it. (Amy, 15 years old, with a 5-month-old)

The majority of these young women were fiercely determined to be a good parent and wanted to give their child the best. They talked about how they tried to weigh up advice from professionals and their mother when making decisions about the baby's care. The following example was a response to the question 'So when it came to weaning, who did you take advice from?':

I asked my mum and I asked my next-door neighbour and I asked my health visitor and I looked at all those books which mum has about bringing babies up on a vegetarian diet, I looked at all of those. So I just sort of took advice from all of them. (Geana, mother of a 6-month-old)

Though the majority were currently receiving state benefits, many saw this as a temporary measure and described a desire to return to, or to continue in, education, in order to gain the training and qualifications that would enable them to get well paid employment:

Now I have got something to work for in school. I have got more reason to knuckle down to classes because I have got a baby to provide for now I am older. (Ellie, aged 15, with a 5-month-old)

All the women in the study were asked questions which aimed to ascertain how well health professionals such as midwives, health visitors and general practitioners had met their needs. A mixed response was received. The young mothers seemed to appreciate those professionals who did not talk down to them, did not condemn them for becoming pregnant, had time to listen and answer questions and who had a warm and caring approach. A number of women discussed how they had failed to attend antenatal classes because they feared the reaction of the older women at the class, others had enjoyed their antenatal care and felt they had been accepted by the older group members.

Few young mothers who were outside education appeared to have contact with other parenting teenagers. Many were enthusiastic about the idea of getting together with other young mothers to discuss experiences and share advice. Likewise, few grandmothers appeared to have contact with other parents of teenage mothers, and they were also enthusiastic about getting together with others who had shared similar experiences. Though support groups for young mothers are relatively common, the authors are unaware of any such meetings for grandparents taking place in the UK.

DISCUSSION

Just some of the issues arising out of the research we have conducted have been presented here, but it is apparent that the findings have clear implications for professionals working with young parents and their families. Some of these will be discussed below. What is clear is that there is much variation in the role played by the grandmother and in the extent to which she shares the parenting task. Many of these women wanted to be, or felt they needed to be, involved and many had grown very attached to their grandchild. Though the young mothers differed in their response to this, most were grateful for their mother's help and acknowledged the importance of her support.

Having presented evidence relating to how young women experience teenage motherhood we hope the validity of our initial statement will be apparent: the experiences of young mothers, and the relationships that they are involved in, do vary greatly. It is clear that simplistic negative images of young mothers are misplaced. Young mothers do not form a simple homogeneous group and the problems they face are often the same as those facing older mothers. Some women adjust well to their new role, others find it much more difficult or even impossible. Some women are able to be independent, others need to rely heavily on the support of those around them. What is obvious, however, is that becoming a parent during the teenage years does not immediately condemn a young woman to a life of welfare dependence and her child to abuse and neglect as some politicians and some sections of the media would have us believe. Support, as in other areas of social life, does appear crucial to a young mother's experience of having a child. The form this support can optimally take differs from woman to woman. The research discussed has, however, illustrated the importance of looking at the wider family when studying, or working with, young mothers and their children.

There are no easy solutions to the problems that young parents experience. Though co-residence with the child's grandparents may be advantageous for some young families, this is not the case for others. For some, involvement of the father in parenting may be beneficial; for others, it is not. Many of the findings from the research appear, at first, to be ambiguous and contradictory. Recent research has begun to offer useful insights. However, many areas remain to be addressed and many questions are yet unanswered. Future in-depth and longitudinal research is necessary to clarify many of the points we have discussed. There is a need to develop further understanding of the factors that are protective for young mothers and their children. Research that starts from listening to descriptions given by the young women themselves, rather than imposing explanations must be a priority.

Key points for caregivers

- Young people should be given the knowledge they need to avoid unwanted pregnancies. They should have easy access to contraceptive advice and provision, and should be given advice on techniques for introducing and using contraceptives.
- Young women, pregnant and parenting teenagers all need practical, balanced and truthful information on which to base their choices at every stage. It should not only present the professional viewpoint but should draw upon information given by young women who have experienced the realities of teenage parenthood. This material should be widely available so that as many women as possible have access to it. It should be in a form that the young women will be able to understand and make use of.
- Efforts should be made to make health care and advice-giving forums as young parent 'friendly' as possible. Antenatal classes for young women only, have been shown to increase attendance during this important phase. Where this is not workable, classes and clinics should be made as attractive to these women as possible.
- Health care personnel and policy should take a perspective which goes beyond the mother–child relationship. They should look at the family relationships surrounding the young mother and where appropriate should include the baby's grandmother or other principal carers in any interventions. Support to the grandmother may benefit the young mother and her child, as well as the grandmother.
- Professionals working with young families should, wherever possible, work to support and help maintain stable relationships with, and continued input from, the child's father. Many young men could usefully benefit from training in preparation for fatherhood.
- Throughout all work with young mothers and their families the importance of considering variation between them should be stressed. For example, in some instances co-residence is associated with positive factors and in other cases it is associated with negative. Any preconceptions about young mothers, their families and their lifestyles may be counterproductive.

REFERENCES

Abraham C, Sheeran P 1994 Modelling and modifying heterosexuals' HIV-preventative behaviour: a review of theories, findings and educational implications. Patient Education and Counselling 23: 173–186
Babb P 1993 Teenage conceptions and fertility in England and Wales, 1971–91. Population Trends 74: 12–22
Barth R P, Schinke S P, Maxwell J S 1983 Psychological correlates of teenage motherhood. Journal of Youth and Adolescence 12(6): 471–487
Birch D 1987 Are you my sister mummy? Youth Support, London
Breakwell G, Fife-Schaw C 1992 Sexual activities and preferences in a United Kingdom sample of 16 to 20-year-olds. Archives of Sexual Behaviour 21(3): 271–293
Brooks-Gunn J, Chase-Lansdale P 1991 Children having children: effects on the family system. Paediatric Annals 20: 467–481
Burghes L, Brown M 1995 Single lone mothers: problem, prospects and policies. Family Policy Studies Centre, London
Chase-Lansdale L, Brooks-Gunn J, Paikoff 1991 Research and programs for adolescent mothers: missing links and future promises. Family Relationships 40: 396–404
Chase-Lansdale L, Brooks-Gunn J, Zamsky E 1994 Young African–American multigenerational families in poverty: quality of mothering and grandmothering. Child Development 65: 373–393
Clark E 1989 Young single mothers today: a qualitative study of housing and support needs. National Council for One Parent Families, London
Cooley M, Unger D 1991 The role of family support in determining developmental outcomes in children of teen mothers. Child Psychiatry and Human Development 21: 217–234

Dawson N 1994 The 1994 survey of educational provision for pregnant schoolgirls and schoolgirl mothers in the LEAs of England and Wales. School of Education, University of Bristol, Bristol

Department of Health 1992 Health of the nation. HMSO, London

Department of Health 1994 On the state of public health. HMSO, London

East P L, Felice M E 1996 Adolescent pregnancy and parenting. Erlbaum, Hillsdale, New Jersey

Furstenberg F 1981 Implicating the family: teenage parenthood and kinship involvement. In: Ooms T (ed) Teenage pregnancy in a family context. Temple University Press, Philadelphia, pp 131–164

Furstenberg F F, Crawford A G 1978 Family support: helping teenage mothers to cope. Family Planning Perspectives 10: 322–333

Furstenberg F F, Brooks-Gunn J, Morgan P 1987 Adolescent mothers in later life. Cambridge University Press, New York

Furstenberg F F, Brooks-Gunn J, Chase-Lansdale P L 1989 Teenage pregnancy and childbearing. American Psychologist 44: 313–320

Hudson F, Ineichen B 1991 Taking it lying down: sexuality and teenage motherhood. Macmillan, Basingstoke

Ineichen B 1986 Contraceptive use and attitudes to motherhood among teenage mothers. Journal of Biosocial Science 18(4): 387–394

Lask J 1994 Parenting in adolescence. ACCP Review and Newsletter 16(5): 229–236

Macdonald I, Skuse T 1996 Intention to become pregnant and contraceptive use amongst a sample of teenage and adult mothers. Educational and Child Psychology 13(1): 69–80

Moore S, Rosenthal D 1993 Sexuality in adolescence. Routledge, London

Ooms T 1981 Teenage pregnancy in a family context. Temple University Press, Philadelphia

Office of Population Censuses and Surveys 1996 Population trends 84. HMSO, London

Office of Population Censuses and Surveys 1997 Birth statistics 1995. HMSO, London

Oyserman D, Radin N, Benn R 1993 Dynamics in a three-generational family: teens, grandparents, and babies. Developmental Psychology 29(3): 564–572

Phoenix A 1991 Young mothers. Polity, London

Schofield G 1994 The youngest mothers. Avebury, Aldershot

Sharpe S 1987 Falling for love: teenage mothers talk. Virago Press, London

Simms M, Smith C 1986 Teenage mothers and their children. DHSS Research Report 15. HMSO, London

Spieker S, Bensley L 1994 Roles of living arrangements and grandmother social support in adolescent mothering and infant attachment. Developmental Psychology 30(1): 102–111

Unger D, Cooley M 1992 Partner and grandmother contact in black and white teen parent families. Journal of Adolescent Health Care 13: 546–552

Voran M J 1991 Grandmother social support to adolescent mothers: correlates of support and adolescents' satisfaction. Unpublished Masters dissertation, University of Virginia, USA

Wakschlag L S, Chase-Lansdale P L, Brooks-Gunn J 1996 Not just 'Ghosts in the Nursery': contemporaneous intergenerational relationships and parenting in young African–American families. Child Development 67: 2131–2147

Wellings K, Field J, Johnson A M, Wadsworth J 1994 National survey of sexual attitudes and lifestyles. Penguin, London

Werner B 1988 Fertility trends in the UK and in thirteen other developed countries, 1966–86. Population Trends 51: 18–24

Winn S, Roker D, Coleman J 1995 Knowledge about puberty and sexual development in 11–16 year-olds: implications for health and sex education in schools. Educational Studies 21(2): 187–201

FURTHER READING

Hudson F, Ineichen B 1991 Taking it lying down: sexuality and teenage motherhood. Macmillan, Basingstoke

Phoenix A 1991 Young mothers. Polity, London

Sharpe S 1987 Falling for love: teenage mothers talk. Virago Press, London

Index